Learning Disability and other Intellectual Impairments

Learning Disability and other Intellectual Impairments

Meeting Needs Throughout Health Services

Edited by

Louise L. Clark
King's College London

and

Peter Griffiths
King's College London

John Wiley & Sons, Ltd

Other Wiley Editorial Offices

John Wiley & Sons Inc., 111 River Street, Hoboken, NJ 07030, USA

Jossey-Bass, 989 Market Street, San Francisco, CA 94103-1741, USA

Wiley-VCH Verlag GmbH, Boschstr. 12, D-69469 Weinheim, Germany

John Wiley & Sons Australia Ltd, 42 McDougall Street, Milton, Queensland 4064, Australia

John Wiley & Sons (Asia) Pte Ltd, 2 Clementi Loop #02-01, Jin Xing Distripark, Singapore 129809

John Wiley & Sons Canada Ltd, 6045 Freemont Blvd, Mississauga, Ontario, Canada, L5R 4J3

Wiley also publishes its books in a variety of electronic formats. Some content that appears in print may not be available in electronic books.

Anniversary Logo Design: Richard J. Pacifico

Library of Congress Cataloging-in-Publication Data
Learning disability and other intellectual impairments / edited by Louise L. Clark, and Peter Griffiths.
  p. ; cm.
  Includes bibliographical references and index.
  ISBN 978-0-470-03471-2
  1. Learning disabled–Medical care–Great Britain.   2. Learning disabled–Services for–Great Britain.   3. Learning disabilities–Nursing–Great Britain.   I. Clark, Louise L.   II. Griffiths, Peter, RMN.
    [DNLM: 1. Learning Disorders–nursing–Great Britain.   2. Community Mental Health Services–Great Britain.   3. Health Services Needs and Demand–Great Britain.   WY 160.5 L438 2007]
  RC570.5.G7L43 2007
  362.196'85889–dc22

                                                                                    2007025155

British Library Cataloguing in Publication Data
A catalogue record for this book is available from the British Library

ISBN 978-0-470-03471-2

Typeset in 10/11pt Bembo by SNP Best-set Typesetter Ltd., Hong Kong
Printed and bound in Great Britain by Bell & Bain, Glasgow
This book is printed on acid-free paper responsibly manufactured from sustainable forestry in which at least two trees are planted for each one used for paper production.

Contents

Editors

Louise L. Clark is the lecturer in Intellectual Impairment at the Florence Nightingale School of Nursing and Midwifery, King's College London. She is responsible for the coordination of education in this subject throughout the school, at both under- and postgraduate levels as well as for Diploma students studying generic nursing courses. Louise also has an interest in leadership and the management of change within the NHS and has been involved extensively in this process in previous posts in both learning disability and mental health services; she is involved in the teaching of this subject to postgraduate students and is a Business Fellow of KCL Business Ltd. She is widely published in the field of intellectual impairment and mental health, particularly in relation to education in this area for generic nurses.

Professor Peter Griffiths is director of the UK Department of Health's policy research programme's National Nursing Research Unit at King's College London. The National Nursing Research Unit has conducted extensive research into the careers and working lives of learning disability nurses in the UK. His own research has focused on nursing-led services and advanced and specialist practice roles in chronic disease management and intermediate care. He has written extensively on evidence-based practice and has written and commissioned many systematic reviews on clinical topics as commissioning editor of the *British Journal of Community Nursing's* 'mini-reviews' series (until 2006) and elsewhere. He is deputy editor of the *International Journal of Nursing Studies* and an associate editor of the journal *Evidence Based Nursing*. His experience of learning disability is that of many in mainstream practice: relatively frequent encounters with clients which provoke awareness of the limitations of his own knowledge.

Contributors

The contributors to the book are from a variety of health backgrounds, predominantly medicine and nursing, and a variety of relevant specialties. They have a wealth of experience in the care of people with all forms of intellectual impairment within their own specialist areas as well as in mainstream NHS services in general.

Dr Louise Barriball, Senior Lecturer, FNSNM,* King's College London.

Dr Catherine Bryant, Consultant Physician, King's College Hospital, London.

Louise Clark, Lecturer in Intellectual Impairment and Mental Health, FNSNM,* King's College London.

Garry Diack, Senior Lecturer, Department of Health, Psychology & Social Care, Manchester Metropolitan University, Manchester.

Dr Howard Cohen, General Practitioner, Elizabeth House Surgery, Warlingham, Surrey.

Professor Peter Griffiths, Director of the National Nursing Research Unit, King's College London.

Allan Hicks, Lecturer in the Care of Older Adults, FNSNM,* King's College London.

Steve Higgins, Senior Tutor, Institute of Psychiatry, King's College London.

Alison Hobden, Lecturer in Primary Care, University of Liverpool.

Michael Kelly, Mental Health Practitioner, Central & North West London Mental Health NHS Foundation Trust.

Elizabeth Lewry, Community LD Nurse. States of Jersey.

Dr Karen Lowton, Senior Lecturer, Institute of Gerontology, King's College London.

Ian Noonan, Lecturer in Mental Health, FNSNM,* King's College London.

Dr Simon Mills, Barrister at Law and General Practitioner, Dublin, Ireland.

Emma Ouldred, Dementia Nurse Specialist, King's College Hospital, London.

Mary O'Toole, Lecturer in Mental Health, FNSNM,★ King's College London.

Mike Reid, Lecturer–practitioner, FNSNM,★ King's College London, South London and the Maudsley NHS Foundation Trust.

Dr Robert Winterhalder, Consultant Psychiatrist, Bromley PCT and Honorary Lecturer, Institute of Psychiatry, King's College London.

Dr Theresa Wiseman, Lecturer and Head of Palliative Care, FNSNW,★ King's College London.

★ FNSNM : Florence Nightingale School of Nursing and Midwifery.

Foreword

This book concerns the provision of health care to people with intellectual impairments within the 'mainstream'. This includes people whose intellectual impairment is acquired at or before birth, in early childhood or later in life through degenerative processes or acute injury. In the United Kingdom this primarily means care provided in general practices, community health services and acute hospitals within the National Health Service.

It is almost 50 years since the normalization movement began to offer the prospect of fuller lives, as citizens, to people with learning disabilities and began to move away from a norm of institutional care. Yet through the contradictory gains and losses of community care too little progress has been made in building a robust social model of support. Too many people are placed in lonely and segregated settings and joint working between health and social services, despite some positive examples, has not surmounted the obstacles caused by the different mindsets and interests of the key statutory agency partners. Meanwhile a number of factors, including ageing of the population, mean that there are many other people with conditions such as dementia and long-term mental health problems whose intellectual impairments result in similar barriers to accessing quality services.

In 2001 the UK government outlined a plan to significantly alter the provision of support to people with learning disabilities in the white paper *Valuing People: A New Strategy for Learning Disability for the 21st Century*. Since then there has been a renewed determination to build strong local systems that remove obstacles to people living ordinary lives and also make available skilled support to help people manage the reality of their disability. Despite significant progress a key weakness has been a failure to develop the necessary skills, understanding and attitudes in mainstream health services and practitioners. Key attributes of learning disability make this more difficult for practitioners and practice managers. This text argues that there are common obstacles to delivering care to all people with intellectual impairments.

Interactions take more time; communicating can be different and difficult; it is more important to know the person when they are well in order to understand the nature of any difficulty that is emerging. Many practitioners seem to have been socialized into thinking that they could not work with people with learning disabilities and avoid the issue by maintaining that specialist training and understanding are needed and that really this population should be managed and treated by specialists. For other groups the challenge of providing quality care is barely recognized at all. The net result is that ordinary – never mind excellent – local health services are few and far between for people with intellectual impairments and there is a risk of leaving their health needs more poorly met than under the earlier segregated system.

As this book was being written a series of scandals were being investigated in NHS provision. The Mencap campaign 'Treat Me Right' and the 2007 follow-up 'Death By Indifference' exposed the terrible human consequences of the failure of health services to grasp the challenge of providing care to people with learning disabilities. Many cases of 'age discrimination' within NHS care are associated with those experiencing intellectual impairment resulting from dementia. There is an increasing recognition that physical health needs of many people with long-term mental health problems are not properly met because of ongoing intellectual impairments even when symptoms of mental illness are controlled. Stories of missed diagnoses, under-investigation and failure to offer appropriate treatments abound. It is necessary that we are now robust in demanding a new openness from people working within and responsible for these systems. It means facing the challenges and finding solutions.

We welcome this book with its contributions from practitioners and academics who are determined to shine a light into this unsatisfactory situation. A number of the arguments made are uncomfortable for those of us who have advocated a social model of care based on a social model of disability. The editors are unconvinced that the current strategy is sufficient and the contributions illustrate that we are losing, not developing, core skills within the NHS. Underlying the argument is the recognition that in abandoning the medical model of care the potential for discrimination in the field of health care has been increased. Of course this is consistent with the social model of disability which identifies disability with discrimination against those with impairment. But the architects of the social model of care may have failed to grasp the importance of general health needs in shaping quality of life and neglected the need to tackle institutional discrimination within health services as they rightly argued that the medical model should not define people's lives.

The contributors to this text survey the political and organizational contexts, and are little impressed. They are polemical in challenging readers to think critically about the reality of people's lives and rigorous in their analysis in order to maintain a focus on what can be done to move forwards. The authors maintain a focus on NHS values of excellence and accessibility that fit well with the current agenda and suggest models within current strategy that they feel will safeguard the best interests of this population. As more than one in fifty of our fellow citizens lives with a learning disability and many more experience other intellectual impairments at some point in their lives the natural injustice of the current position is obvious. However uncomfortable it makes us feel, this book challenges us to clarify our thinking and develop systems to provide – in reality – the quality of service this group deserves.

Professor Ian Norman, Head of the Mental Health Section & Head of Graduate Research Studies, Florence Nightingale School of Nursing at King's College London

Des Sowerby, Joint Director, Learning Disability Kent County Council and NHS

CHAPTER 1
AN INTRODUCTION TO INTELLECTUAL IMPAIRMENT

Louise L. Clark and Peter Griffiths

This is a book about the provision of health care to people with intellectual impairments. The scope of this book is difficult to define because it is intended to fill a gap whose boundaries are not clearly defined. It aims to enhance the knowledge base of those who encounter people with intellectual impairment in general healthcare settings in order to equip them with the skills needed to deliver high quality health care to these patients. Health policy in many developed countries now dictates the use of mainstream healthcare services for all or most people with intellectual impairment. Specialist provision is kept to a minimum. Previously, many people with intellectual impairments were cared for in 'specialized' long stay hospital institutions for people with learning disabilities, mental illness and the chronically physically impaired (especially long stay wards for the elderly). Although current health policy has laudable aims it does have implications for the knowledge base required by doctors, nurses and allied health professionals in order for them to care effectively for these patients in both primary care and acute settings.

Thus this book covers a range of issues including prevalent physical and mental health problems, because they are often unrecognized, and some of the challenges, including communication and behaviour. General healthcare staff may not feel confident in dealing with this client group even though the requisite skills are often those they deploy every day with other client groups. This is both a specialist book for general healthcare staff and a guide to issues arising in the general healthcare setting for specialists. Although transition from child to adult services is touched upon in Chapter 5, this book largely relates to adults who have intellectual impairment and is not aimed at health professionals who are involved in the care of children as a specialism. The reason for this is twofold. Firstly, because we needed to put some limits to the potential scope of the book – which is vast. Secondly, we recognize that although problems are legion and provision patchy the issues raised here have often been better addressed in child health services because of the prevalence of conditions leading to developmental disorders. Thus we felt

Learning Disability and other Intellectual Impairments, Edited by L.L. Clark and P. Griffiths
© 2008 John Wiley & Sons, Ltd

the priority was to address adult services. Within these limits this book attempts to break down the barriers between the various specialties concerned with intellectual impairment in all its aspects and aims to arm health professionals with the transferable skills and knowledge that may be utilized when delivering health care.

WHAT IS 'INTELLECTUAL IMPAIRMENT'?

The umbrella terminology of intellectual impairment refers to the impairments of intellect that are found in those traditionally labelled as having a developmental or acquired learning disability but also people who have dementia, long-term mental illness which has negatively affected cognition, acquired brain injury, and individuals who have low intelligence and poor coping skills (sometimes coupled with mental health problems). There are also other people who may come into the category of intellectual impairment for a variety of less common reasons, some of which will be alluded to throughout this book. They are a heterogeneous group but contain individuals who have much in common across a number of spectra which transcend the traditional categorizations. In addition, attention is given here to those individuals who live their daily lives with unrecognized intellectual impairment. This is an expanding group who, like those whose impairment is recognized, face obstacles in getting access to good quality health care because of their impairment.

Their complex social, medical, behavioural and psychological problems present a challenge to generic healthcare staff. In many countries, including the United Kingdom, United States of America, Australia, Canada and the Scandinavian countries, there has been a commitment made to provide health care within mainstream, generic, services. What remains of specialist services are frequently reduced to low status 'Cinderellas' and they too share many common themes, which include insufficient funding and staffing levels coupled with the problem of low staff morale and perceived inferiority compared to 'high tech' specialties (Clark, 2006).

A shift from the medical model towards a social care approach may have compounded this attitude. Attempts to celebrate intellectual impairment as simply a variant of the human condition may perversely have exacerbated this problem as the need for specialist knowledge is downgraded and disregarded. Given the future agenda, which sees the demise of or further cutbacks to learning disability services (DH, 2001), fewer people will receive specialist services. But even though, as a group, people with intellectual impairment are no longer defined by access to specialist services there is still a need for identification of their problems. A broader terminology is required to ensure that specialist knowledge is not lost because it is recognized as only applying to a diminishing client group restricted to those with the most severe problems.

A myriad of terms has been employed to describe various groups of individuals who are affected by intellectual impairment. Both professionals and society have influenced the labelling process and confusion over such terminology is evident. The general public and health professionals are often uncertain as to which terminology to adopt, on occasion for fear of appearing either ill-informed or insulting as terms acquire social stigma. We choose to use the terminology 'Intellectual Impairment' throughout this book in order to highlight the necessity of a broader view that does not just relate to what is traditionally known as 'learning disability'.

This terminology also makes it clearer that there is much in common with those who would not be classified as experiencing a condition categorized as 'mental retardation' using the International Classification of Diseases-10 (ICD-10) system. Whatever the cause of the intellectual impairment, many of these individuals share a consequent lack of service provision, coupled with a shortfall in specialist skills and knowledge among many of those caring for them. Although this book relates to the broader concept of intellectual impairment, much of the research referred to comes from the field of learning disability because this is where the most work has been done. However, much of this work is applicable across all groups who have intellectual impairment. The following sections briefly consider further the core groups that fall under the broad umbrella term of intellectual impairment.

LEARNING DISABILITY AND PERVASIVE DEVELOPMENTAL DISORDERS

The term 'learning disability' has been much in vogue in recent years replacing terms such as mental subnormality and, latterly, mental handicap or retardation. *Valuing People: A New Strategy for Learning Disability for the 21ˢᵗ Century* (DH, 2001) states that learning disability includes:

- a significantly reduced ability to understand new or complex information, to learn new skills (impaired intelligence);
- a reduced ability to cope independently (impaired social functioning);
- a disability that started before adulthood, with a lasting effect on development.

This definition covers a broad spectrum of individuals with impairments resulting from numerous causes including genetic or chromosomal abnormalities such as Down syndrome, prematurity or hypoxic brain injury acquired at birth.

The number of people who fall within this spectrum is imprecise but *Valuing People* (DH, 2001) estimates that there is a prevalence of about 25 per 1000 population, which equates to approximately 1.2 million people in England who have a mild/moderate learning disability. They surmise that there are roughly 210000 people with severe and profound learning disabilities (65000 children and young people, 120000 adults of working age and 25000 older adults). Predictions are also made in the document that these figures are set to increase by about 1% per annum for the next 15 years for a variety of reasons which include increased life expectancy, the growing numbers of children with complex and multiple disabilities who survive into adulthood, and a sharp rise in the number of children who have autism in conjunction with learning disabilities. With a multiethnic population (especially in inner city areas where services are most stretched) there is also an indication that the figures will rise due to the prevalence of such conditions among some minority ethnic populations of southern Asian origin (DH, 2001).

The term 'learning disability' was applied to individuals at a time of 'political correctness' in the United Kingdom and it could be argued that it belittled the seriousness of the condition that many people endure as part of their daily lives. The term itself bears too many similarities to the educational construct of 'learning difficulties' and many people who had those conditions (such as dyslexia) felt that their issues were not understood by professionals and the public alike. Owing to the shift in service provision that has seen the closure of the institutions and day services (McIntosh and Whittaker, 1998), coupled with a social model of care in the community, people with learning disabilities are now expected to lead a 'normal' life, frequently receiving only limited specialist services whilst their often complex health issues are now placed firmly in generic care.

A pervasive developmental disorder is a group of conditions characterized by abnormalities in social functioning, communication and repetitive behaviour. They include conditions across the autistic spectrum including Asperger's syndrome, Rett's syndrome and other childhood disintegrative disorders. These conditions often do appear hand in hand with a learning disability associated with low IQ but this is not always the case. Such conditions have common features whereby initial development is entirely normal but there then follows a loss of previously acquired skills in several areas. A loss of interest in the environment is usually present and autistic-like behaviours around social functioning and communication become apparent. Many would also refer to learning disability per se as a developmental disorder especially in the case of children where the term 'global developmental delay' is the terminology of choice.

ACQUIRED BRAIN INJURY

Headway, the national organization for people with acquired brain injury, claim that each year a million people in the UK will attend hospital having sustained some form of traumatic brain injury and 12000 of those will require long-term care. Headway estimates that there are 170000 people in the UK suffering from the long-term effects of severe brain damage. In addition to this number it is surmised that there are even greater numbers of people who have had either moderate or mild brain injuries and who experience long-term problems. Rehabilitation for many of these patients may often prove both expensive and time consuming and ideally requires the expertise and skills of trained nurses in order to achieve optimum recovery. However, this is not an option in an overstretched and underfunded healthcare system. Patients' families and carers also need support and long-term help although, as with learning disabilities, there is little specialist provision. In addition to trauma, many disease processes cause injury to the brain of which probably the most prevalent is stroke, which is a leading cause of disability that is frequently associated with long-term intellectual impairment.

The long-term effects of acquired brain injury may include changes of personality, challenging behaviour, epilepsy, sensory and mobility issues, poor memory, loss of concentration and problem-solving skills in addition to mental health problems and depleted cognition. Studies by Franulic et al (2004) and Engberg and Teasdale (2004) found that people still continued to experience high levels of psychosocial difficulties 10 to 15 years following their injury. Although some studies have suggested that community-based rehabilitation may improve outcome several years following injury (Cicerone et al, 2004; Svendsen et al, 2004; Powell et al, 2002), such services are frequently not available. Long-term provision for acquired brain injury is often lacking, with many patients receiving no more than three months' post-injury acute health care in the UK (Braine, 2005) with similar issues arising in many insurance-based healthcare systems. Continuing care is generally provided though social care services either at home or in private nursing homes.

DEMENTIA

More than half a million individuals in England and Wales are affected by various types of dementia, with up to 165000 new cases diagnosed every year (Matthews and Brayne, 2005; MRC CFAS, 1998). By the age of 75 the point prevalence of dementia and dementia subtypes is approximately 10% and thereafter the prevalence doubles with every five years of increasing age. By age 85 it is estimated that 40% of the total population are affected (Cantley, 2001). Dementia may be the result of a variety of causes including age-related conditions such as Alzheimer's and multi-infarct dementia and those such as alcohol-related dementias and Creutzfeldt-Jakob disease (to name but two), which affect younger age groups. Many of these patients have additional medical problems and those who have mild cognitive impairments are more prone to dementia as are those who have Down syndrome.

The impact of cognitive impairment on daily living is now used as a major criterion for differentiating between mild cognitive impairment and dementia, although it is recognized that impairment of complex daily living skills is already present before the conventional threshold of dementia is reached (Perneczky et al, 2006). Recognition of a decline in cognition if someone already has a more marked intellectual impairment is extremely problematic and is often confounded where an individual is already in a care home. Anecdotal evidence would also suggest an acceptance of the situation especially in the case of older people or those with Down syndrome.

For the general population people with dementia are seldom cared for within NHS institutions, except in the most serious of circumstances. Elderly mental illness units (EMIs) are at a minimum and even specialist outpatient services can be hard to access. Nursing homes which have a low ratio of qualified to unqualified nursing staff are often the only option for patients in the final stages of these illnesses.

MENTAL HEALTH PROBLEMS

Cognition may be adversely affected in individuals who have severe and enduring mental health problems. Akin to those people known to have other forms of intellectual impairment, community care may leave them vulnerable and receiving only minimal support. Many of these individuals remain victims of the 'revolving door' phenomenon whereby they regularly require admission to acute mental health services owing to an inability to control long-term mental illness (primarily psychosis) for whatever reason. They may struggle with the basic activities of daily living, and have diminished coping and social skills in addition to a series of complex medical and emotional conditions. These frequently remain unaddressed because of cognitive impairment and mental health status.

Some of this group may use substances or alcohol as a form of 'self-medication' and by the very nature of their condition have difficulty engaging with services. The substance misuse may in itself worsen intellectual impairment. Basic survival needs such as housing, clothing, food and benefits are often problematic let alone the procurement of health care; some are also homeless. Accurate figures for the number of people who fall into this category are not officially identified by services, some have never been known to services and there are no estimates given for those who have suffered cognitive defects as a result of their mental health problems.

Mental health services regularly see patients with borderline undiagnosed intellectual impairment. These are often complicated owing to the additional psychiatric symptoms, which have a tendency to add complexity to the assessment, treatment and care management process due to diagnostic overshadowing.

Psychological adversity, parental socioeconomic class, high rates of unemployment, unstable family background, abuse and neglect are major contributory factors to mild intellectual impairment (Farrington, 2000). Holland et al (2002) state that there is a relationship between antisocial and criminal behaviour and the presence of intellectual impairment. The authors claim that there are two distinct groups of people that fall into this category. The first is those who are known to learning disability services. However, the numbers involved are low, although some crimes go unreported or unpunished owing to the attitude of the police, relatives and care staff, who may choose to turn a blind eye. The second group is somewhat larger in number. They are generally socially disadvantaged, have mental health problems (which are often compounded by substance abuse) and intellectual impairment that has been previously undiagnosed. Many will have just above the level recognized as qualifying for a classification of learning disability but owing to other problems their level of adaptive functioning may mean that they have poor coping skills and subsequently function at a much lower level (Box 1.1).

Several studies have looked at the presence of people with intellectual impairment in prison and other forensic settings. The mean IQ of convicted prisoners as a group is below average and many are intellectually disadvantaged in addition to having mental health problems, substance abuse and/or personality disorders. Studies from the UK, USA and Australia show that although those who are significantly intellectually disadvantaged are over-represented throughout the criminal justice system, it is not certain whether or not they would fulfil the criteria for an ICD diagnosis of intellectual impairment or learning disability (Holland *et al*, 2002).

BOX 1.1　　　GREG

Greg is a 23-year-old man who was admitted for assessment to an acute mental health unit in central London having been detained under Section 2 of the Mental Health Act (1983) after he had initially exhibited bizarre and aggressive behaviour in a shopping centre that morning. He was unkempt and it was assumed that he had probably been sleeping rough. His past history was difficult to obtain; however, some weeks later staff were able to piece together some aspects of his past.

Greg was the third of six siblings who were born and brought up in Glasgow in a low-income family, his father was in and out of prison for a variety of reasons including grievous bodily harm. Social workers had expressed concern that when the father was at home there were several instances that indicated that both mother and the children were victims of domestic violence, but this was never proven conclusively and mother continued to do her best to bring up the family on state benefits.

Greg regularly played truant from school where he failed to excel and was often in trouble for bullying other children. By the age of nine he had his first police caution for shoplifting. There then followed a series of warnings and cautions by the police until finally he was sent to a young offenders unit at the age of 16. He served nine months of his sentence. Once back at the family home he failed to find long-term employment as he would never arrive on time for work, or not appear at all. He continued to be involved in petty crime and in addition began to use a variety of substances on a regular basis. This situation continued for some years, punctuated with another spell in prison, this time for grievous bodily harm following a fight in a pub after he had drunk a large amount of alcohol. This time prison life was almost unbearable for him. He was regularly bullied and subsequently was treated for depression. ➤

On his release he went back to Glasgow until the death of his mother when the family home fragmented. Greg moved to London and was homeless within a few weeks after he fell out with one of his sisters who was allowing him to sleep on her sofa. His substance abuse continued and was funded by petty crime and begging. Greg had been living in this manner for six months when the police detained him under section 136 of the Mental Health Act (1983) and ultimately brought him to a mental health unit. Mental health assessment indicated the presence of a possible psychosis, which responded well to treatment and was considered to probably be associated with the high levels of cannabis that he had been using for some years. Greg could barely read or write and old records showed that he had an IQ of 79, but it was felt that his adaptive functioning level was much lower owing to his mental health problems and poor coping skills. ■

INCLUSION AND NORMALIZATION

The concept of community inclusion (and its forerunners) was the most important revolution underpinning reform of long-term care services for much of the second half of the twentieth century. Although focus has often been on mental health and learning disability services, similar principles have been adopted throughout health services especially in the other 'Cinderella' services, such as rehabilitation and care of older people.

The term 'normalization' in this context first emerged from Denmark in 1959 as part of the Mental Retardation Act. It was initially used to describe the creation of 'an existence as close to normal living as possible'. Wolfensberger (1972) defined it as 'the means which are as culturally normative as possible in order to establish and/or maintain personal behaviours and characteristics which are as culturally normative as possible' (p.28). His commitment to the eradication of the institutions was to mirror this stance. For Wolfensberger the isolation from the wider community that characterized institutional care established a subculture of deviants whereby devalued people often behave in accordance with the deviant label that society has assigned to them. In turn he surmised that this behaviour serves to strengthen society's existing stereotypical beliefs, thus reinforcing them. He later withdrew the term 'normalization', in preference for social role valorization, which emphasized the importance of citizenship and the development of individuals' self-worth as a result of belonging and being accepted by the wider community. Today we would perhaps term this as inclusion or integration.

However, this 'inclusion' in relation to health care is potentially problematic for both primary care and acute services owing to both the inaccessibility of services for people with impairments and the relative lack of expertise of professionals working within them. Some have argued that the concept of normalization and its successors is essentially a professional philosophy, which treats people as a homogeneous group and fails to recognize individuality (Gilbert, 1993). To identify two contrasting examples: people with severe and enduring mental health problems will have different issues from the client with a vascular dementia, as will those who have a mild learning disability compared with a person with profound learning disabilities and an organic behaviour disorder. Coupled with such problems are the complexities of physical health needs that may be syndrome-specific or otherwise and can be difficult to diagnose owing to communication problems, professionals' lack of knowledge and skills in this area in addition to poor accessibility of services or diagnostic overshadowing.

Szivos (1992) claims that whilst much good has come from inclusion, there are aspects which must be questioned. Inclusion presumes that assimilation into mainstream society works and indeed that this is necessarily a good thing. It makes the assumption that in order to be valued by society the disadvantaged person is able and willing to aspire to society's norms. Yet social comparison theory emphasizes how people often choose to interact with people who are similar to themselves in terms of ability and experience because the comparisons of self-evaluation are less challenging (Festinger, 1954). In relation to those with an intellectual impairment one must question the assumption that the random dispersal of such individuals into communities will necessarily lead to them feeling more 'valued' and 'normal' (Szivos, 1992) although the forced institutionalization of a previously independent person is equally unlikely to enhance self-esteem by enforcing reference to an impaired group.

Since the gradual closure of the long-stay institutions there has been increasing emphasis on a person-centred approach towards life planning and a mainstream community model of living for all. This integration includes services meeting health needs, both mental and physical. For many people with acquired causes of intellectual impairment, the shift to community care in the 1990s moved the locus of care away from long-stay hospitals while locating an increased amount of care in private nursing homes or, in the case of mental health problems, hostels. For people with learning disabilities in England and Wales *Valuing People* (DH, 2001) represents a further drive towards the philosophy of inclusion, community presence and participation by advocating that all areas of these people's lives are as reflective of the general population as possible. Whilst the document does acknowledge that there are a 'small' number of people who require specialist services the emphasis is very much on community integration and the use of generic health services with support.

The closure of the long-stay hospitals has also led to the formation of 'tokenistic deinstitutionalization'; group homes, particularly for those with known learning disabilities, and hostels for those with severe and enduring mental health problems. Many of these individuals are living with people that they would not normally choose to be with and with whom they share no common interests. The movement from the institutions meant the loss of lifelong friendships that had often been present since childhood as many individuals were dispersed throughout communities. Rejection by the community may lead to lowered self-esteem and further isolation of the person with intellectual impairment if there is not an understanding by the general public of these conditions as well as an acceptance of them. Ignorance and fear exacerbate the problem.

There is a need for literacy in the public in relation to mental health disorders and Jorm (2000) concludes that many members of the public cannot recognize specific disorders, or signs of psychological distress. He also argues that much of the information available to the public is misleading and needs to be improved if people who have mental health problems are going to receive the necessary support that they need from their local community. The same may well apply to the health services that form part of that community since professionals are not immune from common prejudices and, in relation to intellectual impairment, receive very little training.

MAINSTREAM HEALTH SERVICES AND PEOPLE WITH INTELLECTUAL IMPAIRMENTS

Any debate surrounding the use of mainstream health services in the provision of an inclusive approach to care must incorporate the suitability of such services to provide adequate care. People with intellectual impairment in general access mainstream health services in the same manner that everyone else does so there is some urgency to address outstanding issues of both knowledge and attitudes to care. The barriers and challenges to secondary health care for people with intellectual impairments are numerous and include limited education and training of health-care professionals in this area, the perceived risk of challenging behaviour for other patients and issues surrounding communication problems (Access to Acute Network (Secondary Care) 2002; Mencap, 2004).

As already suggested the general public are not alone in their attitude towards and lack of knowledge of people with intellectual impairments. *Treat Me Right!* (Mencap, 2004) recently highlighted some of the problems that mainstream health service professionals have in the care of these patients. Their findings relate largely to physical health in patients with known learning disabilities, however, many issues raised are extremely pertinent to all groups who have intellectual impairment. Their recommendations include training and education for all health professionals, and an end to health inequalities.

In the past psychiatrists in the institutions cared for both the mental and physical health of their patients. These clinicians developed skills in the management of more common conditions such as epilepsy, depression, dementias, endocrine and behavioural disorders. In more recent times general practitioners and clinical assistants worked alongside these psychiatrists providing general medical care and consequently developed their own skills with these groups of people. Local district general hospitals offered continuity of specialist input including dental, gynaecology and orthopaedics often on site. Although this was far from a perfect state there is now a danger that many of these particular skills will be lost (Asprey *et al*, 2004). People with intellectual impairment must now register with local general practitioners many of whom do not have any special interest in the subject and have been ill-prepared to deal with some of the complex mixtures of physical, psychiatric, emotional and behavioural problems.

Research through the 1990s studied the attitudes of nurses towards patients with learning disabilities in the general hospital environment (Slevin, 1995; Murray and Chambers, 1991; Barr, 1990) and revealed a general lack of knowledge and understanding of this patient group with shortfalls in education and training being considered a contributory factor. This is a situation that has not improved over the last decade (Mencap, 2004). There is more recent evidence that staff working in general psychiatry perceive that they lack both the knowledge and skills needed in order to care for patients with intellectual impairments (Chaplin, 2004).

Throughout the latter part of the last century it was still questioned as to whether people with intellectual impairment were capable of developing the psychological process that could lead to mental illness (Winokur, 1974; Gardner, 1967; Schneider, 1959). However, in the UK The Health of the Nation (DH, 1992) recognized that those individuals with known learning disabilities were in fact more prone to health problems, including that of their mental health. Mental health problems among those who have intellectual impairments are now recognized to be more prevalent than in the general population (Deb *et al*, 2001; Doody *et al*, 1998; Patel *et al*, 1993). Various factors have been cited as being contributory towards this vulnerability including the actual damage to the brain, epilepsy, repeated loss or separation issues, poor coping mechanisms and lack of social skills, communication difficulties and family problems (Fraser and Nolan, 1995).

But people with severe intellectual impairment have low rates of generic psychiatric service use. Staff identify that they lack the education, knowledge and skills needed to care for these patients when they are occasionally admitted. A review of previous studies showed that this group of people may not fit into general psychiatric services at all (Chaplin, 2004). Conditions including organic behaviour disorder will seldom be seen in the mainstream acute psychiatric environment so it is unrealistic for us to expect generic mental health professionals to either recognize, diagnose or successfully manage them.

With clinical governance at the heart of much healthcare policy, the use of mainstream services for people with intellectual impairments must yield a high standard of quality service in an environment of clinical excellence, research and development (DH, 1997). In terms of the achievement of 'best value' for this patient group the 'improvement' currently means the demise of specialist services in favour of mainstream services where this group of people may be lost and ignored because of lack of expertise. This book aims to remedy this by beginning to fill the gap created by the demise of specialist services.

CONTENTS OF THE BOOK

Steve Higgins and Mary O'Toole analyse the range of health needs of people who have intellectual impairment in Chapter 2. Some of the more common physical and mental health problems are identified, as are more general health concerns. Genetic disorders (including some of the more frequently observed behavioural phenotypes), ageing and health for people with intellectual impairment are also discussed.

In Chapter 3 Garry Diack and Howard Cohen draw on their wide community experience of people with intellectual impairment in order to encourage health professionals to examine their generic communication and assessment skills in the light of examination of need for the individual. They encourage the reader to critically appraise communication methods and to understand the value and appropriateness of such in meeting the needs of people with intellectual impairment and to consider what factors are relevant in order to improve the process.

Recognition is given to the anxiety generated for health professionals with only general health training. Similarities and differences between individuals with and without intellectual impairment are explored in detail with the emphasis on effective communication and non-judgemental approaches. Garry and Howard deliver pertinent advice in the area of communication and it is a paramount element of this chapter as it encourages practitioners to utilize their existing skills to good effect in the care of patients who have intellectual impairment.

Chapter 4 examines intellectual impairment from the primary care perspective. Louise Barriball, Allan Hicks, Howard Cohen and Liz Lewry use their expertise to guide the reader through some of the challenges that the primary care practitioner encounters in relation to this group. Opportunities and barriers are explored in relation to healthcare delivery and examples of good practice are highlighted. The implications for joint working across primary care with its various subgroupings are explored, as are individual and organizational learning needs in relation to intellectual impairment. The writers support their work with case studies and examples of good practice, they make recommendations for the future of this speciality within primary care.

Karen Lowton, Theresa Wiseman and Ian Noonan guide us through chronic and enduring illness in people with intellectual impairment in Chapter 5. They introduce us to clients who have intellectual impairment in addition to chronic and enduring health problems. Through them they illustrate key points such as the underlying themes of the continuous assessment process, good communication and the ongoing process of effective care delivery. The importance of lay carers in the long-term management of chronic conditions is amplified as are issues surrounding the provision of support for these and other non-health professionals. Palliative care and bereavement are also discussed.

In Chapter 6 Emma Ouldred and Catherine Bryant consider dementia in both the general population and in those whose existing intellectual impairments render them more prone to dementia. They explore the implications of increased longevity for all populations but especially those with congenital intellectual impairments. Emma and Catherine identify the various forms of dementia, the risk factors for such conditions and their incidence, discussing barriers to service provision. Assessment of dementia is discussed as is the management of such conditions and the impact that dementia may have on carers.

Ian Noonan and Karen Lowton utilize the patient journey from accident and emergency (A&E) department in Chapter 7, through the assessment process, admission and discharge home. Detailed exploration is provided throughout on the practical aspects of assessment and intervention through three patient case studies who present with contrasting physical and mental health problems. They explore the types of emergency that people with intellectual impairment may present with and help the reader to study ways in which they can improve how they work with these individuals. Problems with various aspects of communication in an emergency context, in relation to the explanation of procedures and consent, are visited. Assessment of both pain and distress are described in some detail and some new solutions found in addition to how to assess and treat cases of self-harm and self-injury. The management of disturbed or challenging behaviour in the acute environment is also discussed and inter-professional liaison is addressed as is the importance of clinical supervision in case management and review in the care of people with intellectual impairment.

The assessment and management of the intellectually impaired patient in the acute mental health environment is scrutinized by Mary O'Toole, Mike Reid and Rob Winterhalder in Chapter 8. They describe some of the problems encountered by the mental health professional in relation to people with intellectual impairment when they receive acute care. The trio apply a bio-psychosocial approach to both the assessment and care management processes and refer to some of the complexities of diagnostic overshadowing. Interventions are studied as are some of the ways that traditional generic approaches may be adapted for use with patients who have intellectual impairments. The ongoing argument of the suitability of generic mental health services for these patients is discussed and some solutions suggested.

Chapters 9 and 10 focus on specific approaches to treatments. Rob Winterhalder gives a description of the psychopharmacological issues involved in prescribing for people with intellectual impairments in Chapter 9. Michael Kelly takes us on a journey through some of the main causes of challenging behaviour in Chapter 10, its presentation and ways to assess and overcome it and illustrates this with case studies. Rob uses a practical approach to the reasons why prescribing for people with intellectual impairment differs from that of the general population. Michael refers to government guidelines on the management of challenging behaviour and highlights the absence or insufficiency of the risk assessment process in relation to challenging behaviour in many health environments. He discusses the management through medication of challenging behaviours and its use and misuse. The management of challenging behaviour in residential homes for both formal and informal carers is explored and suggestions are made for staff training and support in this area. Michael critically examines the use of physical interventions for people with intellectual impairments and provides an insight into some of the associated issues.

Chapter 11 reflects on many of the legal and ethical issues that have been touched upon throughout the book. Alison Hobden and Simon Mills examine some of the wider implications relating to people who have intellectual impairment and discuss the appropriate legislation especially in relation to consent. They discuss the various types of consent and its interplay mental capacity using relevant cases that have come before the courts. They refer to pertinent case law throughout and also punctuate the text with relevant case studies.

In the final chapter Peter Griffiths, Rob Winterhalder, Allan Hicks and Louise Clark explore contrasting views on the future of intellectual impairment services. Rob and Louise apply a dialogue in order to show that professionals working together in the speciality can also disagree. This follows an introduction to the commissioning of services, underlying philosophy and service models. The need for joint working across the health, social and voluntary sector arenas and the problems that arise with this is discussed in some detail. A case study introduces us to Doris who is a 50-year-old woman who has Down syndrome, psychosis and dementia. Doris's assessment and care are detailed as are some of the issues that become problematic with her care and the appropriate service provision that she should receive. The care programme approach is applied to Doris and the reader is led to understand both the necessity and the process of such an approach and the future of such a tool in the overall management and care of people with intellectual impairment. Chapter 12 concludes with proposals and recommendations for the future shape of service provision, education and training following the discourse between somewhat opposing stances.

REFERENCES AND RECOMMENDED READING

Access to Acute Network (Secondary Care). (2002) *Supporting People with a Learning Disability on Admission to Hospital*. Shrewsbury: Shropshire Primary Care Trust.

Asprey T, Francis R, Tyrer S, Quillman S. (2004) Patients with learning disability in the community have special medical needs that should be planned for. *British Medical Journal* 318:476–7.

Barr O. (1990) Knowledge and attitudes towards people with mental handicap living in the community. *British Medical Journal* 301:1379–81.

Bhui K, Aubin A, Strathdee G. (1998) Making a reality of user involvement in community mental health services. *Psychiatric Bulletin* 22:8–11.

Braine ME. (2005) The management of challenging behaviour and cognitive impairment. *British Journal of Neuroscience Nursing* 1(2):67–74.

Cantley C. (ed.) (2001) *A Handbook of Dementia Care*. Buckingham: Open University Press.

Chaplin R. (2004) General psychiatric services for adults with intellectual disability and mental illness. *Journal of Disability Research* 48(part 1):1–10.

Cicerone KD, Mott T, Azulay J, Friel JC. (2004) Community integration and satisfaction with functioning after intensive cognitive rehabilitation for traumatic brain injury. *Arch Phys Med Rehabil* 85:943–50.

Clark LL. (2006) What's in a name? Transfer of skills across the Cinderella services. *British Journal of Neuroscience Nursing* 1(5):161–2.

Deb S, Thomas M, Bright C. (2001) Mental disorder in adults with intellectual disability: prevalence of functional psychiatric illness among a community-based population between 16 and 64 years. *Journal of Intellectual Disability Research* 45:495–505.

Department of Health. (1992) *Health of the Nation.* London: DH.

Department of Health. (1997) *The New NHS: Modern, Dependable.* London: DH.

Department of Health. (2001) *Valuing People: A New Strategy for Learning Disability for the 21ˢᵗ Century.* London: DH.

Doody GA, Johnstone EC, Sanderson TL, Owens DG, Muir WJ. (1998) 'Propfschizophrenie' revisited: Schizophrenia in people with mild learning disability. *British Journal of Psychiatry* 173:145–53.

Edwards N. (2003) Promoting mental health and well-being. In: Edwards N, Lennox N, Holt G, Bouras N (eds). *Mental Health in Adult Learning Disability.* Queensland: University of Queensland.

Engberg AW, Teasdale TW. (2004) Psychological outcome following traumatic brain injury in adults: a long-term population-based follow-up. *Brain Injury* 18:533–45.

Farrington DP. (2000) Psychosocial causes of offending. In: Gelder MG, Lopez-Ibor JJ Andreasen (eds). *New Oxford Textbook of Psychiatry* 2. Oxford: Oxford University Press, 2029–36.

Festinger L. (1954) A theory of social comparison processes. *Human Relations* 7:117–40.

Franulic A, Carbonell EG, Pinto P, Sepuleveda I. (2004) Psychological adjustment and employment outcome, 5 and 10 years after TBI. *Brain Injury* 18:119–29.

Fraser W, Nolan M. (1995) Psychiatric disorders in mental retardation. In: Bouras N (ed.). *Mental Health in Mental Retardation: Recent Advances and Practices.* Cambridge: Cambridge University Press.

Gardner W. (1967) Occurrence of severe depressive reactions in the mentally retarded. *American Journal of Psychiatry* 124:386–8.

Gilbert T. (1993) Learning disability nursing: from normalisation to materialism – towards a new paradigm. *Journal of Advanced Nursing* 18(5):1604–9.

Holland T, Clare ICH, Mukhopadhyay T. (2002) Prevalence of 'criminal offending' by men and women with intellectual disability and the characteristics of 'offenders': implications for research and service development. *Journal of Intellectual Disability Research* 46(1):6–20.

International Classification of Mental Health and Behavioural Disorders. ICD-10 (1994) *World Health Organization.* Geneva: Churchill Livingstone.

Jorm AF. (2000) Mental Health Literacy. Public knowledge and beliefs about mental disorders. *British Journal of Psychiatry* 177:396–401.

Matthews FE, Brayne C, Medical Research Council Investigators. (2005) The incidence of dementia in England & Wales: findings from the five identical sites of the MRC CFA Study. *PloS Med* 2:e193.

McIntosh B, Whittaker A. (1998) *Days of Change.* London: King's Fund.

Mencap. (2004) *Treat Me Right! Better healthcare for people with a learning disability.* London: Mencap.

The Mental Health Act. (1983) London: HMSO.

MRC CFAS. (1998) Cognitive function and dementia in six areas of England & Wales: the distribution of MMSE and the prevalence of GMS organicity level in the MRC CFA study. The Medical Research Council Cognitive Function & Ageing Study (MRC CFAS). *Psychological Medicine* 28:319–35.

Murray M, Chambers M. (1991) Effect of contact on nursing students' attitudes to patients. *Nurse Education Today* 11:363–7.

Patel P, Goldberg D, Moss S. (1993) Psychiatric morbidity in older people with moderate or severe learning disability (mental retardation) Part 2: The prevalence study. *British Journal of Psychiatry* 163:481–91.

Perneczky R, Pohl C, Sorg C, Hartmann J, Komossa K, Alexopoulos P, Wagenpfeil S, Kruz A. (2006) Complex activities of daily living in mild cognitive impairment: conceptual and diagnostic issues. *Age and Ageing* 35(3):240–5.

Powell J, Heslin J, Greenwood R. (2002) Community based rehabilitation after severe traumatic brain injury: a randomised controlled trial. *Journal of Neurology and Neurosurgical Psychiatry* 72:193–202.

Schneider K. (1959) *Clinical Psychopathology.* New York: Grune & Stratton.

Slevin E. (1995) Student nurses' attitudes towards people with learning disabilities. *British Journal of Nursing* 4(13):761–6.

Svendsen H, Teasdale TW, Pinner M. (2004) Subjective experience in patients with brain injury and their close relatives before and after a rehabilitation programme. *Neuropsychological Rehabilitation* 14: 495–515.

Szivos S. (1992) The limits to integration? In: Brown H, Smith H (eds). *Normalisation: A Reader for the Nineties*. London: Routledge.

Winokur B. (1974) Subnormality and its relation to psychiatry. *Lancet* 2:270–3.

Wolfensberger W. (1972) *The Principle of Normalisation in Human Services*. Toronto: National Institute on Mental Retardation.

CHAPTER 2
MEETING THE HEALTH NEEDS OF PEOPLE WITH INTELLECTUAL IMPAIRMENT
Steve Higgins and Mary O'Toole

STUDY AIMS:

1. To explore the complexity of healthcare problems experienced by people with intellectual impairment.

2. To understand some of the difficulties experienced by people with intellectual impairment in accessing treatment.

3. To study some of the more common conditions experienced by people with intellectual impairment.

4. To examine the relationship between physical and mental health problems of people with intellectual impairment.

Recently in the UK the development of Health Action Planning (DH, 2002) has required health providers to complete a plan outlining the health needs of all individuals with learning disabilities, which can then be used as a baseline of information for health professionals when an individual is referred for assessment or consultation. Similar health action plans for those with severe and enduring mental health problems are also available under the Care Programme Approach (CPA), which originally came into being as a form of discharge planning associated

Learning Disability and other Intellectual Impairments, Edited by L.L. Clark and P. Griffiths
© 2008 John Wiley & Sons, Ltd

with the Mental Health Act (1983), although the focus here is predominantly on mental health issues. The single assessment process for older people aims to fulfil the same role for the comprehensive health and social care needs of that group which also includes many with intellectual impairment.

These initiatives recognize the extent of previously unmet needs and the challenges in delivering comprehensive services in the face of complex impairments including intellectual ones. Despite these initiatives, unmet healthcare needs remain a major issue for many (Mencap, 2004). A number of reasons have been identified for this disparity between health needs and the provision of health care for people across the range of intellectual impairments. In a review of prevalence studies, Jansen *et al* (2004) identified that all previous comparative studies showed that people with intellectual impairment have higher rates of most physical and mental health disorders compared with the general population. This is not surprising given the bio-psychosocial impact of intellectual impairment, whatever its cause, on an individual and their everyday functioning.

These 'excess' health problems emerge from both internal and external risk factors and can result in specific as well as systemic health problems. If left unidentified or untreated, some health problems may result in secondary conditions which may compound the original condition.

BARRIERS TO ASSESSMENT, DIAGNOSIS AND TREATMENT

Accessing primary healthcare services remains problematic for people with intellectual impairment (Jansen *et al*, 2004; Lennox and Kerr, 1997), despite having higher rates of healthcare needs. Indeed, this client group will frequently be faced with a number of barriers which operate at a number of levels when attempting to access services.

Client-related barriers involve some of the problems surrounding communication and identification of health needs, atypical presentation and atypical responses to treatments as well as difficulties in diagnostic overshadowing, the use of self-medication and the monitoring of the effectiveness of treatment.

As a function of their intellectual impairment some people can experience various difficulties identifying and communicating their health needs. They can have problems in recognizing that some of the symptoms that they may be experiencing are health-related and therefore they may not inform others of their problems. In addition, the person may have problems in localizing areas of pain or in understanding that the pain they experience is something that is related to their health. Even if the person does recognize they have a health need, they may experience difficulty in both expressive and receptive communication. This will undoubtedly affect their ability to communicate their concerns regarding their health needs to professionals or carers.

People with mild intellectual impairments may not have the support of professional carers and will be expected to initiate contact and use health services without support. This may be problematic for some, especially those with learning disabilities, as they are a particularly suggestible and acquiescent group, unlikely to assert themselves with professionals and therefore they are more dependent on professional facilitation of their consultation than would otherwise be expected (see Chapter 3). They may also have difficulty complying with treatments owing to reading problems and difficulties with recall and receptive language skills. Thus they may not follow instructions on medication dosage, be unable to assess if treatments have been effective, or to know if they are experiencing side effects.

People with severe or profound intellectual impairment are almost wholly dependent on others to identify their healthcare problems as their ability to communicate pain or illness may be reduced to the expression of challenging behaviour. This may be misinterpreted as part of their impairment and not as a function of experiencing pain or discomfort (this issue is discussed in more detail in Chapter 10).

'Clinician/professional' barriers relate to a lack of the necessary knowledge and skill regarding intellectual impairment among professionals, as well as a limited understanding of health issues in this client group, including required modification in the assessment, treatment and monitoring of health status that may affect them. Many healthcare professionals display 'layperson' levels of understanding of intellectual impairment and may reflect the prejudicial views that permeate society, particularly towards those who have milder forms of intellectual impairment who may not be supported by social care services.

A number of studies have assessed the attitudes and knowledge of primary healthcare staff including GPs and district nurses/practice nurses and it would appear that there is growing recognition amongst these professional groups that they should be providing care for people with intellectual impairment (Melville *et al*, 2005). Indeed, the majority of primary care professionals identify a lack of confidence and competence in meeting the health needs of people with intellectual impairment (Melville *et al*, 2005).

In response to such deficits information and training material has been developed, aimed at primary healthcare professionals. For example, the Getting Better (Band, 1997) video is a resource for health professionals conducting consultations with people with intellectual impairment, outlining some of the difficulties facing both the patient and professional and providing simple and effective strategies to improve the consultation process. Hardy *et al* (2006) have recently produced some basic guidance points for nurses working in primary health care who are supporting patients with intellectual impairments, in this case specifically aimed at people with learning disabilities although potentially of wider utility. Likewise, Bouras *et al* (2000) have also produced guidance for GPs and other primary health professionals in the assessment and treatment of mental illness in people with intellectual impairment. (Further discussion on training issues can be found in Chapter 8.)

Organizational barriers are largely concerned with the accessibility of primary care services and issues such as the additional time often needed in the consulting room for patients who have intellectual impairments. Historically, care for people with intellectual impairment fell within the remit of specialist services, usually on hospital-based campuses. Following the process of community integration, funding for care moved to the remit of social services for most people with intellectual impairment. Moreover, as they were not initially considered as requiring any specialist health care, the bulk of their healthcare needs were deemed the responsibility of general practices. Similarly, mental health and intellectual impairment services were funded separately resulting in much confusion over who should be providing mental health care for people with intellectual impairments for other reasons.

Small community health teams for people with learning disabilities (but not for the other groups of people with intellectual impairment) emerged in the 1980s. Their original role was to provide a specialist, multidisciplinary assessment and treatment service for a wide range of health needs such as psychology, speech and language therapy, occupational therapy, specialist nursing and psychiatry These teams currently have a remit of facilitating access to generic healthcare services for their client group and provide health promotion with much of their specialist work now performed within generic health services (DH, 2001).

The role of healthcare professionals specializing in people with intellectual disabilities has come under question several times and their role has subsequently been transformed many times over the past decade. There has been increased recognition by the government that accessibility to services remains problematic and initiatives have been developed to attempt to resolve some of these inequalities (e.g. Health Action Plans, DH, 2002; the 'Greenlight Toolkit', National Institute for Mental Heath, 2004). Despite these initiatives, the fact remains that people with intellectual impairment often have multiple and chronic healthcare needs that are either undiagnosed or untreated and the government's clear view is that this is the responsibility of both mainstream NHS and primary care services, with specialist service input only where essential.

The length of appointment times for people with intellectual impairments in both primary care and acute services requires a degree of flexibility. General practices are under pressure to see as many patients as possible and this can limit the average time spent with each patient. People with intellectual disabilities not only have difficulty understanding complex language and expressing themselves, but may also be very sensitive to social situations. The presence of a healthcare professional within the health setting is likely to be stressful and possibly intimidating to a person with intellectual impairment, and sitting in the waiting room may in itself prove too frightening, sometimes resulting in the person not even getting as far as going into the consulting room for their scheduled appointment. Fear, anxiety and stress may exacerbate communication difficulties and result in acquiescent and suggestible behaviour. Mencap (2004) recommends extended and more flexible appointment arrangement times for people with learning disabilities because of the difficulties they can experience – this should also include any individual who has an intellectual impairment for whatever reason.

A final area of concern regarding organizational barriers is the very idea of intellectual impairment itself. The present tripartite definition of learning disability being an Intelligence Quotient (IQ) below 70, onset under age 18 years, and presence of significant impairment of adaptive functioning is not an inclusive enough definition. Anyone who cannot adequately demonstrate that they meet all three criteria may be denied access to any specialist services despite presenting with many similar needs as people who do meet the definition. People with autistic spectrum disorders or pervasive developmental disorders such as Asperger's syndrome may not have a reduced IQ though they may well be severely disabled in their everyday functioning. Similarly, those who have sustained brain damage beyond the age of 18 years may also have many similar healthcare needs as those whose brain damage occurred before the age of 18 years.

There is also a large group of people who have low intellectual functioning but who are considered 'borderline' in terms of intellectual impairment. These people can usually function reasonably well; however, when healthcare or social problems emerge they can have difficulty coping with the stress or complexity of the situation. They find the navigation of health services problematic and as a result generally receive poor quality services as the level of support that they need is often not recognized. This has recently led some authors to advocate for a change of definition and more inclusive approach to provision of enhanced support (Clark, 2006).

BOX 2.1 — STEPHEN

Stephen is a 24-year-old man who acquired a brain injury two years ago as the result of a serious blow to the head whilst boxing. Following three months in hospital he was discharged home to his parents. He has very limited verbal ability and can only say six words which include 'drink, mum, dad and bed' and his use of these is inconsistent and takes a great deal of effort. Stephen has to be assisted with all his skills of daily living including feeding, washing, dressing; he is incontinent of urine, is chronically faecally impacted and has limited use of both his arms and legs. He can no longer walk; he is therefore confined to a wheel chair for most of the day and has limited stimulation. Social services provide help in the form of a carer who helps Stephen's mother to bath him twice a week and the district nurse comes twice a week to give him an enema, otherwise there is no support.

Over a two-day period Stephen seems to have become agitated and anxious, he moves his head from side to side and rolls his eyes, he attempts to bang his head on any nearby object including the back of his wheel chair and the wall. His mother mentions this to the district nurse when she next visits and the nurse says that she thinks it is probably a 'form of challenging behaviour due to Stephen's brain injury'.

Consider other causes of Stephen's agitated state and think what other questions the nurse should have asked before making her 'snap diagnosis'. ◼

Consider the scenario in Box 2.1. Stephen has experienced a sudden and quite dramatic change in behaviour over a two–day period. When such a change occurs the reason very often has an underlying physical health cause, something as simplistic as an ear, urinary tract or dental infection. In a situation like this it is essential for an urgent referral to a medical practitioner who can then make a full and thorough physical assessment. Given Stephen's past history of an acquired brain injury more serious neurological conditions cannot be ruled out.

The presentation of behaviour like this, which may also be cyclical over a period of months, may be due to organic behaviour disorder which is understood to be a biological psychiatric condition resulting in the characteristic of violence and self-injury. It affects many people who have intellectual impairments, usually those who are more profoundly intellectually disabled. It is a question of debate among psychiatrists as to whether or not the condition conforms to the requirements for the term 'psychosis' and obviously Mental State Examination (MSE) is virtually impossible. There is no distinct category within either ICD-10 or DSM 1V. However, many patients who are suspected of having this condition are medicated using risperidone and there is a consequential ethical debate surrounding this practice.

There is also a possibility that Stephen could be suffering from some form of seizure activity and once the most basic of physical causes for his agitation have been eliminated it may be necessary to investigate this as a possibility.

The nurse should have asked about other possible changes in Stephen's behaviour:

1. Has there been a change in his sleep pattern?

2. How does his appetite appear, is it reduced?

3. Does he seem hot to the touch?

4. What is his urine like? Does it seem to be more concentrated? Does it smell?

5. Does he urinate immediately after one of these episodes of head-banging?

6. Does he show excessive distress when having his teeth cleaned?

A few simple biometric measurements may have also proved useful at this juncture, for example temperature, pulse and blood pressure readings and a simple look in the ears for any outward signs of infection.

The nurse was quite wrong to dismiss Stephen's sudden change in behaviour as 'challenging', sadly this is not an uncommon label that is applied to people with intellectual impairments. Stephen's behavioural change could literally be due to almost any condition and without the patient being able to articulate the symptoms it makes the process of diagnosis extremely difficult. In addition, it is a reason why people with intellectual impairments often have their health needs seriously and sometimes fatally neglected (Mencap, 2007).

BARRIERS TO HEALTH PROMOTION AND PREVENTIVE CARE

Access to information and health promotion is another area of concern for people with intellectual impairments. The use of complex and sometimes 'medical language' may cause confusion for an individual and thus accessible information is an important aspect not only of health promotion but also of treatment and compliance issues. There is now an increasingly good range of material available for use in primary care services that present information in an accessible style, for example leaflets provided by the Elfrida Society (see reference list for web contact details). These leaflets are designed to be used both during a consultation and as well as a resource for the individual to take away with them. Others resources include the Books Beyond Words series which covers a range of health-related issues such as *Going to the Doctor* (Hollins, Bernal and Gregory, 1996) and are helpful for use during the consultation.

Access to health screening and health checks is routinely recommended for certain people in the community such as breast and cervical screening for women. Despite this, women with intellectual disabilities are less likely than the general population to receive cervical screening and similarly they are less likely to be offered breast examination or mammography appointments. Similarly, as this group have complex health needs, annual health checks should be offered routinely to identify unrecognized health problems so the burden of identification is not solely on carers who may have little healthcare knowledge. This relies on medical records to identify which patients have an intellectual impairment.

The identification of people with borderline intellectual impairments can allow practices to plan care in a more proactive way. Hospitals and primary care services have a duty of care to their patients and must also fulfil their legal obligations by ensuring that individuals with special support needs have them in place so that they can access the health services equitably. *Tackling Health Inequalities* (DH, 2003) identifies the use of health audit as a means to achieve greater equity of access for a range of people including those with intellectual impairments and places responsibility on primary care to develop and implement such strategies at a local level. Mencap (2004) highlights inquiries into premature death of people with intellectual impairments due to a failure to properly assess need and offer appropriate care.

SYNDROME-RELATED HEALTH NEEDS

Comorbidity is high in people with intellectual impairment. Many disorders are inter-related, some as primary disorders, others emerging systemically and as a consequence of a primary disorder. Additionally, illness may be the result of either internal or external lifestyle factors. Here we identify physical health needs according to bodily system with separate sections on mental illness and behavioural disorders. We recognize that this is a largely artificial categorization as bodily systems impact on each other as well as on an individual's mental health and any resulting behavioural problems. Practitioners must avoid the use of a 'tunnel-vision' approach to assessment and case management in order to capture the full extent of an individual's health status.

GENETIC DISORDERS

A number of genetic disorders lead to intellectual impairment. These are numerous and detailed and their description is beyond the scope of this chapter (there is a list of accessible texts and resources at the end of the chapter). The general issues will be discussed and a focus on one or two more common conditions will be offered to illustrate the range of health implications for genetic disorders associated with intellectual impairment.

Genetic disorders may result in a wide range of physical, mental and behavioural problems as a result of specific phenotypes. Phenotypes are physical, mental or behavioural disorders that are associated with the genetic syndrome itself. Physical phenotypes relate to the physical features associated with a syndrome, such as the epicanthic eyelid folds and cardiac problems which are present in people with Down syndrome or the microcephaly, broad-based nose and micrognathia associated with cri-du-chat syndrome. Behavioural phenotypes are forms of behaviour/mental illness specifically associated with particular disorders, such as insatiable appetite, skin picking and temper outbursts seen in Prader-Willi syndrome, the abnormal sleep pattern seen in Smith-Lemli-Opitz syndrome, or the inappropriate smiling or laughter seen in people who have Angleman's syndrome.

Down syndrome (which is the most common chromosomal/genetic abnormality) is strongly associated with intellectual impairment as well as a wide range of both physical and mental healthcare problems including cardiovascular abnormalities, lung and respiratory disorders, muscular hypotonia and endocrine disorders including most commonly hypothyroidism. In terms of mental health disorders it is closely associated with Alzheimer's disease, often with an earlier onset than that seen in the general population, from middle age onwards. The condition is also associated with depression as well as hypothyroidism, this is a classic example of diagnostic overshadowing as the symptoms of the two conditions are similar and present a challenge to the inexperienced practitioner, especially as the two may coexist and be complicated by the individual's intellectual impairment.

The main issue of concern in these cases is that medical disorders tend to co-occur and promote the development of further disorders so that clinical presentation and management is often extremely complex. Similarly, just because a behaviour may have a genetic predisposition there may be a wide variation in its expression. Genetically caused behavioural disorders are sometimes open to modification depending on early childhood intervention, family support and education. Such early intervention can reduce the impact of behavioural phenotypes by instilling therapeutic interventions in order to prevent a predisposition becoming a serious and entrenched 'challenging' behaviour.

It is also crucial to remember that those affected by these syndromes are also at risk of disorders affecting the general population such as those associated with ageing. Practitioners should refer to the excellent resources listed at the end of the chapter for specific detail on other syndromes.

PHYSICAL HEALTH

NEUROLOGICAL DISORDERS

Major areas of neurological dysfunction affecting people with intellectual impairments include epilepsy and other types of seizures. This has long been presumed to be associated with the actual damage to the brain. Damage to the brain also has a part to play in the development of schizophrenia and organic behaviour disorder, these conditions also occurring much more commonly in people with intellectual impairments than in the general population.

Seizures are closely associated with increasing severity of intellectual impairment (whatever the aetiology) with up to 50% of people diagnosed with severe intellectual impairment experiencing seizures. Whole population studies for people with intellectual impairment are few, but the prevalence rate of active epilepsy is thought to be around 20% (Forsgren et al, 1990). This compares to a general population rate of active epilepsy of about 1% with around a quarter of new cases appearing in older adults (Sander et al, 1990). Such seizure onset is most likely associated with organic disorders such as dementia. These commonly occur in adults with Down syndrome and late onset seizures are strongly linked to the development of Alzheimer's dementia in these people.

Ryan and Sunada (1997) found undiagnosed or untreated epilepsy was the most common physical cause underlying the behavioural disturbance in people with intellectual impairment referred for psychiatric evaluation. The full range of seizure disorders are seen, though more associated with intellectual impairment are drop attacks (atonic), atypical absence, myoclonic and tonic seizures, partial and generalized seizures also occur. Status epilepticus, whereby seizures occur in rapid succession to the extent that recovery of consciousness between episodes does not occur, is also seen. Hyperpyrexia develops, coma deepens and permanent brain damage may occur due to anoxia. It is generally associated with infections, metabolic disorders or the withdrawal of anticonvulsants. Status epilepticus is an emergency medical condition and may not be easy to detect because presentation can be behavioural (as in stereotypies) or with cognitive signs with the person appearing psychotic.

Management of epilepsy will involve the prescribing and administration of medication. Healthcare professionals should ensure that clients and their carers are aware of dosage, potential side effects and the dangers of stopping medication against medical advice.

Although some identify environmental causes for self-injury in people with intellectual impairment (e.g. Iwata et al, 1982) a number of authors consider neurobiological aetiology as equally important. Dopamine, seratonin and opioids are all cited as contributors to self-injury in some individuals. It is certainly believed that there is some neurochemical involvement in the onset of self-injurious behaviour, particularly so for those individuals who have profound and multiple disability or specific genetic disorders (such as Lesch–Nyhan and cri–du–chat syndromes).

SENSORY SYSTEMS

Visual impairment

There is a strong association between intellectual impairment and visual impairment with studies showing high prevalence rates in children with learning disabilities (Warburg *et al*, 1979). Twenty to thirty per cent of adults with learning disabilities have moderate visual impairment and 1–5% have severe visual impairment or blindness (Beange *et al*, 1995). In people with severe and multiple physical and intellectual impairment the prevalence rates are greater than 50% (Warburg, 2001).

As with the general population, the problem increases with age. Janicki and Dalton (1998) found in their large scale studies that as people with learning disabilities age, the reported prevalence of visual problems increases from 17% (age 35–39 years) to 34% (age 60–69 years) and 53% (age 80–89 years). Common causes of visual impairment in people with learning disabilities include senile cataracts, optic nerve atrophy, retinitis pigmentosa and congenital cataracts which differ from the variety often seen in older adults in that they usually occur further into the eye itself, as opposed to as an outer film.

Ocular disorders are particularly common in people with Down syndrome including blepharitis, strabismus, keratoconus, cataract, nystagmus and high myopia. Blepharitis or inflammation of the eyelid may result in a sticky discharge, redness and swelling of the eyelids and conjunctiva. This occurs frequently in people with Down syndrome unless proactive action is taken, therefore simple daily hygiene may prevent long-term serious damage to the eyes. Age-related cataracts also appear prematurely in people with Down syndrome – usually from the age of 40 years onwards thus earlier regular assessment by an ophthalmologist is advisable. Myopia can also commonly occur in Down syndrome but management through spectacle use may be complicated by concordance issues particularly when the severity of an individual's cognitive ability means that they do not understand the rationale for wearing spectacles. Finally, Brushfield spots, which are small white spots on the iris, are a common phenomenon in Down syndrome, they are a harmless feature and do not cause any visual impairment.

People with acquired brain injuries and damage such as cerebrovascular accident (CVA) frequently have sensory problems that stem from the neurological damage. Visual disturbances such as field deficits, blurring and double vision can cause major functional impairments which are often hard to identify in the face of complex impairments in cognition, expression and comprehension.

Auditory impairment

There is a high prevalence of hearing impairment in people with intellectual impairments, especially in people with learning disabilities but also among older people with dementia. Yeates (1995) studied a sample of 500 adults and found that 40% had sufficient hearing impairment to warrant some amplification intervention. In addition, 64% of people with Down syndrome in the sample were affected by hearing loss. Hearing loss compounds problems with communication and can make an individual appear more disabled (Williams, 1982) exacerbating the person's ability to interact with others, but it may also colour the views of carers towards the individual's capabilities and thus their expectations and interactions with the individual.

In addition to Down syndrome, there are other rarer forms of genetic disorders that are also associated with hearing impairment, similarly a range of pre- and postnatal causes of intellectual impairment that can also affect auditory functioning. For example, infections such as rubella, meningitis, toxoplasmosis and cytomegalovirus have both cognitive and sensory effects. Postnatal causes such as prematurity, birth anoxia and hyperbilirubinaemia due to rhesus incompatibility can cause both intellectual impairment and sensory disability in infants.

During childhood, chronic otitis media is a common cause of hearing impairment in children with and without intellectual disabilities. It is known that children with intellectual impairments may find it problematic to communicate an ear infection to others, for instance they may bang their head against a wall or exhibit other forms of perceived 'challenging behaviour' in order to communicate their discomfort. This may also be the case in adults with intellectual impairments who have ear infections; the danger here is that if the condition is ignored irretrievable damage may result.

CARDIOVASCULAR SYSTEM

Cardiovascular disease is commonly reported, Van den Akker *et al* (2006) found 14% of people with intellectual impairment in their study were diagnosed with cardiac diseases and, similarly, coronary artery disease accounted for between 14% and 20% of deaths in people with intellectual disabilities (Hollins *et al*, 1998) making coronary heart disease the second highest cause of death for people with learning disabilities.

Cardiovascular problems are associated with genetic causes of intellectual impairment as well as lifestyle factors for all groups of people with intellectual impairment. Congenital heart defects are associated with a number of common genetic conditions with both Williams and Fragile X syndromes displaying a range of congenital cardiac abnormalities. Congenital heart defects are common in people with Down syndrome, occurring in around 50% of births, and may affect their risk of developing hypertension and stroke.

Lifestyle factors associated with intellectual impairment also lead to the development of cardiovascular disease. These typically involve a poor diet high in fat, sugar and calories coupled with a sedentary lifestyle which increase the likelihood for the development of hypertension and obesity. Individuals with mental health problems are also more likely to smoke cigarettes than the general population whilst the long-term use of psychotropic and anti-epilepsy drugs may contribute further to lethargy and obesity.

ENDOCRINE SYSTEM

Disorders that cause disruption to cerebral and organ development and function are also likely to involve endocrine function and it is therefore expected that disorders of these systems should occur at a higher prevalence in people with intellectual impairment. Lifestyle factors may also have endocrine consequences, obesity in people with intellectual impairment being an example. Similarly, treatment for other associated disorders may have consequences for the endocrine system, such as the use of anticonvulsants. Below we will consider a range of these issues including thyroid disease, diabetes, hypogonadism, and the menopause.

Thyroid disease

Undiagnosed thyroid disease is a common reason for people with intellectual impairment to be referred for particularly common complications of Down Syndrome. evaluation (Ryan and Sunada, 1997). Both hypo- and hyperthyroidism are particularly common complications of Down Syndrome. Thyroid dysfunction is a common complication of Down syndrome. Hyperthyroidism is marked by behavioural and emotional changes, often with an increase in activity, and increased irritability. In contrast hypothyroidism can be marked by symptoms reminiscent of mild depression though weight gain is usual.

Diabetes

Diabetes is a common complication of obesity and as high rates of obesity and poor lifestyle are found among people with intellectual impairment, they are also at risk of developing diabetes. Prader-Willi syndrome, which has a phenotypic association with satiety dysfunction, will normally result in obesity in affected individuals. Secondary complications of diabetes and subsequent problems such as retinopathy, neuropathy and vascular disease can occur, particularly if diabetes has been poorly controlled or there have been extensive delays in diagnosis. Given the general poor health status of this client group and the barriers evident in diagnosing their physical and mental disorders they are at risk of receiving poor healthcare treatment for diabetes. Delayed diagnosis is problematic with many early signs and symptoms being labelled as 'behavioural'.

Careful monitoring and specifically targeted health education is indicated in this client group. It is likely that people with intellectual impairment will be less able to recognize and communicate symptoms of hyper- and hypoglycaemia and adhere to an appropriate diet than the general population. Problems of communication and comprehension will also present challenges in communicating preventive lifestyle advice and strategies for managing established disease.

REPRODUCTIVE SYSTEM

Hypogonadism is relatively common in both males and females with genetically caused intellectual impairments and can be difficult to manage. A lack of aggression in adult males and absence of menarche (and a reduced subsequent risk of pregnancy) in females may be supported by carers; however, hypogonadism can lead to adverse health effects such as obesity and osteoporosis which require management.

Undescended testes can lead to an increase in the risk of testicular cancer and commonly occurs in males with intellectual impairments of a genetic origin such as Down Syndrome.

Amongst the more common disorders the problem is particularly common in men with Down syndrome. Testicular examination should be a routine part of physical examination as it is unlikely males with intellectual impairments will be able to perform these reliably themselves.

Natural hypogonadism or menopause may be treated by hormone replacement therapy (HRT) in women with intellectual impairment. There are benefits in reducing osteoporosis and post-menopausal symptoms. The use of HRT may be considered particularly for affected younger women although there are increasing concerns about adverse cardiovascular outcomes which means that HRT may only be suitable where symptoms are severe. Many women with intellectual impairments go through the menopause without being able to communicate any symptoms that they may have. This is also a time when 'challenging behaviour' may escalate and it is helpful to keep a record of when periods occur, their duration and if they have become heavier than normal. It is generally only in extreme cases of menorrhagia where an appointment with the GP is made. Close questioning relating to symptoms such as 'hot flushes', 'night sweats', sexual discomfort and associated mental health problems should take place in a manner most appropriate to the woman if menopause is suspected. McCarthy and Millard (2003) highlight two important points. First, the confusion for women that much terminology can cause – for example, 'stopping periods' was associated variously with menarche, pregnancy, and each menstrual cycle. Secondly, many women may have health beliefs that are at odds with the general population, for example one woman believed that eating red food would make her period commence. They wisely suggest the use of pictures with women, in order to convey the messages more precisely.

Consider the scenario in Box 2.2. Charlie and Nicolette's marriage is currently under stress and this could be addressed with counselling, however, such services are often few and far

BOX 2.2   NICOLETTE

Nicolette is 47 and has been married to Charlie for 10 years. They met when they were inpatients in a psychiatric ward and now live largely unsupported in the community. Their income comes from state benefits, neither has a named social worker, Charlie comes under the 'duty' system. Charlie's CPN arranges to visit him about once every two weeks as Charlie is not good at keeping clinic appointments, however, he is seldom there when the nurse arrives.

Charlie has a diagnosis of schizophrenia which is somewhat unstable largely due to the fact that he doesn't comply with his medication regime. This sometimes necessitates admissions into hospital under the Mental Health Act. Although Charlie attended mainstream school and there is no history of any early intellectual impairment his cognition has certainly been affected over the years, probably due to his schizophrenia and long-term use of both cannabis and alcohol. Charlie is not subject to the Care Programme Approach (CPA) at either the Enhanced or Standard level. He is unemployed and now spends his days drinking and smoking with like-minded friends and shows little interest in much else in his life; this upsets Nicolette.

Nicolette has a mild learning disability which has never been considered sufficient enough to warrant the provision of services. She has suffered from serious bouts of depression and two suicide attempts in the past which have necessitated hospital admission; her GP currently manages her mental health problems. She has in the past been employed in basic and mundane jobs that she has not managed to hold on to due to her depression, poor time-keeping and a feeling that she would rather be at home with Charlie!

Over the last few months Nicolette has been sleeping badly and sweating profusely during both the day and at night. She has had episodes of tearfulness and has lost her temper with Charlie on several occasions, she is suffering from very heavy periods which occur on a three-weekly basis and last for about 10 days – she is bleeding for most of the time. Charlie has started to sleep on the sofa due to a combination of Nicolette's disturbed sleep pattern and the apparent change in her personality, the relationship has broken down.

Nicolette is admitted to an acute medical ward following another suicide attempt, this time she took an overdose of sertraline (which she is prescribed) and paracetamol following a large amount of alcohol.

The Duty Psychiatrist visits her and performs an assessment the next morning; he asks about her psychiatric history and establishes that she has never suffered from any serious medical condition or undergone surgery. He discharges her home in the belief that the attempt on her life was not a serious one and had been largely induced by alcohol. She has been issued with a psychiatric outpatient appointment for two weeks' time and a brief letter is sent to her GP.

What are the issues in this case and how can they be resolved? ■

between for individuals with some of the issues present in this case. Named social worker involvement is essential for Charlie at this stage and more structured input from his CPN would also be indicated in order to stabilize his own situation and that of the marriage. Nicolette would probably benefit from a referral to the Community Learning Disability Team which is adept at dealing with complex mental and physical health issues in people with intellectual impairments. However, this is unlikely to happen as she has never been known to learning disability services even though her level of adaptive functioning given her low IQ coupled with ongoing depression means that she is coping at a far lower level than that of the general population. The only feasible option is that of a named community psychiatric nurse (CPN) who may not be conversant with some of the physical problems that she is experiencing.

It is likely that Nicolette is experiencing signs and symptoms of the menopause, and due to her level of intellectual impairment she may not be aware of what the menopause is or what it entails. The symptoms alone may lead her to believe that she is ill with a serious disease which could compound her anxiety and add to her already emotional and depressed state. Many women suffer from some sort of mental health crisis during the stages of the menopause. The breakdown in her relationship with Charlie, coupled with his abuse of substances and unstable mental health status, will only compound the situation.

It is essential when performing a mental health assessment that a full history is obtained and it is vital that in women of all ages information is obtained on menstrual history and current menstrual bleeding patterns. All practitioners should be aware of the impact that disturbed menses and the menopause may have on the emotional status of women. Nicolette may also be sleep deprived and could be anaemic. The GP may consider a gynaecological referral in order to exclude the presence of a more serious condition before deciding on a course of treatment. Referrals to a gynaecologist should not be avoided because of 'behavioural problems'. It is known that cancers of the uterus, cervix and breasts in women with intellectual impairments are often detected later than they are in the general population making adequate treatment impossible.

Teenagers with intellectual impairment will need careful and sensitive advice around the onset of menstruation as well as practical guidance on use of sanitary protection and hygiene issues. Women with intellectual impairment have long had their health needs ignored and this includes acknowledgement of them as sexually active. Ignorance and denial amongst health professionals remain rife with denial of both consensual sex and sexual assault of women with intellectual impairments together with a reluctance to test for sexually shared infections or cervical screening (Langan *et al*, 1994) places them at risk of chronic sexual health and reproductive problems.

The rate of uptake for cervical screening for women with intellectual impairments ranges from 8% to 16% compared with uptakes of 85–88% amongst women generally (Band, 1998; Stein and Allen, 1999).There are several reasons including:

- a concern by the person's carer, be they informal or paid, that a cervical smear test or mammography will be traumatic and uncomfortable for the person concerned;

- a sometimes mistaken belief by carers that the person that they care for is not sexually active so does not need a smear test;

- the fear of such procedures instigating challenging behaviours.

Women with intellectual impairments are often unable to check their breasts regularly for lumps and this is not something that is generally performed by care staff. The same situation is seen in males having checks for testicular cancer.

URINARY SYSTEM

Evidence suggests that people with intellectual impairment are more prone to urinary tract infections. A number of reasons have been suggested including generally poor hygiene and incontinence as well as insufficient fluid intake. Continence training can be problematic in this client group. Simple strategies have been identified that may improve the situation including prompting clients to use the toilet every two hours, as well as ensuring privacy and a pleasant environment. As with the general population, clients should be encouraged to drink at least two litres of clear fluid per day to prevent dehydration and promote general good health.

It is important when any routine visit is made to the GP that the older patient with intellectual impairment is asked about his micturition habits and if there has been any change in them. For men in particular, who are at risk of prostate problems, the presence of nocturia, discomfort due to incomplete voiding of urine, or 'dribbling' may go unnoticed by carers or may not be communicated by the patient due to embarrassment.

MUSCULOSKELETAL PROBLEMS

Many musculoskeletal disorders are secondary to severe and multiple disabilities though lifestyle factors such as the sedentary lifestyle of people with intellectual impairment, obesity, inadequate nutrition and endocrine problems may also lead to problems. Jaffe *et al* (2005) investigated factors that increased the risk of low bone mineral density in people with intellectual impairment in a sample of 211. They found the main factor associated was a lack of mobility. Postmenopausal women were also at high risk, especially those who were prescribed enzyme-inducing anticonvulsant medications. Center *et al* (1998) found that age, small body size, Down syndrome and hypogonadism were the clearest risk indicators in a group of intellectually impaired adults with a mean age of 35. They also found an association of low bone density and fractures in females with intellectual disability but not in males.

Fractures in people with intellectual impairment may occur because of a combination of lower bone density and the risk of falling associated with other conditions such as epilepsy, cerebral palsy and accidental falls. Compounding this is the difficulty of identifying fractures particularly if the individual has a severe learning disability and cannot communicate discomfort or pain to carers who may not be sensitive to such issues.

People with severe and multiple disability and those who have cerebral palsy as well as muscle degenerative disorders can experience a number of associated problems that result in muscular deformities and wider systemic health problems. Spinal deformities include kyphosis (outward curvature), scoliosis (left/right curvature) and lordosis (lumbar or cervical inward curvature). Deformity of limbs and the skeletal system is a result of two main effects, gravity and abnormal movement patterns. Gravitational effects are seen in those with no or limited leg movement, particularly those with hypotonia, resulting in the characteristic 'windswept' appearance; if untreated this can become severe and result in hip dislocation.

For those with abnormal or little movement, particularly people who have more severe spasticity, joints and bones can become pulled out of shape owing to under- and over-tension in different muscles, similarly those with little movement may gradually become 'fixed' in the positions they primarily adopt. Such deforming forces may affect not only the musculoskeletal system but also internal organs and these people are at increased risk of skin and tissue breakdown which may be represented in the form of pressure-related sores. Poor handling techniques by carers may also be a contributory factor particularly if families and care staff do not use, or have access to, lifting and handling equipment.

ORAL CARE

The epidemiology of oral disease in people with intellectual impairments remains unclear though generally as a group they seem to have greater and more complex oral healthcare needs and a poorer oral health status than the general population (Shapira *et al*, 1998). A number of factors may be involved including: institutionalization; socioeconomic status; competence in completing oral care; dependency on carers to meet oral care needs; concomitant disorders; medication side effects; and lack of professional expertise with this client group in the dental professions.

Residual build-up of plaque bacteria can lead to a range of oral diseases including dental caries and periodontitis both of which are linked to diet and poor hygiene. People with intellectual impairment may require specific skills training to improve oral hygiene competence. Similarly the carers of dependent individuals will also require adequate training in tooth brushing and oral hygiene techniques. This is particularly so when individuals have severe intellectual impairment or advanced dementia as these people are unlikely to understand the need for carers to clean their teeth or the process by which oral hygiene is achieved resulting in resistance to oral hygiene attempts by carers.

Poor technique and client resistance may help to explain the occurrence of both dental and tooth brushing phobia observed in this population. If the person cannot understand why a carer is pushing a plastic toothbrush into their mouth, coupled with poor carer technique, it is easy to envision how physical trauma to the mouth and psychological trauma to the client can occur, both of which will compound poor oral hygiene and care. Often the use of an electric tooth brush may improve the situation and many people with intellectual impairment prefer them, although this is not always the case in people who have autism who may dislike the vibrations of the brush.

However, there may be more to the problem than the challenges of maintaining adequate dental hygiene. Zigmood *et al* (2006) report the findings of a 10-year, longitudinal study investigating the effectiveness of a preventive dental care programme for adults with Down syndrome. In a comparison with a matched, non-intellectually impaired group they found that people with Down syndrome suffered greater prevalence, increased extent and severity of periodontitis, including tooth loss, despite the similar dental care treatments provided for both groups, including training, supervision and follow-up of carers for the disabled group. The authors concluded there may be factors other than dental hygiene and care that affect periodontitis in people with Down syndrome. Gingival overgrowth occurs as a result of a number of reasons, particularly in the side effects of certain medication, especially phenytoin. This can then lead to secondary problems such as gingivitis, dental caries and speech and functional impairment.

People with intellectual disabilities are less likely to receive dental restoration as a treatment option with higher rates of edentulism (absent teeth) apparent in this group. This can lead to the ongoing problems associated with gum resorption over time, particularly in the elderly who thus require ongoing dental checks as resorption can lead to ill fitting dentures and difficulties in chewing hard foodstuffs.

Oral disease is also related to other systemic diseases seen in people with intellectual impairment. Chronic gum disease is shown to have an association with both cardiovascular disease, cerebrovascular disease and diabetes through the causative bacterial pathogens of gum disease entering the blood stream and lungs through aspiration (especially common in people who have Down syndrome). Both osteoporosis and chronic gum disease result in loss of bone density on the alveolar bone support of the teeth increasing the risk of tooth loss particularly in postmenopausal women. In both types 1 and 2 diabetes there is an increase in gum disease likely through vascular changes and reduced immune system response as a result of diabetes.

NUTRITION AND FEEDING PROBLEMS

People with severe and multiple disability are commonly reported to experience feeding problems. These range from bulbar palsies affecting the chewing and swallowing of food, to psychogenic vomiting, reflux, regurgitation and behavioural disorders such as hyperphagia, anorexia and pica alongside secondary physical features such as constipation, abdominal distension and in more severe cases of pica medical emergencies such as bowel perforation. The latter stages of dementia are also associated with multiple feeding problems, including those of 'forgetting' how to eat.

Hypotonia occurs in a number of syndromes (cri-du-chat and Prader-Willi syndromes). This can make chewing and swallowing more difficult and the aspiration of foodstuffs more likely. Hollins *et al* (1998) found that asphyxia related to foodstuffs was responsible for 1.87% of deaths of people with learning disabilities in their UK study, The main risk factors were dysphagia, behavioural factors such as poor eating technique (cramming of food) and physiological factors, for example premature loss of bolus in the pharynx (Samuels and Chadwick, 2006). Samuels and Chadwick (2006) identified that the risk of asphyxiation was present in 71% of a group of people with learning difficulties who had dysphagia.

Pica, the chewing, eating and ingestion of non-foodstuffs is prevalent amongst some people with severe intellectual impairments including those in the latter stages of dementia. Some pica is clearly linked to addiction such as the chewing of cigarette ends whilst other forms have no clear function. However, those who engage in pica are at an increased risk of choking, poisoning, tissue damage via corrosive material, bowel impaction and bowel perforation. These risks are compounded as affected individuals usually have severe communication difficulties and symptoms of ill health may only manifest as challenging behaviour and may not be identified as an urgent medical condition.

Good nutrition is an important factor in maintaining health. There is an increased vulnerability to poor nutritional status in people with intellectual impairment as they commonly experience a number of related problems including feeding difficulties, reliance on carers, poor oral hygiene, metabolic disorders, reduced mobility and altered growth patterns influencing both food intake and nutritional absorption. This range of different oral health and dietary problems coupled with the dependency of many on others places them at risk of obesity and undernourishment.

Obesity amongst people with intellectual impairment is at extremely high levels and significantly higher than in the general population. The main factors influencing this are their dependency on others to provide nutrition and inadequate exercise and physical activity, again closely associated with care environments. Additionally, this obese group can also suffer from nutritional imbalance due to the poor quality of their diet. Undernourishment more typically occurs in people with multiple disability or dysphagia who may depend on others to feed them.

Both nutritional states result in longer-term secondary health problems with increased risk of congestive cardiac failure and other cardiovascular disorders in the obese group and reduced bone density and risk of bone fractures in the undernourished person. Both conditions also affect the immune system and make individuals more susceptible to opportunistic infections that may go unnoticed. In both instances adequate health promotion and the involvement of appropriate health professionals can alleviate these problems and prevent secondary disorders from developing.

Oesophageal abnormalities can add to the problems with gastric reflux a not uncommon problem especially in those with learning disabilities (Halpern *et al*, 1991).

There are two further dietary problems, both associated with genetic disorders. Some genetic disorders require dietary control to reduce or prevent deterioration of the phenotypes in the person. Two examples are phenylketonuria (PKU) and galactosaemia both of which require restricted diets. Phenylalanine diets in PKU patients are associated with cognitive and adaptive decline and often severe intellectual impairment if untreated. The second dietary complication occurs in satiation problems such as hyperphagia as seen in the genetic disorder Prader–Willi syndrome. The insatiable appetite associated with the syndrome can result in severe obesity requiring both behavioural modification and direct environmental interventions such as locking fridges and cupboards.

BOWELS

People with intellectual impairment are more prone to bowel disorders than the general population. This is for a variety of reasons including a lack of exercise, a poor diet that is low in fruit and fibre and dehydration. Many people with intellectual impairment, especially those attending day services or in staffed group homes, receive limited fluids, often at 'set times'. Constipation is common and may result in challenging behaviour, often in the form of 'rooting and smearing' (see Chapter 10) as the person may be unable to communicate their distress. Changes in bowel habit may not be communicated or noted by care staff and there is a danger of the early signs and symptoms of bowel cancer being overlooked. People with intellectual impairment may not have high standards of hygiene and therefore they are more prone to both gastrointestinal upsets and threadworm.

CIRCADIAN DISORDERS

There are a range of sleep disorders including insomnia, difficulty initiating sleep, difficulty maintaining sleep, unrefreshing sleep, hyper-somnia and narcolepsy, breathing-related sleep problems, sleep schedule problems, nightmares and sleep terrors, sleepwalking/talking, periodic limb movements, enuresis, tooth grinding and rhythmic movement problems.

Sleep disorders, prevalent amongst people with intellectual disabilities, have a wide aetiology. They can be associated with mental health problems, other medical disorders such as epilepsy, medication, sensory deficits and a number of specific disorders including autism, cerebral palsy and Tourette's syndrome. Quine (1992) found 80% of parents of children with developmental disability reported significant sleep problems and that these often continue into adulthood.

Sleep problems can be associated with conditions such as the hyperkinetic disorders which include attention deficit hyperactivity disorder (ADHD). The medications that treat these conditions can also cause sleep disorders, for example dexamfetamine and methylphenidate which are stimulants that are given in low doses. Other medications may also affect sleep, such as thyroxine, phenytoin for epilepsy and anticholinergics (which are often used to treat the extrapyramidal effects of antipsychotic medication), as well as common drugs such as beta-blockers and bronchodilators.

Chronic sleep disturbance may well affect an individual's adaptive functioning. This is of particular concern as people with intellectual impairment already experience compromised adaptive functioning skills and the ability to learn new skills. Emotional consequences are also seen in terms of a poorer tolerance to frustration and changes in routines which can result in the increase of pre-existing challenging behaviour (Durand *et al*, 1996). For those living with their families their sleep disturbance may also affect the emotional health of the other family members and contribute to the high rates of depression seen in parents and carers of those who have sleep problems.

SEXUAL HEALTH

The sexual health of people with intellectual disabilities is an area that has received little attention or research. Taboos and prejudice regarding the sexuality and sexual behaviour of this group have resulted in both increased vulnerability and denial that abuse can occur. They also lead to limited access to sexual health services.

People with intellectual impairments are at an increased risk of sexual abuse with rates ranging from 25% to 88% (Chamberlain et al, 1984; Hill, 1987). Sobsey (1994) found that physical abuse was also a feature in 40% of sexual abuse cases reported. This subject is discussed in greater depth in Chapter 10.

People who have intellectual impairment, especially those that have learning disabilities, tend to be acquiescent. This may result in lack of understanding or assertiveness to take sexual health precautions to minimize their risk of sexually shared infections and pregnancy. This is particularly relevant for the men and women with mild and borderline intellectual impairments involved in prostitution. Lung and Chen (2006) found 11.8% of female prostitutes had either full or permutation of the gene associated with Fragile X syndrome and 35.1% were found to have a mild or borderline intellectual impairment.

The denial of sexuality and sexual behaviour of people with intellectual impairments has led to denial of not only sexual health services but also primary healthcare activities such as cervical screening in women. The premise being that if they have no sexuality they will not be sexually active and therefore not require cervical screening. These professional stereotypes belie the evidence of both consensual and non-consensual sexual behaviour prevalent amongst people with intellectual disabilities.

There is a tension between government policy which promotes sexual behaviour in people with intellectual impairment (DH, 2001) and an individual's level of disability and adaptive functioning level which leads most people with intellectual impairment to be classed as vulnerable adults (Clark and O'Toole, 2007).

INJURIES

People with intellectual impairment appear to have at least twice the risk of sustaining accidental injuries when compared with the general population (Sherrard et al, 2004). However, some disorders associated with intellectual impairment such as epilepsy are associated with even higher accidental injury risks. People with intellectual impairments are predominantly at risk of accidental injury at home with 75% of injuries sustained at home compared with 33% in the general population. There appears to be a developmental relationship with the injury types occurring commonly in people with intellectual impairment similar to those seen in children without intellectual impairment. This suggests that it is factors directly relating to reduced intellectual functioning that contribute to these injury risks.

Common injuries seen include asphyxia and drowning leading to death (Sherrard et al, 2001), falls and asphyxia associated with increased hospitalization (Sherrard et al, 2001) and falls, transport injury and burns leading to attendance at accident and emergency and general practice clinics. Given the increased risks of accidental injury, Sherrard et al found surprisingly little literature on accident prevention aimed at either people with intellectual impairment or their carers.

The physical abuse of vulnerable people is also a significant problem. Verdugo *et al* (1995) found that 11.5% of children in their sample had been subject to maltreatment with physical neglect (98%) and physical abuse (36%) being the most common forms reported. The types of physical abuse are varied though it may only be the most serious incidents that are identified. Perlow and Latham (1993) in a two-year survey of residential care homes found 21 instances of recorded client abuse involving slapping, punching, twisting arms behind the client's back, one resulting in fracturing the person's arm, throwing chairs at clients, pulling hair and in one case kicking a client in the face. These were serious incidents but it may well be the number of less severe or apparent forms of physical abuse is unknown as the Verdugo *et al* (1995) study suggests.

MENTAL HEALTH

There has been a gradual realization and acceptance that people with intellectual impairments experience the same range of mental disorders as do the rest of the population (Borthwick-Duffy, 1994) despite widespread belief, which persisted into the second half of the twentieth century, that they were incapable of supporting the psychological process that could lead to mental illness. Indeed, there is now a general consensus that not only do people with intellectual impairments experience the same mental disorders but also the prevalence of mental disorder in these individuals is significantly higher. Some of the biological factors such as genetic disorder and physical illness associated with mental health problems have already been discussed and this section concludes by looking at the overlap between physical and mental illness.

BIO-PSYCHOSOCIAL CAUSES AND PRESENTATION OF MENTAL ILLNESS

The relationship between epilepsy and mental health problems is controversial and there is no clear consensus about the relationship between seizures and mental illness. Certainly direct association is unlikely with some authors suggesting that what looks like mental illness is more likely explained as epiphenomena of seizure activity (Reid, 1985). However, it is possible that psychosocial consequences of epilepsy such as learned helplessness and parental overprotection could lead to emotional problems later in life. Undiagnosed physical illness can also have an apparent impact on mental health. Ryan and Sunada (1997) undertook a large scale survey of people with intellectual impairment who were referred for psychiatric evaluation. They found that high numbers had at least one underlying physical disorder that was impacting on the individual's mental state. The most common undiagnosed disorders included epilepsy and thyroid disorders.

Neurochemical theories of mental disorder such as serotonin and dopamine theories can also be used to explain the higher occurrence of mental disorder as these pathways can be disrupted in the presence of brain damage. Psychosocial factors also impact on mental health. Childrearing practices coupled with society's prejudicial views of disability can permeate an individual's life and promote the development of a 'disabled personality' characterized by overdependence, acquiescence, low self-esteem and helplessness that is more a reflection of society's treatment of a person than their underlying disability (Zigler and Burack, 1989). Finally in the age of social integration many people with mild intellectual impairment live independently and can become socially isolated (Reiss and Benson, 1984), suffer stigma and be vulnerable to all forms of abuse in their search for reciprocal human contact.

Box 2.3 illustrates how the atypical presentation of mental illness in some people with intellectual impairment can make diagnosis difficult. Atypical signs of mental illness are not always recognized by professionals. They can present with less florid and different symptoms from those of the general population as a function of their disability. Psychotic symptoms may be less marked such as the person saying that others 'don't like them' which could be representative of persecutory ideas.

BOX 2.3   EDMOND

Edmond is a 22-year-old man who lives with his parents and two sisters in a small rural village. He suffered from meningitis when he was 10 years old and was left with a moderate learning disability and some degree of hearing loss. He attended a special school following his diagnosis and for the last three years has made the 40-mile round trip to the nearest day centre which his mother takes him to twice a week.

Edmond has always had a happy disposition and likes to be around people; he wanders around the village and people are always glad to stop and have a chat with him.

Over an eight-week period Edmond started to isolate himself; he stated that Mrs Murphy who runs the post office hated him and is planning to kill him; he refused to leave the house and would not attend his day placement which he used to love. Finally Edmond's mother went to see Mrs Murphy whom Edmond has known and liked all his life. Mrs Murphy was very distressed by Edmond's accusations and stated that she had never even had a cross word with him. Following this Edmond's mother asked the GP to visit Edmond; the GP claimed that the cause of Edmond's problem was probably behavioural in origin and it would 'sort itself out'. Six months later Edmond was finally prescribed citalopram as his behaviour had not improved and the GP thought he might be depressed. Counselling was not offered as the GP felt that the counsellor that he used was ill-equipped to cope with someone who had an intellectual impairment and there were no specialist services available.

Once taking citalopram Edmond's behaviour became increasingly bizarre and a year after first being approached with the problem the GP finally referred Edmond to a psychiatrist at the local Mental Health Trust. The psychiatrist who assessed Edmond had no experience of people with a diagnosis of both learning disability and mental health problems and felt ill-equipped to deal with the case. After a series of inaccurate diagnoses and ineffectual treatment regimes Edmond was finally diagnosed with schizophrenia four years after his initial contact with the GP. He complied with his medication plan and returned to being his old self within a few months.

Consider the complications that diagnostic overshadowing may present to the practitioner in the patient who has both an intellectual impairment and psychosis. ■

Simpler forms of psychosis, as seen in people with intellectual impairment, can easily be over-looked by professionals who may expect more pronounced and complex persecutory ideation. To the inexperienced or non-expert practitioner the process from assessment to diagnosis may be fraught with obstacles. The person's disability may also influence their ability to express some of the abstract and complex ideas that are seen in many mental disorders and to communicate them effectively to others (intellectual distortion). Some symptoms such as depersonalization require an understanding of complex abstract concepts which may be difficult for the individual to express. The experience of stress can affect the individual and result in a decompensation in their mental state (cognitive disintegration). This can result in emotional and behavioural stress reactions that make the person appear chaotic but are in fact a function of a stress reaction. Mental illnesses may result in the emergence of new forms of challenging behaviour but more likely are simply a change in the rate and pattern of a person's pre-existing challenging behaviour.

Consider Box 2.4. In Martin's case, referral for a psychiatric evaluation because of his behaviour shows that staff are thinking in a limited way. They have seen changes in behaviour and

---

BOX 2.4   **MARTIN**

Martin is a 53-year-old man with a moderate learning disability. He also has a diagnosis of lupus which is thought to cause him some arthritic pain. He lives in a residential home with two other men with learning disabilities and has lived there for over eight years. He has regular day activities but has been refusing to attend these recently; staff also feel increasingly concerned about taking him into the community because of his behaviour.

He was referred following an incident of aggressive and disturbed behaviour. He has progressively deteriorated over the past four weeks and will sometimes shout and act bizarrely, including rubbing and masturbating through his trousers and urinating in inappropriate places The staff think he may be experiencing a psychotic episode. He has attacked a new member of staff by pushing her down the stairs and kicking her and disturbs the home both during the day and at night prompting an urgent referral. Staff say that when they try to calm him down, he doesn't always seem 'to all be there'. His behaviour is described as out of character for him as he is described as usually a quiet and easy natured individual.

Identify the health and social factors that could be affecting Martin, this should help identify areas for further clinical assessment.

Martin has been referred for psychiatric evaluation, why do you think that the staff have done this and what may be the consequence of such a referral? ■

are presuming these are related to his mental health. A number of other bio-psychosocial factors may equally be affecting his behaviour and warrant investigation.

Investigation into his lupus status may reveal he is experiencing pain and appropriate management may help relieve the behavioural symptoms that are a response to pain. Similarly, rubbing and incontinence of urine may be a symptom of urinary tract infection. This should be investigated, including the possibility he has a sexually transmitted disease. If this is the case sexual health inquiry into the nature of his sexual relationships, whether consenting or abusive, should take place. Finally the presence of new staff may cause problems for him as they may have difficulties communicating effectively with him resulting in deterioration in his behaviour. Thus by taking a broader bio-psychosocial perspective a wider range of areas for investigation and possible interventions can be identified.

Physical disorders affecting neurological, endocrine and metabolic systems can have a direct or primary effect on the development of mental illness in a range of conditions such as brain tumour and hypothyroidism, and also through the side effects of treatments such as medication (e.g. digoxin), that is prescribed for physical disorders. Physical disorders can also have a secondary effect in the form of emotional reactions to a debilitating physical illness that may also contribute to mental illness. Disorders that result in compromised functioning in mobility and sensory functioning can lead to adjustment problems and reactive depression. Sensory impairment (both visual/auditory) may increase the risk of mental illness through the psychosocial consequences on the individual. Other physical disorders can mimic symptoms of mental illness as in the case of untreated hypothyroidism mimicking symptoms of depression. Finally, other factors may exacerbate the symptoms in pre-existing mental illness such as cannabis use in people diagnosed with schizophrenia, which is not uncommon in people with mild or borderline intellectual impairment. Some mental disorders can have a primary effect on physical health as a result of, for example, the toxic effects of alcohol in alcohol dependency, and the toxic side effects of psychotropic medication. Symptoms of mental illness can also present physically and somatically, such as feeling pain or tremor especially in people with intellectual impairment who may complain of physical symptoms owing to their inability to effectively communicate emotional distress.

RESPONSE TO TREATMENT

Medication, particularly psychotropic medication, is prescribed at a higher rate in people with intellectual impairments than the rest of the population. This increased rate of psychotropic medication is not wholly explained by the prevalence of mental illness seen in this group and it is thought large numbers of people are prescribed medication to control so called 'challenging behaviours'. The pharmacokinetics of medication, that is the interaction of drugs in relation to the brain, can be disrupted in people with intellectual impairment due to underlying brain damage or developmental abnormality. This can affect the absorption and synthesis of both prescribed and recreational drugs in this population. As a result this group appears to be more sensitive to adverse reactions, and toxicity associated with many medications. Similarly, this can affect the therapeutic doses in this group with research showing they may require lower doses to achieve therapeutic effect.

The greater risk of side effects and sensitivity is further compounded by a reduced ability to recognize and report the development of side effects to professionals making the use of medication monitoring systems all the more pertinent when supporting this client group and their carers. Polypharmacy is also common, with multiple medications prescribed for both physical and mental disorders in the same individual. Haw and Stubbs (2005) reviewed the use of psychotropic medication in people with intellectual impairment and found that polypharmacy was the norm (67.9%) in the sample and that nearly half the sample was prescribed at least one off-label psychotropic (46.4%). For a more in-depth discussion on psychopharmacology see Chapter 9.

People with intellectual impairment are often dependent on others to assist them with daily living. This includes the compliance and monitoring of prescribed medication regimes, therefore carers are paramount in ensuring medication efficacy. With this in mind Rasaratnam *et al* (2004) investigated carers' attitudes using the Rating of Attitudes to Medication Scale (RAMS). They included both informal and professional carers in their samples and found that family carers tended towards more negative views of medication, in particular towards psychotropic drugs, than professional carers (46% v. 11%). The efficacy of therapeutic treatment options to support individuals with intellectual impairment is limited and non-compliance rates in both chronic medical conditions and psychiatric disorders are high. Rasaratnam *et al* (2004) argue that there are several reasons for non-compliance which include negative carer views but also the complexity of some medication regimes for people with intellectual impairment.

CONCLUSION

This chapter has attempted to raise awareness of the health needs of people with intellectual impairment which are often complex and multiple. There are a number of individual, carer and organizational factors that interact with intellectual impairment which in turn raise barriers to health care. Physical and mental health needs are caused by biological, psychological and social factors that often interact and can cause specific health problems but can also result in the development of other systemic disorders. Healthcare professionals need to be aware of their own prejudice and limitations of knowledge when providing care for people with intellectual impairments. The government white paper, *Valuing People* (DH, 2001) sets out a policy direction whereby primary care and acute services should undertake the responsibility of providing health care for people with intellectual impairment. In order to achieve this aim, healthcare professionals need to be adequately educated to understand the complexities of caring for these patients. The use of a systematic and comprehensive approach to assessment and therapeutic interventions is essential as well as seeking support from intellectual impairment specialists where available.

REFERENCES, RESOURCES AND RECOMMENDED READING

Band R. (1997) *Getting Better: a training pack to help people with learning difficulties get the best out of their GP.* Brighton: Pavilion.

Band R. (1998) *The NHS – Health for All? People with learning Disabilities and Health Care.* London: Mencap.

Beange H, McElduff A, Baker W. (1995) Medical disorders of adults with mental retardation: a population study. *American Journal of Mental Retardation* 99:595–604.

Borthwick-Duffy SA. (1994) Epidemiology and prevalence of psychopathology in people with mental retardation. *Journal of Consulting and Clinical Psychology* 62(1):17–27.

Bouras N, Holt G, Day K, Dosen A. (2000) *Mental Health in Mental Retardation: The ABC for Mental Health, Primary Care and Other Professionals.* 2nd edn. World Psychiatric Association.

Center J, Beange H, McElduff A. (1998) People with mental retardation have an increased prevalence of osteoporosis: a population study. *American Journal on Mental Retardation* 103:19–28.

Chamberlain A, Rauh J, Passer P, McGrath M, Burket R. (1984) Issues in fertility control for mentally retarded female adolescents: I. Sexual activity, sexual abuse and contraception. *Pediatrics* 73: 445–50.

Clark LL. (2006) Intellectual impairment: a forgotten speciality. *International Journal of Nursing Studies* 43:525–6.

Clark LL, O'Toole MS. (2007) Intellectual impairment and sexual health: Information needs. *British Journal of Nursing* 15(11):604–6.

Crawford P. (1997) Epilepsy and learning disabilities. In: S Read (ed.) *Psychiatry in Learning Disability*. Saunders: 380–98.

Department of Health (1983) *The Mental Health Act*. London: The Stationery Office.

Department of Health (1996) *Health of the Nation: A Strategy for People with Learning Disabilities*. London: The Stationery Office.

Department of Health (2001) *Valuing People: A New Strategy for Learning Disabilities for the 21st Century*. London: The Stationery Office.

Department of Health (2002) *Action for Health: Health Action Plans and Health Facilitation: Detailed Good Practice Guidance on Implementation for Learning Disability Partnership Boards*. London: Department of Health.

Department of Health (2003) *Tackling Health Inequalities: A Programme for Action*. London: The Stationery Office.

Durand VM, Gernert-Dott P, Mapstone E. (1996) Treatment of sleep disorders in children with developmental disabilities. *Journal of the Association for Persons with Severe Handicaps* 21:114–22.

Forsgren L, Edvinsson SO, Blomquist HK, Hejibel J, Sidenvall R. (1990) Epilepsy in a population of mentally retarded children and adults. *Journal of Intellectual Disability Research* 6:234–48.

Halpern LM, Jolloey SG, Johnson DG. (1991) Gastrooesophageal reflux: a significant association with central nervous disease. *Journal of Pediatric Surgery* 26:171–3.

Hardy S, Woodward P, Woolard P, Tait T. (2006) *Meeting the Health Needs of People with Learning Disabilities: Guidance for Nursing Staff*. Royal College of Nursing: London.

Haw C, Stubbs J. (2005) A survey of off-label prescribing for inpatients with mild intellectual disability and mental illness. *Journal of Intellectual Disability Research* 49(11):858–64.

Hill G. (1987) Sexual abuse and the mentally handicapped. *Child Sexual Abuse Newsletter* 6:4.

Hogenboom M. (2001) *Living with Genetic Disorders Associated with Intellectual Disability*. London: Jessica Kingsley.

Hollins S. (2003) Counselling and psychotherapy. In: W Fraser, M Kerr (eds) *Seminars in the Psychiatry of Learning Disabilities*. 2nd edn. Gaskell: London, 186–200.

Hollins S, Bernal J, Gregory M. (1996) *Going to the Doctor*. Royal College of Psychiatrists, London: Gaskell.

Hollins S, Attard MT, Frunhofer N, McGuigan S, Sedgwick P. (1998) Mortality in people with learning disability: risks, causes, and death certificate findings in London. *Developmental Medicine and Child Neurology* 40:50–60.

Iwata BA, Dorsey MF, Slifer KJ, Bauman KE, Richman GS. (1982) Toward a functional analysis of self-injury. *Analysis and Intervention in Developmental Disabilities* 2:3–20.

Jaffe JS, Timell AM, Elolia R, Thatcher SS. (2005) Risk factors for low bone mineral density in individuals residing in a facility for people with intellectual disability. *Journal of Intellectual Disability Research* 49(6):457–62.

Janicki MP, Dalton J. (1998) Sensory impairments among older adults with disability. *Journal of Intellectual and Developmental Disabilities* 23:3–11.

Jansen DEMC, Krol B, Groothoff JW, Post D. (2004) People with intellectual disability and their health problems: a review of comparative studies. *Journal of Intellectual Disability Research* 48(92):93–102.

Langan J, Whitfield M, Russell O. (1994) Paid and unpaid carers: their role in and satisfaction with primary health care for people with learning disabilities. *Health & Social Care* 2:357–65.

Lennox NG, Kerr MP. (1997) Review: Primary health care and people with an intellectual disability: the evidence base. *Journal of Intellectual Disability Research* 41:365–71.

Lund J. (1985) Epilepsy and psychiatric disorder in the mentally retarded adult. *Acta Psychiatrica Scandinavica* 78:369–74.

Lung FW, Chen PJ. (2006) Fragile X syndrome in adolescent prostitutes in Southern Taiwan. *Journal of the American Academy of Child and Adolescent Psychiatry* 42(5):516–17.

McCarthy M, Millard L. (2003) Discussing the menopause with women with learning disabilities. *British Journal of Learning Disabilities* 31:9–17.

Melville CA, Finlayson J, Cooper SA, Allan L, Robinson N, Burns E, Martin G, Morrison J. (2005) Enhancing primary health care for adults with intellectual disabilities. *Journal of Intellectual Disability* 49(3):190–8.

Mencap (2004) *Treat Me Right! Better Healthcare for People with a Learning Disability.* London: Mencap.

Mencap (2007) *Death by Indifference.* London: Mencap.

National Institute for Mental Health (2004) *Greenlight for Mental Health.* London: NIMH.

Perlow R, Latham LL. (1993) Relationship of client abuse with locus of control and gender: A longitudinal study in mental retardation facilities. *Journal of Applied Psychology* 78(5):831–4.

Pary R. (1993) Mental retardation, mental illness and seizure disorders. *American Journal of Mental Retardation* 98(Supplement):58–62.

Quine L. (1992) Severity of sleep problems in children with severe learning difficulties: description and correlates. *Journal of Common and Applied Social Psychology* 2:247–68.

Rasaratnam R, Crouch K, Regan A. (2004) Attitude to medication of parents/primary carers of people with intellectual disability. *Journal of Intellectual Disability* 48(8):754–63.

Reid A. (1985) Psychiatric disorders. In AM Clarke, ADB Clarke, JM Berg (eds) *Mental Deficiency: The Changing Outlook.* New York: Free Press, 291–325.

Reiss S, Benson B. (1984) Awareness of negative social conditions among mentally retarded, emotionally disturbed outpatients. *American Journal of Psychiatry* 141(1):88–90.

Ryan R, Sunada K. (1997) Medical evaluation of persons with mental retardation referred for psychiatric assessment. *General Hospital Psychiatry* 19:274–80.

Samuels R, Chadwick DD. (2006) Predictors of asphyxiation risk in adults with intellectual disabilities. *Journal of Intellectual Disability Research* 50(5):362–70.

Sander JW, Hart YM, Johnson AL, Shorvon SD. (1990) National General Practice Study of Epilepsy: newly diagnosed epileptic seizures in a general population. *Lancet* 336:1267–71.

Shapira J, Efrat J, Berkey D, Mann J. (1998) Dental health profile of a population with mental retardation in Israel. *Specialist Care in Dentistry* 18:149–55.

Sherrard J, Tonge B, Ozanne-Smith J. (2001) Injury in young people with intellectual disability: descriptive epidemiology. *Injury Prevention* 7:56–61.

Sherrard J, Ozanne-Smith J, Staines C. (2004) Prevention of unintentional injury to people with intellectual disability: a review of the evidence. *Journal of Intellectual Disability Research* 48(7):639–45.

Sobsey D. (1994) Sexual abuse of individuals with intellectual disability. In: A Craft (ed.) *Practice Issues in Sexuality and Learning Disabilities.* London: Routledge.

Stein K, Allen N. (1999) Cross sectional survey of cervical cancer in women with learning disabilities. *British Medical Journal* 318:641.

Van den Akker M, Maaskant MA, van den Meijden RJM. (2006) Cardiac diseases in people with intellectual disability. *Journal of Intellectual Disability* 50(7):515–22.

Verdugo MA, Bermego BG, Fuertes J. (1995) The maltreatment of intellectually handicapped children and adolescents. *Child Abuse Neglect* 19:205–15.

Warburg M. (2001) Visual impairment in adult people with moderate, severe, and profound intellectual disability. *Acta Ophthalmologica Scandinavica* 79:450–4.

Warburg M, Rattlief J, Kreiner-Moller J. (1979) Blindness among 7700 mentally retarded children in Denmark. In Smith V, Keen J (eds) *Visual Handicap in Children.* London: Heinemann Medical Books.

Williams C. (1982) Deaf not daft: the deaf in mental subnormality hospitals. *Special Education: Forward Trends* 9:26–8.

Yeates S. (1995) The incidence and importance of hearing loss in people with severe learning disability: the evolution of a service. *British Journal of Learning Disabilities* 23:79–84.

Zigler E, Burack JA. (1989) *Personality Development and the Dually Diagnosed Person. Research in Developmental Disabilities*, Vol. 10:225–40.

Zigmood M, Stabholz A, Shapira J, Bachrach G, Chaushu G, Becker A, Yefenof E, Merrick J, Chaushu S. (2006) The outcome of a preventive dental care programme in the prevalence of localized aggressive periodontitis in Down's syndrome individuals. *Journal of Intellectual Disability Research* 50(7):492–500.

Internet Resources

Books Beyond Words
http://www.rcpsych.ac.uk/publications/booksbeyondwords.aspx

Estia Centre
http://www.estiacentre.org/freepub.html

Elfrida Society
Ordering information leaflets:
http://www.elfrida.com/publications.htm

Contact a Family
http://www.caf.org.uk

Society for the Study of Behavioural Phenotypes
http://www.ssbp.co.uk

CHAPTER 3
EFFECTIVE COMMUNICATION

Garry Diack and Howard Cohen

STUDY AIMS:

1. To encourage all health professionals to examine their communication skills in the light of the needs of people with intellectual impairment.

2. To examine some of the more common issues related to communication deficits.

3. To examine how communication styles and organization of care may be adapted for use with people who have intellectual impairment.

The shift of care away from specialized institutions to community healthcare settings means that most health professionals now see people with intellectual impairment in their daily work. Van Loon *et al* (2005) identified multiple concerns regarding the quality of medical care that people with learning disabilities, in common with others with intellectual impairments, receive. Their work highlighted that communication difficulties were one of the main issues affecting the provision of adequate appropriate health care. Lennox *et al* (1997) identified the principal problem as that of eliciting information from the patient. The taking of an adequate, let alone comprehensive, medical history proved to be difficult. A further issue was the failure to follow 'doctor's orders', suggesting a two-way communication deficit and failure to achieve concordance. They also identified the relative inexperience of the majority of primary and secondary care practitioners in engaging with people who have intellectual impairment.

Although some advocate integrated care as a method of removing barriers to accessing health services (Jansen *et al*, 2006) such solutions are not universally implemented and cannot cover the full spectrum of care encounters. The communication must in part be met by a detailed examination of communication strategies between 'generic' health professionals and people with

Learning Disability and other Intellectual Impairments, Edited by L.L. Clark and P. Griffiths
© 2008 John Wiley & Sons, Ltd

BOX 3.1	GP'S THOUGHTS

It is a busy morning at an inner-city general practice and the next person that you as the GP are due to see is a middle-aged man who has an intellectual impairment as the result of a stroke. His communication is very poor and he has a tendency to forget what he is trying to say in the middle of a sentence. Many of his comments are very sexually inappropriate. You don't know him well, although you have seen him around the surgery in the past, what are your immediate thoughts? ■

intellectual impairment. The role of specialists, for example community learning disability nurses, in bridging the gap should not be underestimated but their availability is limited and restricted to only a subgroup of those with intellectual impairment.

This chapter aims to identify issues that lie behind communication difficulties and to identify strategies to improve communication in encounters between professionals and people with intellectual impairments. Communication is a complex process made more challenging in circumstances where there are constraints on time and manpower. As an introduction to this chapter let us examine the scenario in Box 3.1.

Many health professionals may feel a sense of unease at the prospect of a consultation with an individual who has an intellectual impairment. Whilst priding ourselves on our professionalism to offer the best quality care to every client regardless of race, gender, class or intellectual ability, the reality is the consultation is likely to be longer, more difficult and somewhat stressful. Education and training often do not seem to prepare health professionals adequately for this role leaving them feeling inadequate and ineffective.

Such anxieties are entirely reasonable and reminiscent of some of the feelings of apprehension that often pervade the early days of patient care. Experience, knowledge and practice have made many health professionals at ease in the consultation over time, but further work needs be done to help them to become more relaxed in what can sometimes be a challenging consultation. Most health professionals do possess the necessary skills and insights to work effectively with clients regardless of intellectual ability, but often fail to have the confidence to recognize them. The following case study will help to illustrate this.

Consider the scenario in Box 3.2. Nigel is no more technically competent an optician than his colleagues but he certainly was able to make a more effective connection with his client and achieve a more satisfactory outcome. He brought an attitude to his consultation that explored ways in which to connect with Jake, and at the level that Jake was willing and able to cope with. Jake was at the centre of the consultation, he set the pace and Nigel worked accordingly, whilst being relaxed enough to do what he could, accepting of the time this took and the compromises required. Nigel did not prejudge how Jake should behave at the optician but accepted the reality and worked with it.

Did Nigel learn his approach? Probably not in any formal way, experience and past mistakes may have shaped Nigel's style. By modelling himself on other colleagues he may have enhanced it. It is, however, possible that Nigel possessed an intrinsic characteristic which dictated his approach, that of respect of Jake's right to be treated as an individual irrespective of his disability.

BOX 3.2   JAKE

Jake is a teenager with a learning disability and autism. He has some expressive language and reasonably good receptive understanding. He gets anxious in new situations, which often leads him to be noisy and to use repetitive behaviours such as hand flapping and blowing. His level of social functioning is roughly equivalent to that of a three-year-old child.

His parents and siblings are all short-sighted. Family concern that Jake may also be short-sighted has prompted a number of attempts to visit the optician for an eye test. Several visits to different opticians have ended in abandoned consultations. The opticians have themselves become anxious and flustered. Jake's lack of understanding has been taken as an unwillingness to cooperate; a natural wariness of the new situation, the lights, the equipment viewed as an impossible hurdle to cross.

Success, however, occurred on the fifth attempt with a different optician, Nigel. Jake was just as anxious, just as noisy as before but the optician was not distracted or dissuaded from his task. His demeanour was friendly and relaxed, he seemed to have all the time in the world (even though he didn't). Jake, whose interest was taken by the electronic controls of the examination chair was encouraged by Nigel to make a game of the chair controls which led on to playing with the lights, the eye test charts, the ophthalmoscope and eventually enough of an examination to confirm that against all the odds Jake was in fact long-sighted. ■

Nigel also was sufficiently self-confident to apply his general communication and consultation skills to an unusual and unfamiliar situation. Observing Jake's behaviour and level of communication, Nigel was able to adapt the consultation to make it meaningful and appropriate to Jake.

Most health professionals have been patients or carers at various times of their lives and can readily conjure up the feelings engendered by good or bad experiences. Some reflection on such encounters is helpful in defining the features of the kind of consultation that should be aspired to. Research on satisfaction with the consultation identifies a number of consistent components, such as accessibility, competence of the practitioner and a suitable physical environment (Trumble *et al*, 2006). That is to say, the patient wants to be able to see a clinician who knows what he or she is doing at a time and place which is appropriate to the issue. However, the perceived demeanour of the clinician is of crucial importance. A polite, friendly and courteous approach is important as a marker that the clinician has recognized and valued the patient as an individual worthy of respect.

The extreme opposite of our idealistic consultation, is the gruff, 'off hand', bored clinician, slumped in a chair, avoiding eye contact and looking at the computer screen. Interrupting the patient, prejudging and stereotyping on appearance may compound this. From the client's point of view the appointment has probably been hard to get and the wait has been overlong because the clinic is running late. To add insult to injury the waiting area is often cold (or hot), crowded and uncomfortable.

Before a consultation there is a complex process of decision making on the part of the patient. Personal coping mechanisms are employed, lay networks consulted. The patient often arrives at the consultation with a set of beliefs and concerns about their problems, the expectation being to explore them with the clinician and gain a deeper understanding as well as the benefit of the health professional's experience and expertise. Together the two experts in the room, the patient (expert in themselves) and the clinician (expert in their discipline) will reach a common understanding which should help to establish what the next stage of the patient journey or treatment plan may be.

Recognition that the patient has feelings, concerns and anxieties, hopes and aspirations is a prerequisite to respecting them as an individual. The difficult step for many of us is to accept that these feelings may differ greatly in nature and intensity from our own. The ethical imperative of respecting the autonomy of the individual should feature strongly and vulnerable individuals are predominately autonomous people whose views demand respect. The conflicting duty to avoid harm should only be given precedence in extreme situations.

Clinical practice should naturally follow from this ethical or moral standpoint. Structures and organizations should be geared towards meeting the needs of vulnerable individuals as they would for clients without a disability. The development and maintenance of consultation skills that are effective with people who have intellectual impairment is essential. This aspiration does, however, challenge the system, as inevitably the demand on time and resources to meet the needs of a vulnerable individual may greatly exceed that of the standard consultation.

COMMUNICATION AND THE ASSESSMENT OF NEED

Individuals with intellectual impairments represent a significant part of the caseload of all healthcare practitioners. Effective communication with all our clients should be considered as a core competence for all professionals and worthy of our time and attention. Consultations with clients who have intellectual impairments are challenging and sometimes anxiety provoking, but they can be also be joyful and immensely rewarding experiences.

A formal, structured process of inquiring as to the potential needs of a person with intellectual impairment has significant merits and attractions. It goes some way towards compensating for that person's lack of ability or motivation to seek help or healthcare advice and may be a start in the process of addressing long-term health inequalities; it also helps the non-specialised practitioner to be comprehensive in their inquiry. Having a structure can go some way to alleviating some of the practitioner anxiety discussed above, allowing rehearsal of important areas and gathering supporting materials and resources.

The needs assessment model can be criticized as being potentially rigid and has the aim of meeting more the needs of an organization than those of the client. This criticism needs to be aimed at the quality of the needs assessment programme and the skill of the practitioners who deliver it rather than of the underlying concept. In a patient or client-centred approach, the assessment tool can at most be treated as a tool, rather than a rule, allowing flexibility and adaptability.

The assessment of a person's needs is often undertaken in the context of meeting an immediate need and perhaps the assessor will have an unconscious initial idea of the outcomes. Placing the client at the centre of the consultation is both ethically desirable and practically effective. Being willing to adapt generally applicable consultation skills to match the level of functioning of the individual requires a willingness and confidence on the part of the practitioner. As with all individual skills, improvement can come from formal education, modelling on more experienced practitioners and by trial and error

POWER AND AUTHORITY IN COMMUNICATION

For many people there are a number of times in a week when they acquiesce to something that is expected of them and a number of times in which they will unconsciously comply with someone else's wishes, directions or requests. It may well be that after the event they stop and think 'actually, I didn't really want to do that', 'I didn't want to give that' and 'I didn't want to say that'. A uniform, a position in a company, or someone who is in a particular office, can represent a mantle of authority for many. There are numerous other examples of the various tokens that indicate that others have authority over us. In addition to this there is the risk that the communicator who does not have a cognitive impairment will assume that the problem and the deficit lies with the person who does. This is particularly likely in situations such as medical consultations or interactions with acute care where arguably the doctor, nurse or the allied professional is actually operating within what could be perceived to be their territory, with all the attendant notions of power that go with this.

When someone enters a hospital as a patient the process of disempowerment, albeit unintentionally, begins and within a short space of time the person is dispatched to a bed and asked to get undressed and fill in various forms. The beds are all exactly the same, they are usually fairly uncomfortable and surrounded by all the attendant hospital paraphernalia such as medical gas outlets and nurse call buttons. Before surgery the patient is undressed and given a gown that usually has just two ties at the back and they are expected then to walk around, maintaining what dignity they can under the circumstances. All the power and control rests with the health professionals who will be dressed in their habitual uniforms carrying the symbols of power and authority such as stethoscopes, thermometers, watches, clipboards and files. The patient rapidly loses autonomy and any feelings of control over the situation thus becoming amenable to suggestions that they should do a number of different things, for example, 'Can you give me a sample in this bottle?', 'Can you just pop yourself on the bed and I will have a look?', 'Can you just lift up your gown so I can listen to your chest?'. The patient usually complies because those in authority have demanded it.

Such communication problems are frequently misconstrued as being solely a result of the person's intellectual impairments, However, it is often the unthinking actions of others that render the impairment disabling in the act of communication. McConkey et al (1999) undertook research around the issue of communication in residential and day service settings. They concluded that staff communicating with people who had intellectual impairments were not being proactive in facilitating effective communication. The principles described here are equally applicable within a clinical practice setting where people may resort to language use that has its derivation in their own clinical lexicon.

It is worth giving some consideration to the aspect of the skill of listening rather than merely asking the questions, listening to what is being said and what is being presented by the patient. Buszewicz et al (2006) discuss the importance of attentive listening skills in helping to build a trusting relationship between the patient and the medical practitioner.

COMPLEXITY OF LANGUAGE AND HIDDEN MEANINGS

Morgan (1996) identified the need for practitioners to have considerable self-awareness of the ways in which they communicate their behaviour and the style of communication, the voice prosody, the tone of voice, the clarity of the message and the use of simile and metaphors. Many people with intellectual impairments will use literal interpretation, especially those on the autistic spectrum. Consider the scenario in Box 3.3. John has heard some comments made about Rose, these are:

'She bit my head off.'

'She jumped down my throat.'

John fails to appreciate the metaphor of the statements. He has a very real fear that this is what she is going to do. She is actually going to bite his head off or jump down his throat and he is extremely agitated and nervous for the next few days until the situation is explained to him. Of

---

BOX 3.3   JOHN

John has a learning disability and lives in a group home with three other people supported at any one time by three members of a staff team (18 of them in total). One of these staff members, Rose, is the house manager and at times is felt by her staff to have a particularly authoritarian management style.

John is sitting on the sofa in the living room and the television is on but he is not particularly interested in the programme that is on; two of the care staff are standing in the kitchen, drinking coffee and chatting within earshot of John who is next door.

The staff members are talking about an incident that happened with Rose, the manager, the previous evening when she arrived unannounced to undertake an audit and took the staff by surprise. During the course of the audit, Rose expressed dissatisfaction with a number of aspects of record keeping. At this point John overhears one of the staff saying to the other, 'Yep, Rose bit my head off last night, absolutely bit my head off!', and the other staff member responds by saying 'Well, it was only two or three weeks ago that she jumped down my throat so I know what you are talking about!'

John hears this and processes the information accordingly. The following day, Rose arrives at the house for a morning shift, she knocks and goes into John's bedroom and asks him if he wants a cup of tea and some breakfast; John is extremely agitated and nervous and refuses to get out of bed or speak to Rose at all. ■

particular note here is the fact that, on this occasion, the mistake was recognized. It may be the case that often people will be unaware of any miscommunication. In such cases there may well be a long period of anxiety and confusion for the person with an intellectual impairment.

This case study (Box 3.4) illustrates issues related to the use of language within a hospital setting.

EXERCISE

Engage in a conversation with someone and take note of how many times you use metaphors, similes and colloquialisms. Some examples are given below but it would be instructive to consider the frequently used examples from your own experience.

- Metaphor: e.g . . . 'now we're cooking'

- Simile . . . e.g. 'as light as a feather'

- Colloquialism: . . . e.g. 'sorted!'. ■

An additional feature of communication patterns between people who have intellectual impairments and those that care for them is that a lot of communication can tend to be quite directive in content rather than being communication on a reciprocal social basis (Prior *et al*, 1979). People are used to being told, instructed, requested or directed how to perform and have a limited experience of reciprocal interactive communication.

A further problem, which has to be considered, is the use of body language, intonation, facial expression and exaggeration in order to convey a point. Hogg *et al* (2001) discuss the issue of affective behaviour, particularly with regard to how an individual with intellectual impairment and associated communication difficulties will respond to those who care for them. The authors describe some of the affective communication styles which range from facial expression to convey anger, sadness and pleasure, to body movements. There is, however, a considerable difficulty in interpreting correctly what type of affective communication is being presented.

For example, if a doctor is interviewing a prospective patient with intellectual impairment as a candidate for surgery and is explaining the procedures, smiling and nodding by the patient may be assumed to indicate agreement and understanding. They may in fact be responding to some other aspect or indeed simply indicating deference to the presumed authority. The onus is on the person who is communicating the information to try and be aware of the possibilities for interpretation. Another example of this is where capacity to consent is questioned (for a further discussion see Chapter 11).

BOX 3.4	CLIVE

Clive is a 49-year-old man who has schizophrenia; he has a long history of abusing alcohol. As a result of his condition he has intellectual impairment and suffers from confusion. He has been admitted to hospital for abdominal surgery. He has had a number of opportunities to discuss his surgery with his CPN, and there was an extensive process of seeking consent. On the night before the operation Clive has been told that he will be fasting from midnight and initially there is some trepidation about fasting because he does not understand this to be going without food, he understands this to be something to do with running very fast.

This issue is resolved very quickly but the next morning he gets up and expects his breakfast and has to be reminded that he is not having any. Following this Clive is told that he is going to theatre in 10 minutes and to 'pop the gown on'. Clive starts to think about the time that he went to the theatre a few years ago to see a play and naturally is very joyful thinking that he is off to the theatre when in fact what is meant is the operating theatre. Another particular issue is the concept of time: 10 minutes. For example, we are very used to using notions of time to explain actions or potential actions, but the actual use of time isn't particularly concrete. For example:

'I will see you in a minute'
'Can you do something for me?'-'Yeah, just give me a minute'
'In a bit'
'See you later'.

We rarely actually mean specifically a period of 60 seconds or precisely 10 minutes. It is a notional concept which conveys the idea that it will happen some time soon. The understanding of the time period referred to is context-dependent and each person in the dialogue has an implicit understanding of the parameters. However, a person with intellectual impairment may well construe it absolutely pedantically or may fail to understand and think that it is going to happen imminently. ■

ENHANCING THE CLINICAL ENCOUNTER WITH INDIVIDUALS WITH INTELLECTUAL IMPAIRMENT

There is a case to be made for a 'positive discrimination' in favour of people with intellectual impairment in clinical practice. As with all such *positive* discriminations the aim is to deliver the same quality of experience that others take for granted. As discussed elsewhere their health needs are greater, there has been a longstanding adverse health inequality to be addressed and the process of consultation is more complex and demanding. Essentially in order that our services do not disadvantage them, changes need to be made.

One possible alteration could be to routinely offer extended appointment times to people with intellectual impairments. It could be questioned whether the setting aside of double (or triple) appointment times in a busy surgery as a routine for someone with intellectual impairment represents a fair (or just) allocation of limited resources. Such judgements are difficult and need to vary over time in response to the whole picture of the service. The balance of a demand-led service, as opposed to a needs-led approach, is of particular importance with a group of people who often lack the capacity to demand. However, there are good and long established precedents for such approaches, such as child health services and more latterly mental health services. Enhanced provision for the needs of children is so much a part of culture that it is not questioned; in time, enhanced provision for vulnerable adults must also be the norm.

If it is accepted that vulnerable individuals deserve the same respect in healthcare provision as others without disability, approaches can be set against the satisfaction criteria described above.

ACCESSIBILITY

It must be considered how client friendly any organization is for individuals who have intellectual impairment. The process of making an appointment, turning up on time and in the right place is a fairly complex process. Whilst accepting many such appointments are made and managed by an individual's carers the raising of staff awareness of the differing needs of vulnerable individuals and encouragement of a level of tolerance and flexibility might be helpful. If the patients themselves are given the opportunity to practise the process then this will help in the reduction of anxiety and will also help in the development of new skills. Breaking down the information into small fragments and simple commands can be helpful.

CLINICAL COMPETENCE

The general competence of the clinician is a key prerequisite of a successful outcome to any consultation; a good grounding in the care of people with intellectual impairment will enhance this and at the same time will arm the clinician with confidence. Case discussions within teams which focus on certain aspects of the care of people who have intellectual impairment can help to identify the likely recurrent themes which emerge and action can be taken where needed.

An example would be the management of chronic constipation which is common in people who have intellectual impairment.

- Identify how this can go unnoticed.
- Consider different presentation in people with intellectual impairment as opposed to the general population.
- How does it affect an individual's behaviour, mood, appetite, etc.?
- Sharing expertise as to dietary interventions or the appropriate use of laxatives would be helpful.

This process demonstrates the need to take general knowledge and skills and to expand and adapt them in the specific circumstances of intellectual impairment.

A good working knowledge is required of specific health needs relating to defined syndromes associated with intellectual impairment. Examples of syndrome-specific health needs can be found in Chapter 2.

PHYSICAL ENVIRONMENT

The physical layout and built environment is increasingly recognised as an important factor in the experience of patients. A comfortable, calming atmosphere can reduce an individual's anxieties and provide a suitable foundation for a successful consultation. Such factors are particularly relevant to people with intellectual impairment. Autistic individuals can find waiting rooms with too bright colours and too many posters overwhelming; their relative inability to filter information leads to increased anxiety in busy environments.

There also needs to be some attention given to the use of symbols and signs around healthcare facilities. A great deal of work goes into helping people with intellectual impairment to recognize standard signs, for example male and female lavatory signs. Advice could usefully be taken to ensure that the signs utilized conform to such standards.

EFFECTIVE COMMUNICATION

As suggested above the basis of good communication in consultations with people who have intellectual impairment lies with the relationships formed. Clinicians should adapt their communication styles in response to the nature of their patients and the circumstances of the encounter. An individualized approach places significant demands on the participants but leads to potentially more effective outcomes in terms of concordance with treatment, re-attendance rates and psychological adjustment (Trumble et al, 2006). The essence of communication can potentially be taken for granted, the significance and meaning of some of the phrases used relies on a common understanding that may be lacking. This understanding is influenced by culture and background, and is often context specific and can change over time. We develop a wider comprehension of vocabulary through both experience and formal education, we also learn the social skills, which allow us to explore and check ambiguities in the course of social interactions.

Poor receptive language skills coupled with an intellectual impairment places many patients at a disadvantage in the consultation. This is compounded by expressive language problems which may prevent a process of checking and clarifying from occurring effectively. The clinician needs to take the responsibility to create the circumstances most conducive to effective communication. The pace of speech and the vocabulary used needs to be considered with care and the clinician must be willing to check comprehension, repeat and summarise at key points. A high level of sensitivity to non-verbal clues is important, the clinician's body language can significantly affect the anxiety levels of the patient, and similarly the clinician must pick up on the client's non-verbal signs of anxiety, confusion or disengagement.

Without the intention to devalue or disrespect the individual with an intellectual impairment, it can be useful to employ the skills which are successful with young children when communicating whilst avoiding patronization, but care should be applied with the phrases and structures that are used. Simple short segments of language work well, as does avoiding strings of commands or questions, and the use of repetition and phrases aimed at checking comprehension is important. Using the individual's name can help keep the attention and focus of the client.

Attention must be given in order to recognize individual rates of comprehension, consideration and responses. In everyday conversation, responses are often rapid and immediate. People who have an intellectual impairment may pause and consider their responses for relatively long periods of time, this can be quite disconcerting, with confusing difficulties in sequencing leading to disjointed conversations.

An awareness of the concrete nature of some clients' understanding and use of language will also be helpful. A tendency to take things literally, especially among high-functioning autistic individuals, can lead to misunderstandings but can also be quite unsettling for the individual. Idiomatic phrases should be used with care, as with slang or colloquialisms, and attempts at humour may backfire! The English used in some of the 'Janet and John' books of the primary school, whilst formal and stilted, is safe, basic and unambiguous. It would be advisable to start consultations using such basic language structures and to judge the client's response and ability; versatility is a recognized attribute of a competent practitioner.

COMMUNICATING WITH OR THROUGH CARERS

One to one consultations with people who have known intellectual impairments are relatively rare in general clinical practice or outpatient clinics, usually a carer is present and contributing. Whether the carer is a relative or a professional carer, the presence of a third person adds whole new levels of complexity to the consultation process. Effective communication with the carer presents its own challenges, as does the communication between the patient and the carer. Attempts by the carer to interpret and represent the patient's experiences, feelings or concerns can only at best be an approximation.

Carers might prejudge aspects of communication, either in the details of the information that is thought to be important or in terms of the desired outcome. This can be a well-intentioned paternalism or affectionate protectiveness, but can occasionally be contrary to the clients' hopes and aspirations and rarely, part of a pattern of poor care of a vulnerable individual. The clinician needs to involve the carer as a valued resource in the consultation, whilst placing the individual at the centre of the process. This once again concurs with the over-riding principle of respecting the value of the individual.

EXTENDING EFFECTIVE COMMUNICATION BEYOND THE CONSULTATION

The face-to-face consultation is only one part of the potential interaction between people who have intellectual impairment and health services. A great deal of health information is delivered in the form of printed material, especially in the field of health promotion. Ensuring that such material is accessible to the full spectrum of clients with intellectual impairment is a challenge, requiring skill and perseverance. A number of health promotion leaflets, prepared especially for intellectually impaired individuals, are available. They are useful in daily practice but are also helpful in providing an example of the style and level of language found to be generally appropriate. Adapting current literature employed in various healthcare settings with these examples in mind then becomes a realistic possibility.

EXERCISE

1. Take a regularly used form or document from your daily practice and consider its appropriateness and comprehensiveness when working with an individual with a moderately severe learning disability.

2. Practise breaking down complex task instructions into single simple commands, (e.g. how to make a cup of tea) with a colleague. Repeat the exercise with a piece of health advice appropriate to your field (e.g. how to take a course of antibiotics). ■

REFLECTION AND PERSONAL DEVELOPMENT

The sociological notion of a 'life-world' that each of us inhabits and from which we unconsciously draw ideas about how to interact with others (Kelleher and Leavey, 2004) is helpful when trying to understand the potential difficulties with communication. In order to achieve effective communication between two individuals it is necessary for each person to share a common understanding of what is actually happening. It is conceivable that whilst the practitioner may have a clear understanding of what it is they are trying to achieve, the person with an intellectual impairment may not. They may well be focused upon the difficulties in getting to the clinic that morning or an incident that happened the previous evening with a support worker or even a preoccupation with the type of aftershave being worn by the doctor. People have a number of potentially conflicting thoughts and personal anxieties that can intrude on our day-to-day interactions, however, most people are able to control thoughts and attend to the task at hand. It may be that a person with an intellectual impairment will struggle with such an idea and be unable to put aside intrusive thoughts.

In any encounter between a professional and a client with intellectual impairment the dialogue will be influenced by the previous experiences of both. Reflection following consultations with people who have intellectual impairment is essential to the development of knowledge and skills in communication. If the clinician's knowledge and understanding of the realities of having an intellectual impairment is limited the clinician might be tempted to assume, even on a subconscious level, that the next consultation will proceed in the same manner.

CONCLUSION

There is of course an implicit message here about maintaining professional competence by accessing appropriate awareness training. Consider the message from the *Once a Day* document (DH, 1999). At least once a day a person with a learning disability would present at a typical healthcare establishment. Add to this the other groups of people who have intellectual impairments and the frequency will be higher.

Bury and Gabe (2004) note that unclear communication can lead to errors in patient care. Each practitioner, doctor and nurse, has a responsibility to their patients to ensure communication is clear and unambiguous. Language is frequently held to be a fundamental cultural system and is an essential component of human life. All cultures develop language and while some people with intellectual impairments may not have spoken language, they will find ways and means by which to communicate. The challenge for professionals is to be able to interpret the subtleties and nuances of body posture, facial expression and other behaviours which are indicative of communication attempts.

Although this chapter has largely discussed communication skills and people with intellectual impairment, much is relevant to the general population too. It is important that practitioners regularly examine and reflect on their own communication skills; complacency must be avoided. However effective a practitioner may be from a technical standpoint, poor communication skills will undermine overall performance.

REFERENCES AND RECOMMENDED READING

Bury M, Gabe J. (2004) *The Sociology of Health and Illness*, London: Routledge.

Buszewicz M, Rait G, Griffin M, Nazareth I, Patel A, Atkinson A, Barlow J, Haines A. (2006) Self management of arthritis in primary care: randomised controlled trial. *British Medical Journal* Oct 28; 333 (7574): 879. Epub 2006 Oct 13.

DH (1999) *Once a Day*. London: NHS Executive.

DH (2001) *Valuing People: A New Strategy for Learning Disability for the 21st Century*. London: Department of Health.

Hogg J, Reeves D, Roberts J, Mudford OC. (2001) Consistency, context and confidence in judgements of effective communication in adults with profound intellectual and multiple disabilities. *Journal of Intellectual Disability Research* 45:18–29.

Jansen DEMC, Krol B, Gruthoff JW, Post D. (2006) Towards improving medical care for people with intellectual disability living in the community: Possibilities of integrated care. *Journal of Applied Research and Intellectual Disabilities* 19:214–18.

Kelleher D, Leavey G. (2004) *Identity and Health*. London: Routledge.

Lennox NG, Kerr MP. (1997) Review: Primary health care and people with an intellectual disability: the evidence base. *Journal of Intellectual Disability Research* 41:365–71.

McConkey R, Morris I, Purcell M. (1999) Communications between staff and adults with intellectual disabilities in naturally occurring settings. *Journal of Intellectual Disabilities Research* 43:194–205.

Morgan H. (1996) *Adults with Autism: A Guide to Theory and Practice*. Cambridge: Cambridge University Press.

Prior M, Minnes P, Coyne T, Golding B, Hendy J, Magilivry J. (1979) Verbal interactions between staff and residents in an institution for the young mentally retarded. *Mental Retardation* 17:65–9.

Trumble S, O'Brien MH, O'Brien M, Hartwig B. (2006) Communication skills training for doctors increases patient satisfaction. *Clinical Governance: An International Journal* 11(4):299–307.

Van Loon J, Knibbe J, Van Hove G. (2005) From institutional to community support; consequences for medical care, *Journal of Applied Research in Intellectual Disabilities* 18:175–80.

CHAPTER 4
PRIMARY CARE SERVICES FOR PEOPLE WITH INTELLECTUAL IMPAIRMENT

Louise Barriball, Allan Hicks, Howard Cohen and Liz Lewry

STUDY AIMS:

1. To study the challenges of meeting the needs of people with intellectual impairment in primary care.

2. To look at examples of good practice that draw on local UK initiatives in order to enhance learning.

3. To investigate how primary care and specialist health and social services can work jointly.

4. To study ways of developing an integrated approach to service planning, assessment, health promotion and facilitation.

Individual patients with a learning disability or other forms of intellectual impairment have the right to utilize the primary care services alongside fellow members of their communities. The expectation that patients with an intellectual impairment will look to primary care for services is, however, a fairly recent development. When the majority of specialized learning disability services were delivered from the large institutions, the general healthcare needs of clients were

Learning Disability and other Intellectual Impairments, Edited by L.L. Clark and P. Griffiths
© 2008 John Wiley & Sons, Ltd

often met by their own healthcare staff. The shift to community-based care has brought with it the expectation that primary care will now deliver the necessary non-specialized health care for all people with an intellectual impairment.

Inevitably this policy shift has not always been translated into everyday practice. The barriers for change have come from both professionals and clients as well as their carers. Professionals often lack the training and experience to feel confident with managing intellectually impaired clients. In addition, primary care organizations have often failed to examine their structures and processes to ensure that they are accessible to clients with an intellectual impairment. When there has been willingness, other seemingly more pressing issues (often in the form of targets dictated by government policy) have sometimes taken precedence over providing a comprehensive approach to meeting the needs of clients with an intellectual impairment which becomes a 'Cinderella Service' (Clark 2005/6).

Clients and their families have often been accustomed to using their specialist services for all aspects of health care. They may have a perception, sometimes correct, that primary care services lack the experience and skills to deal with intellectually impaired clients. The changes needed to alter such beliefs have been slow to evolve. The quality of the experience when primary care services are accessed is a key determining factor in how rapidly trusting and effective relationships are built up. There is something of a 'Catch 22' situation here. Clients and professionals need to encounter each other to build trust and expertise, but neither is confident to do so before the expertise is gained.

Primary care in the UK is a long-established and complex network of agencies and individual professionals, including general practice, dental services, optometry, chiropody, dietetic and health visiting services as well as community specialist teams in areas such as mental health. In addition specialist health and social services for people with learning disabilities operate within the community and are currently provided and coordinated by teams commonly known as the Community Team for People with Learning Disability (CTPLD). A large constituent part of primary care services is general medical practice. Traditionally, general medical practice consists of neighbourhood-based teams of doctors, practice nurses, nurse practitioners and administrative staff. Often other community-based services, such as community nursing, are co-located with general practices.

However, the shift towards care through mainstream services is not without its challenges, not least because weaknesses in the interface between primary care and, for example, the specialist learning disability team can negate responsibility as one service may assume other services have overall responsibility for health improvement.

The potential effects of multiple challenges in the care of the person with intellectual impairment on how well various teams are able to integrate the care can be imagined. In this chapter we explore the perspectives of various primary care providers and identify key drivers for change.

GENERAL PRACTICE

The Disability Rights Commission (2006) recently completed an 18-month study into the primary healthcare problems experienced by people with mental health problems or learning disability. The study revealed that people with intellectual impairments were less likely to receive basic health checks such as cholesterol levels and preventive treatments such as statins compared with their non-disabled peers. The report also highlighted the issue of diagnostic overshadowing where physical conditions are attributed to the mental health problem or the learning disability, and are therefore not investigated. The report calls for action and asks the government to take steps to close the gap including incentives in the GP contract to offer regular health checks for people with learning disabilities or mental health problems (see Box 4.1 for a profile of a general practice's experiences).

BOX 4.1   PROFILE OF A TYPICAL GP PRACTICE

The GP list is a convenient way of picturing the prevalence of intellectual impairment. Translating national statistics into the profile of a typical practice allows the non-specialized health professional to grasp the potential workload they may expect to see. Drawing from the detailed experience of the practice of one of this chapter's authors a rough sketch can be drawn.

The practice serves a population of 5000 patients. The patient group comes from a wide range of backgrounds but comprises predominately skilled manual workers and middle management families. There is a slightly higher than average population of patients in the age group 70 years or above. There are relatively few minority ethnic patients. The practice does not care for any specific residential or nursing units for individuals with a learning disability or intellectual impairment, nor does it take particular responsibility for residential or nursing homes for the elderly.

The practice has identified 20 adult patients with a mild to moderate learning disability and a further seven people with a severe learning disability. Additionally, there are four adults with intellectual impairment due to brain injury or disease. There are also 35 individuals with dementing illnesses of sufficient severity to require care and supervision. Thirteen young people under 18 years of age with a recognized learning disability are known to the practice.

The figure of around 80 patients with intellectual impairment is only a rough estimate. It translates to a rate of around 16 cases per 1000, less than the 25 per 1000 prevalence quoted in Valuing People (DH, 2001). This may reflect the nature of the practice population or the fact that even in a relatively small healthcare organization significant numbers of individuals are not known to the service.

When examining the attendance patterns of intellectually impaired individuals it is noteworthy that attendance rates are not significantly different from other individuals of similar ages, and that a significant proportion of the clinical encounters are generated by the practice as part of structured care programmes. The perception that the consultations are time consuming is borne out in a small scale survey of consultation times, with appointment times averaging out to twice that of the standard ten minute consultation. As with most other patient groups, the additional consultation length is less apparent when the patient and the doctor have already established a working relationship.

Consequently, in planning for the needs of intellectually impaired individuals in the practice setting, it would be advantageous to allow longer appointment times as routine and to endeavour wherever possible to offer a continuity of health professional over time. Whilst this in effect amounts to a form of positive discrimination in favour of individuals with an intellectual impairment, it could be justified in terms of addressing a longstanding health inequality and respecting the particular needs of the individual (Kerr, 2004). It is also a potential way of enhancing the professional's experience, reducing stress and ensuring a satisfactory encounter. ■

The introduction of the Disability Equality Duty in December 2006 should provide a clear framework to ensure that all NHS organizations provide equal opportunities for disabled people, although achieving this in practice requires considerable change. There are examples of worthwhile initiatives that seek to tackle this difficulty. The education of individual practitioners, either within their own disciplines or across disciplines in their locality, is important. The Royal College of General Practitioners, for example, has had a Learning Disability Working Group for a number of years which has promoted good practice and offered education opportunities. Some local health groups, such as Primary Care Trusts (PCTs), have appointed doctors and nurses with specialist interests in intellectual impairment to support practices and promote good care. Specialist community teams have appointed outreach workers to liaise with and support practices and their staff when working with intellectually impaired clients.

Practices have now also been offered incentives in many areas to deliver services more effectively, either through the quality frameworks or through locally enhanced schemes. These schemes recognize the potential additional resource demand on practices and the team, when seeking to meet the needs of individual clients with intellectual impairment. Such an approach is necessary to redress the longstanding health inequalities experienced by the intellectually impaired patient group. It also sends out a clear message that the provision of appropriate primary care services for those with an intellectual impairment is not an optional act of altruism but a core function of a modern service. This mirrors the political intention to address the needs of clients with an intellectual impairment as a matter of right rather than as 'charitable' acts.

It remains to be seen whether primary care has been sufficiently galvanized by these initiatives to rise to the challenge and maintain its response, incorporating it at the centre of its organizational culture. Some of the challenges to the right of people to high quality care are often the result of deep-rooted stereotypes and misconceptions. This is the case for all people with intellectual impairment but perhaps can best be illustrated with the situation facing older people with dementia. This group often suffers from a stigmatizing double jeopardy where not only do they have an intellectual impairment but also suffer stigma associated with ageing (Jenkins and Laditka, 1998). The stereotypes that surround old age have been seen to directly affect how people access services and indeed whether services are seen as necessary. Consider whether it is more acceptable to deny treatment to an older person 'at their age' than for a younger person. Is this always a result of a clinical decision on potential benefit? Until we can be sure of the answer to that question then we will not meet the challenge of seeing care as a right not a privilege.

SPECIALIST TEAMS

The Community Team for People with Learning Disability (CTPLD) may consist of a wide range of specialists, including:

- Community learning disability nurses

- Occupational therapists

- Physiotherapists

- Psychiatrists

- Psychologists

- Social workers/care managers

- Speech and language therapists.

Some teams also contain challenging behaviour specialists, specialist community psychiatric nurses (usually trained in both mental health and learning disability), hearing and visual therapists. In other specialties there are dedicated services for people with mental illness and in some areas older people with dementia or stroke, all with an analogous multidisciplinary composition.

The role and function of specialist teams is ever evolving. In the field of learning disabilities policies such as Valuing People (DH, 2001) have underpinned the practice of consultation and specialist support for services in primary care. The specialist teams aim to work in partnership alongside general practices and other primary care services in delivering health care to people with learning disabilities. A core role of the specialist teams is to advocate the need for individuals to access services with support where needed. They should also take a key role in assisting clients in the full range of health services including access to acute services.

'Once a Day' (NHS Executive, 1999) highlighted the lack of skills primary care practitioners felt they had in working with people with a learning disability or intellectual impairment. It also challenged the way in which community teams function when supporting and facilitating primary care to gain skills to work with this client group. More joint working and stronger links are still needed. Even though the profile of the specialist team is now higher than in the past there is still considerable ignorance and lack of understanding in primary care (Carlson, 2003). There is a danger of the specialist worker functioning in isolation and the links with primary care services being those of a paper trail of referral, assessment and treatment with little face to face contact or rapport.

Examples of good practice include community specialist nurses working alongside practice nurses and general practitioners. Such direct joint working opens the possibility of transference of specialist skills. This can operate as either formal or informal learning. Another example is the specialist counselling psychologist facilitating therapeutic work within the primary care setting. A further benefit of this is a demonstration that services can be integrated and accessible for the service user.

Learning takes place on both a formal and informal basis and opportunities must be created for both. Case studies can be shared along with examples of barriers to the delivery of health care and success in overcoming them for service users. Anecdotal evidence is hugely informative within this process of understanding the needs of individuals with intellectual impairment. This reiterates the need for a person-centred approach which is challenging in the light of the range of different ways in which health services have been developed and designed, with many coming from a tradition of being somewhat prescriptive and rigid in their organization and delivery.

The following sections discuss the various elements that need to be considered when trying to improve healthcare provision for people with intellectual impairment living in the community.

IMPROVING HEALTHCARE PROVISION

There are a number of key challenges to improving the quality of health care for people with intellectual impairment in primary care. Carlson (2003) studied the views of primary care providers and their links with the specialist service. It is clear that significant numbers of primary healthcare professionals are not aware of the role or function of specialist teams for people with learning disabilities. This mirrors previous research by Marshall *et al*, who as early as 1996 highlighted the need for specialist teams to advertise their services in the wider health arena. Terminology can cause problems. The terms used and distinctions between physical disability, learning disability, mental handicap, mental illness and intellectual impairment or disability have all been described as a source of confusion for primary care practitioners. Particularly where a person may have both physical and intellectual impairment, the interface between the teams may cross organizational as well as service culture barriers. Older people with dementia, for example, may have both physical and intellectual care needs which may be met from a PCT or a mental health trust or both. This can cause challenges in terms of communication and effective goal setting.

The need for collaborative working has been discussed for some years. While pockets of good work have emerged there is little standardization. Increasingly specialists have viewed their role as one of facilitation on to mainstream primary care services and not as part of the provision of the service. Indeed, it could be argued that this is the intended future of learning disability services (DH, 2001). However, the understanding is not universally shared in primary care and this can lead to clients not receiving appropriate services as primary care staff presume that services are being provided by the specialist team and vice versa. A classic 'postcode lottery' in provision of health care occurs so that one of the main influences on quality of services for people with an intellectual impairment is where they live. Both provider roles need to be clear to all involved in order to prevent duplication and overlap or, in the worst case scenarios, no health care at all.

Powrie (2001) states that the gaps identified within primary care can easily be filled by collaborative working. This will include closer support and partnership with informal carers as well as the specialist service. With greater recognition of the fundamental work that informal carers do there could be a more inclusive approach towards primary care provision. The key area for collaborative working is within health needs assessment, health surveillance and most importantly health promotion. In addition to this there is a need for effective training and skills development within local organizations. Only then will there be an improvement in the clinical effectiveness and quality of the intellectual impairment/primary care interface.

One approach to improvement is the model of a specialist nurse-led health facilitation team. These are considered to be expert at tapping into existing services and modifying techniques to include people with an intellectual impairment. These specialists can be instrumental in breaking down the barriers faced by clients with an intellectual impairment. The approach focuses on devising protocols for people with an intellectual impairment in accessing acute and primary care services as well as training and development of resources for non-specialist practitioners (e.g. GP resource packs). Sadly there is little but anecdotal evidence for the benefits of such roles. Consequently it can be difficult to secure funds for further developments and existing roles can become vulnerable in times of financial pressure.

In summary, services need to devote some time and effort in joint working and planning, sharing vital skills and knowledge and supporting each other meaningfully. The ideas for practice need to be shared and not 'guarded' by teams and the need to demonstrate efficacy is paramount in bidding for the additional resources needed to fulfil such roles.

HEALTH NEEDS ANALYSIS

There is a strong body of evidence highlighting the fact that clients with all levels of intellectual impairment have significant unmet health needs, both chronic and acute (Hollins et al, 1998). The intellectually impaired patient group has higher rates of coexisting morbidity compared with the general population (Baxter et al, 2006; Kerr, 2004). While some additional morbidity is related to the aetiological process underlining specific conditions (see Chapter 2), it is likely that long-standing health inequalities, particularly poor access to services, is also a contributing factor often compounded by relatively poor socioeconomic circumstances (Nocon, 1994). Yet they are less likely to be afforded health screening and often do not benefit from mainstream health promotion activity (Thompson and Pickering, 2001). There are a number of reasons why needs are not met, including problems gaining consent, the need for support from both formal and informal carers to facilitate uptake as well as communication difficulties, challenging behaviours and difficulties with queuing, waiting and navigating services.

A structured, proactive approach to care such as the Health Action Plan (HAP) (see Box 4.2) affords the opportunity to identify and address comorbidities as well as plan for resources and modify techniques in health surveillance to reflect the individual requirements of clients. As this is a relatively new approach it is likely that, initially at least, significant levels of work will be required. With time it is hoped that the 'catch up' will be completed and the incidence of newly identified disease and uptake of screening services will be closer to those of age matched controls in the non-intellectually impaired population. However, HAPs are not standardized throughout the UK and the level of detail explored may vary quite dramatically from one geographic area to another.

The morbidities identified in HAP assessments cover the range of chronic conditions expected from screening activities in the general population, such as for diabetes, hypertension and hypothyroidism. Cases will also be found resulting from previously underused screening activities for conditions such as breast and cervical cancer. Sensory impairments such as deafness (often due to ear wax) or poor vision are frequently picked up even though not often reported as problems by patients themselves. Skin problems, constipation and obesity are often identified (Baxter *et al*, 2006). However, the HAP is only applicable to people who have known learning disabilities. Currently other groups of people with intellectual impairment are not offered them although the approach could be adapted to all groups. The single assessment process for older people has some similar elements to it and although this is a national programme in the UK substantive implementation and integration into care management is patchy.

In addition to individual HAPs some primary care teams will provide patients who have intellectual impairment with personal health records. These vary in the amount of information given

BOX 4.2 HEALTH ACTION PLANS

A Health Action Plan is a simple tool to be used to map out what a person needs to do in order to stay healthy. It enables individual clients to identify services and support needed to meet their identified health needs (DH, 2001). The approach of person-centred planning should be considered throughout the process of assessment. An example of this is to think about what is important to the individual client by listening and developing a therapeutic relationship. Assisting individual clients to consider what needs to happen in order for services to work together for their benefit is integral to such plans (DH, 2001).

but are a useful tool when there are many different health professionals involved in providing care. It is important that associated conditions such as epilepsy or autism are noted in the personal health record, as are communication difficulties. The person with the intellectual impairment or their carer will keep the record and take it to each of the practitioners or services involved, or to acute hospital services when needed.

It remains to be seen if initiatives designed to foster social inclusion translate into improved and sustained health gains. This poses a significant research challenge, particularly with so many confounding factors influencing outcome. However, as the changes in care are merely a process of normalization bringing people with intellectual impairment in line with the wider population, success should initially be judged in terms of access not health outcomes. The wider question of the beneficial impact of individualized and structured preventive care applies to the entire population.

PUBLIC HEALTH AND HEALTH PROMOTION

The Department of Health (2000) describes Public Health as:

A perspective which encompasses the roots and causes of ill health as well as its treatment . . . an approach which sees health within its overall social and political context, rather than an isolated medical event and looks for solutions in a wider social action, individual empowerment and community development, as well as clinical interventions.

Public health focuses on the need for health to be understood in the wider context of society and not simply as a matter of individual pathologies. Public health is a way of looking at health that combines multiple factors that influence and shape the health of the individual and the community (Thompson and Pickering, 2001).

Within the intellectually impaired community the existence of health inequalities is clear. A public health approach to health care is needed to try to remove barriers to good health that this community faces. The action for primary care and the specialist teams is to try to tackle the causes of these health inequalities through effective health promotion in order to promote positive health along with preventing disease. This can only be achieved when health professionals and individuals have jointly explored the links between their own health and that of the community. This includes the connection between evidence and epidemiological information and the social and economic make-up of the community (Lessof et al, 1998).

Individuals with intellectual impairment are two and a half times more likely to have physical and mental health conditions that warrant medical attention (Van Schrojenstein et al, 2000). There is a significant increase in morbidity mainly attributed to missed opportunities on the part of healthcare professionals. People with a learning disability and intellectual impairment are 58 times more likely to die before they reach the age of 50 than that of the general population (Hollins et al, 1998). While not all of the excess mortality and morbidity is avoidable or attributable to inequalities in provisions, these statistics highlight the need for a more positive approach to health care for clients with an intellectual impairment.

Mainstream services have little expertise or indeed funding in which to develop health promotion services in order to include those needing more support. This can lead to the development of services which effectively (albeit unintentionally) exclude people with an intellectual impairment. For example, older people generally are not seen as 'good customers' for health promotion initiatives. Stereotypes around lack of ability or desire to change may be an influence on this. Add to this some degree of intellectual impairment and inclination to engage with this group of people may decline further. In fact engagement with the person or their carer in this case may well have positive benefits. If physical health is maintained the person with dementia may still be able to visit a place or person they can remember and relate to in a way that is impossible elsewhere. This contact with 'reality' can have great benefit.

Communication is a key factor. Difficulties in communicating must be acknowledged and health promotion needs to take into consideration the way in which health professionals are trained in primary care. The training needs identified by practitioners include disability equality and communication methods (Mental Health Foundation, 1996). This must encompass other factors such as cultural needs, ensuring culturally sensitive health information and tailoring information accordingly. Community learning disability nurses are a frequently untapped resource. Many are skilled at health assessment and intervention, including planned appropriate health promotion for groups and individuals. They should be utilized as consultants, advisers or liaison workers across the primary health care setting.

The Health Care Commission (2005) has funded a three-year strategic plan in order to improve the health of people with a learning disability. This culminated in a strategy whereby from December 2006 a duty of care would be placed on UK public services to promote disability equality. In England, primary care practices must produce a list of patients with a learning disability as part of the Quality and Outcome Framework. There are additional financial gains for primary care services that choose to offer additional services for people with a learning disability. This funding is to provide clinical care which is deemed to be outside of the scope of routine essential services.

These initiatives form the backdrop for the health intervention work undertaken by one of the authors (see Box 4.3). An integral component of the approach adopted for developing and shaping the enhanced service was setting goals and identifying areas for future development. These include better training for service providers in the acute sector and tertiary facilities as well as primary care. The importance of galvanizing support from stakeholders cannot be overestimated

BOX 4.3   ENHANCED SERVICES

The aim of the enhanced service based in one locality includes:

- *ensuring that people with a learning disability have equitable access to primary care services;*

- *ensuring that patients with a learning disability are included in disease registers and practice-based registers;*

- *offering health facilitation, focusing on individualized health assessments and care for service users;*

- *placing an emphasis on health promotion and illness prevention.*

Achieving these aims is sought through a number of specific initiatives including: ➤

- *practice nurse and specialist learning disability nurse working together for health assessments and surveillance in the primary care setting;*

- *integrating health promotion and key referrals where necessary into the health assessment process;*

- *data from health assessments and surveillance forming an integral part of the information technology system;*

- *developing a guide to good practice aimed at increasing both access to services and acting as a learning tool for staff.*

Key stakeholders identified include:

- *primary care teams, GPs, practice nurses and practice managers;*

- *specialist learning disability team and their commissioners;*

- *clients, carers and their families;*

- *local champions such as strategic health facilitators who can lobby local primary care groups;*

- *additional health and well-being services, i.e. dentistry, optometrists, chiropodists, dietitians, sports facilitators and audiology;*

- *information technology departments within the organization;*

- *learning disability partnership boards consisting of service users, commissioners, service managers, advocacy services and carers;*

- *public health departments;*

- *health improvement libraries.*

Key to success:

- *promoting the enhanced service to all stakeholders;*

- *planning strategically;*

- *ensuring that staff training occurs;*

- *collaborating with colleagues across agencies and disciplines;*

- *data monitoring.* ■

as an omission of influence will limit the impact of new initiatives (Jukes and Bollard, 2002; Matthews *et al*, 2002). What is needed for success with such initiatives is not only sufficient resources but also vision on the part of staff that are committed to providing a user-led service, including by those with an intellectual impairment.

CARERS AND THEIR NEEDS

The tendency for whole families to be registered with the same practice in primary care allows an additional opportunity to focus on the needs of carers of intellectually impaired patients as well as the clients themselves. The day-to-day reality of caring for family members with a disability should not be underestimated. The physical and emotional toll is immense. Carers can easily become marginalized and experience the same pervading economic and health inequalities experienced by the clients with intellectual impairment themselves. A cultural expectation of long suffering and not complaining can lead to a degree of self-neglect. Physical and psychological problems can present later than normal, with more adverse consequences. Indeed the shift from formal to informal care in the community requires increased vigilance of the health needs of carers of intellectually impaired clients (Norman, 1998).

A proactive approach to assessing the impact of caring on the health and quality of life of carers is important. Practices need to identify carers and take opportunities to facilitate assessment of their needs. The coincidence of an intellectually impaired individual with ageing carers, such as parents or spouses, means that difficulties will inevitably arise. Box 4.4 outlines a 'typical' case history. Care planning for the routine needs of the carer needs to be coupled with contingency planning for unexpected emergencies. A clear plan can provide reassurance to the carer who might otherwise feel compelled to remain 'on duty' and may avoid delayed presentation of health problems. Primary care professionals may be ideally placed to identify such situations and facilitate an appropriate multi-agency approach to providing solutions.

Box 4.4 also illustrates another challenge to practice. Although life expectancies do not match those of the general population, people with intellectual impairment live much longer than they

---

BOX 4.4   **ROBERT'S CASE HISTORY**

Robert is a 48-year-old man with Down syndrome. Robert is non-verbal, usually placid and amenable, but tends to become restless and irritable if scared or uncomfortable. Robert's health is good, except for a long-term tendency to be constipated. He lives with his Mum (Enid) who is 88 years old. His dad died some twenty years ago. He has an older sister who lives an hour away with her family. He has always lived at home.

Three years ago Enid went into hospital, having fallen and broken her hip. Robert was found an emergency placement for six weeks; he was very unhappy, refused to eat and lost three stone in weight whilst away from home. Since then, Enid has been reluctant to be separated from Robert, fearful that no one else can care for him as she does.

As a primary care practitioner new to the area, you are called to see Robert as his constipation has become more troublesome.

Discuss your initial thoughts and concerns about Robert and Enid.

What would be your plan of action having met them?

What services, available to you locally, would be helpful and how would you access them? ■

did in the past. Consequently there is also an expanding population of elderly parents or spouses who are continuing to care well into old age. As the majority of people with intellectual impairment in the UK live at home with their families the recognition of the needs of older carers specifically should be growing in terms of policy and practice.

ABUSE AND NEGLECT

All health professionals have an important role in the protection of vulnerable individuals from abuse, neglect or exploitation. The definition of 'vulnerable adult' given by the Lord Chancellor's department in its 1997 'Who Decides' report is a person: 'who is or may be in need of community care services by reason of mental of other disability, age or illness and who is or may be unable to protect him or herself against significant harm or exploitation'.

It can be readily seen that a lot of clients who could be defined as having an intellectual impairment fall into this definition, not the least of which are older people with dementia, but while child protection initiatives are required by statute, e.g. The Children Act, adult abuse initiatives are not, although the 2005 Mental Capacity Act does re-emphasise professional responsibilities.

As with paediatric practice, there is a duty of care and practitioners must assure themselves that intellectually impaired clients are being cared for appropriately and safely. When doubts occur immediate action must be taken rather than assuming someone else will deal with the situation. Discussions within teams and across agencies are important and need to be part of the regular working routine. Local referral and advice networks are often less clearly defined than in child protection work, but need to be developed and improved. Multidisciplinary case discussions are often poorly attended by GPs and barriers to attendance should be examined and minimized.

CONCLUSION

This chapter has outlined many of the challenges faced by primary care services in meeting the needs of people with intellectual impairment. It has also outlined the very positive role that primary care can play in promoting positive health, prevention and delivering primary care to a group that currently experiences significant exclusion. The transformation of services of people with intellectual impairment will not be easy.

There is a strong case for the establishment of an intellectual impairment register within primary care teams. This should include all groups of people with intellectual impairment and not just people with known learning disabilities. By identifying an intellectual impairment lead within the team, who can liaise with other agencies, mentor team members, and raise awareness of the needs of intellectually impaired individuals within the practice, a coordinated approach may be achieved. This individual may also collect and commission suitable resources to support the work of the primary care teams, both written and visual. They should also be able to identify the education and training needs for practitioners.

Better links need to be made across primary care services, roles must be clarified especially in relation to the community psychiatric services, specialist dementia services and the community teams for people with learning disabilities. Responsibility for the provision of care for patients who have intellectual impairment often remains unclear to primary health practitioners, as it does to specialist teams, and this is compounded by geographic differences in areas of clinical responsibility.

REFERENCES AND RECOMMENDED READING

Baxter H, Lowe K, Houston H *et al*. (2006) Previously unidentified morbidity in patients with intellectual disability. *Br J Gen Pract* 56:93–8.

Carlson T. (2003) What is the community learning disability? *Primary Health Care* 13(5):37–41.

Clark LL. (2005/6). What's in a name? Transfer of skills across the Cinderella Services. *British Journal of Neuroscience Nursing*. 1(5):214–15.

Department of Health (2000) *Midwives and the New NHS*. London: Royal College of Midwives.

Department of Health (2001) *Valuing People: a New Strategy for Learning Disability for the 21st Century*. London: DH.

Disability Rights Commission (2006) *Equal Treatment: Closing the Gap*. London: DRC.

Health Care Commission (2005) Draft Three-Year Strategic Plan for Assessing & Encouraging Improvement in the Health and Healthcare of Adults with a Learning Disability 2006–2009.

Hollins S, Attard MT, von Fraunhofer N, McQuigan S, Dedgwick P. (1998) Mortality in people with learning disability: Risks, causes and death certificate findings in London. *Developmental Medicine & Child Neurology* 40(1):50–6.

Jenkins CL, Laditka SB. (1998) Double Jeopardy; the challenge of providing mental health services to older persons. *Administration and Policy in Mental Health* 26(1):65–74.

Jukes M, Bollard M. (2002) Health facilitators in learning disability are important roles. *British Journal of Nursing* 11:297.

Kerr M. (2004) Improving the general health pf people with learning disabilities *Advances in Psychiatric Treatment* 10:200–6.

Lessof S, Durnelow C, McPherson K. (1998) *Feasibility Study of the Case for Natural Standards for Specialist Practice in Public Health*. London: NHS Executive.

Lord Chancellors Department (1997) *Who Decides? Making Decisions on Belief of Mentally Incapacitated Adults*. London: The Stationery Office.

Marshall S, Markin D, Myles F. (1996) Survey of GPs' views of learning disability services. *British Journal of Nursing* 5(13):11–24.

Matthews R, Blake P, Hornibrook J. (2002) Health gains through health checks: Improving access to primary healthcare for people with intellectual disabilities. *Journal of Intellectual Disability Research* 41(5): 401–8.

Mental Health Foundation (1996) *Building Expectations: Opportunities and Services for people with learning disabilities*. London: Mental Health Foundation.

NHS Executive (1999) *Once a Day*. London: Department of Health.

Nocon A. (1994) *Collaboration in Community Care in the 1990's*. Sunderland: Business Education Publishers.

Norman IJ. (1998) Priorities for mental health & learning disability nurse education in the UK: a case study. *Journal of Clinical Nursing* 7:433–44.

Powrie E. (2001) Caring for adults with a learning disability. *British Journal of Nursing* 10:928–34.

Thompson C, Pickering S. (2001) *Meeting the Health Needs of People who have a Learning Disability*, 1st edn. London: Balliere Tindall.

Van Schrojenstein Lantman-de Valk HMJ, Metsemakers JF, Haveman MJ, Crebolder HF. (2000) Health problems in people with intellectual disability in general practice: a comparative study. *Family Practice* 17(5):405–7.

CHAPTER 5
TRANSITIONS IN THE AGEING POPULATION

Theresa Wiseman, Karen Lowton and Ian Noonan

STUDY AIMS:

1. To consider the problems experienced and service provision required during transition from paediatric to adult care.

2. To consider the chronic health conditions and care requirements of adults with intellectual impairment.

3. To understand the social, psychological and behavioural issues arising from ageing intellectually impaired groups of people.

4. To explore the issues arising at end of life, and the consequences these have for the individual and their family.

The population with intellectual impairment is ageing, mirroring trends amongst general populations in developed countries. Following a transition from child to adult services, many will increasingly face an extended adult life within which they may benefit from health promoting initiatives. For many, adult life will involve management of long-term conditions. Increasingly people with intellectual impairment will experience age-related disorders and indeed many will acquire their intellectual impairment later in life. All, at whatever age, will potentially move into a phase where care becomes palliative as they near the end of life. This chapter considers health care from this lifespan perspective beginning with the transition from child to adult services.

Although a diverse group, some issues of increasing age and declining health can be considered as common for all (Kerr, 2004). Diversity exists in terms of level of intellectual impairment,

Learning Disability and other Intellectual Impairments, Edited by L.L. Clark and P. Griffiths
© 2008 John Wiley & Sons, Ltd

education and employment achieved, physical and mental health status, social ties and stability of relationships with family and friends, in addition to connections with health and social care services. Increasing age brings a pressing need for health professionals and lay carers to focus on the physical, emotional, psychiatric and behavioural factors that influence adults' health and illness; specifically the prevalence of chronic illness and its implications for long-term management (Bittles *et al*, 2002). When planning acute, long-term management and end-of-life care, it is especially important to consider the levels of support given by family members and other carers, as well as issues of social exclusion and isolation. This chapter considers these issues in the light of ethics, communication practices, assessment and consent.

As a group, people with intellectual impairment have greater mental and physical health needs than the general population, yet they are less likely to be in regular contact with healthcare services at every stage of life (Kerr, 2004). Access to services will initially be influenced by which individuals are already known to services and the ability of lay carers to negotiate the professional care available. This has led to those who are already more socially excluded experiencing difficulty in being referred for appropriate care (Cornford and Cornford, 1999). As a potentially stigmatized group, individuals are more disadvantaged in terms of discrimination and discriminatory practice (Siegrist and Marmot, 2004). Older individuals with existing impairments have higher rates of mental health problems, epilepsy, hearing and sight difficulties, which in turn may cause associated problems for effective communication with both personal and professional carers (Bittles *et al*, 2002). In common with the general population, the prevalence of specific chronic or enduring physical health conditions such as coronary heart disease and diabetes is rising amongst those with intellectual impairment.

NHS mainstream services have not embraced those with intellectual impairment in the past and despite the recent focus of user involvement, individuals continue to face exclusion, or poor quality services (Cook *et al*, 2000). As Clare and Cox (2003) argue, it is possible that people with learning disabilities who have complex needs (either through impaired communication, challenging behaviour, or chronic physical or mental health conditions) are seen by professionals as being too 'difficult' to involve as users of mainstream services, and thus they are excluded and marginalized from treatment and care. This is indeed a phenomenon that may be applied across all groups who have intellectual impairment. As health service provision for ongoing treatment and care is increasingly being focused within community or home care, the exclusion of people with intellectual impairment is likely to worsen.

In examining the causes of differences in health between social groups, Siegrist and Marmot (2004) suggest that attention needs to be paid to the range of opportunities in the individual's social environment that is available to meet their needs of well-being, productivity and positive self-experience. The two aspects of an individual's positive self-experience that are of particular importance for well-being and health, the perhaps the least likely to be achieved by people with intellectual impairment, are self-efficacy (that is awareness of one's own ability to achieve a particular goal) and self-esteem (the sense of one's own dignity or self-worth). Appraisal of self within a social group will affect both self-efficacy and self-esteem.

Social inclusion in society brings health benefits both physically and mentally, yet a multitude of social and environmental barriers exist that prevent those with intellectual impairment from achieving such benefits (Siegrist and Marmot, 2004). Those with intellectual impairment are usually found in the most deprived social groups. Social gradients are known to affect differences in morbidity and mortality, with the poorest health outcomes, highest prevalence of risk behaviours such as cigarette smoking and poor diet, and shortest life expectancies seen in the most disadvantaged social groups. Differences in health outcomes can be attributed to the difference in power held amongst groups – that is, the ability to access and use material resources. More specifically, health status is influenced not only by unchangeable factors such as age and gender, but also by individual lifestyle factors, social and community influences, leisure and working conditions, and the broader socioeconomic and cultural environment (Dahlgren and Whitehead, 1991).

In addressing responsibility for health and well-being, many recent UK government policies imply a 'duty' for individuals to improve or maintain personal health, through edicts including eating five portions of fruit and vegetables a day. For those with chronic disease, government policies promote self-help in disease management, such as the 'expert patient' which aim to equip individuals with the knowledge and skills necessary to manage their long-term conditions within the home, with recourse to a health professional for regular monitoring and help for relapses in the condition. A strategy based upon building individuals' knowledge and skills in managing their own chronic health condition, raises particular challenges for people with intellectual impairment and their carers if it is not to create additional barriers in accessing ongoing health care.

TRANSITION FROM PAEDIATRIC TO ADULT CARE

Although this book does not study paediatric care, it is important to discuss the transition process. For many people with intellectual impairment a significant challenge occurs as they reach adulthood and responsibility for care passes from specialist children's services. Even those without existing long-term conditions move to a stage where 'dependence' is no longer normal, and therefore tension is introduced when negotiating access to care, either because support is removed or adult services do not readily accept the particular needs of people with intellectual impairments. For example, the need to fast track children in accident and emergency (A&E) departments is readily accepted. Suggestions that the same be applied for adults with intellectual impairments are far less likely to be adopted and this certainly does not represent universal current practice.

In taking a life-course perspective to caring, transitional care has been introduced in a variety of models. Multidisciplinary team working has proved to be successful in managing patients with conditions requiring complex intervention, input is essential from all through the transition process. In order to maintain continuity of care, collaboration is essential between all parties, both horizontally (between services within each different age-band) and vertically (between services concerned with children and adults respectively); in addition to inter-agency and inter-professional working. Transition planning should not only involve health issues but also the move from special education to adult services. The move should involve a person-centred approach to life planning. The advent of children's trusts should certainly improve the transition process as they are focused on joint working between the NHS and local authorities. Transition is an extremely difficult time for parents even though the process should have been anticipated and planned for some time. The worries that parents have over transition are numerous and include not only the physical and mental health concerns of their now adult offspring, but those of future housing and employment too. Apart from professionals, parents can often gain an enormous amount of support from other parents who are in the same position. In addition voluntary groups such as Mencap or those focused on specific syndromes (e.g. Down) are extremely useful groups in providing support and contact at any time during the transition process.

BOX 5.1   **DANIEL**

Daniel is a 13-year-old boy who has an acquired brain injury from an accident when he was six years old. He has marked intellectual impairment affecting his speech and his understanding (he is able to understand very simple sentences and commands). He gets very frustrated at times and has behavioural problems. In the last few years Daniel has been getting very erratic with his eating habits. Sometimes he will not eat and becomes aggressive when his carers try and encourage him to eat. ■

In accessing adolescent or adult care, many issues need to be visited. Consent now needs to come from the individual, rather than from the carer or next of kin. Although chronologically the young person has reached adulthood, their mental capacity may not be that of an adult, and a careful balance must be sought between protecting the vulnerable adult, and enabling an individual to decide on treatment preferences. There will be conflicts between individual wishes and health effects (e.g. wishing to choose one's own diet, and the potential for being overweight). It is likely that conflicts of interest between individuals and their carers will arise, for example in areas of sexual health and expression.

Many of the issues are illustrated by the case of Daniel (Box 5.1). Daniel has been complaining of abdominal pain, which is making him extremely restless and aggressive. His mother is very worried about him and has taken him to casualty.

Consider the strategies the triage nurse may take in order to facilitate Daniel's experience in the A&E department.

- How would you support Daniel and his mother at this time?

- Before beginning Daniel's assessment, what issues would you consider relevant and how would you prepare yourself to assess him? (Assessment per se is discussed later in the chapter.)

- Consider the investigations Daniel may need. How might you prepare Daniel and his mother?

HEALTH PROMOTION, HEALTH MAINTENANCE AND THE PREVENTION OF RELAPSE

Health promotion strategies for the general population in the UK are channelled through primary prevention (designed to prevent poor health conditions); secondary prevention (minimizing symptoms to slow or prevent the development of disease); and tertiary prevention, that is treatment and care strategies to limit the health and social impact of a chronic disease or condition (Ewles and Simnett, 2003). In the UK, typical health promotion strategies attempt to promote health and well–being through information campaigns, health surveillance through screening programmes, and providing health care and health maintenance through service provision. People with intellectual impairment are served more poorly than the general population through each of these mechanisms (Clare and Cox, 2003).

HEALTH PROMOTION

Some health problems common to people with intellectual impairment are due to underlying poor daily health practices, such as nutrition (either overweight/obesity or malnourishment); poor hygiene leading to, or exacerbating, skin disorders; and poor dental care leading to dental caries and other oral cavity problems. Indeed, people with intellectual impairment are at higher risk than the general population of two of the most commonly known risk factors for chronic health – that is lack of exercise and poor diet. For example, the majority of adults with Down syndrome are overweight or obese, with very few meeting healthy eating targets (Braunschweig *et al*, 2004), which is likely to have implications for morbidity and mortality. Ensuring good access to primary care services and promotion of health generally, such as healthy eating and regular exercise, are essential for this group of people. Many others face a variety of problems in obtaining adequate and balanced nutrition.

It is likely that the general public has difficulty in reaching the 'five a day' target of fruit and vegetables. Portions, in terms of size and numbers, can be difficult to estimate. Given this, it is an even more unattainable goal for people with intellectual impairments. This situation is compounded by the fact that care staff themselves are often ill informed as to the components of a healthy balanced diet and household budgets are often tight in relation to catering in both the statutory and private social care sectors. All these factors need to be taken into consideration when thinking about promoting health of people with intellectual impairment.

HEALTH SURVEILLANCE

There are also difficulties in accessing, retaining and applying information, and getting help and referral to the relevant healthcare provider. Poor health screening (Nightingale, 2000) and diagnostic overshadowing where features of the intellectual impairment mask ill health have been identified as factors which may lead to delayed diagnosis (Read, 2005). A lack of knowledge and experience among healthcare staff means that individual needs may be unrecognized and subsequently unmet (Read, 2005).

Early detection and management of mental and physical health problems is vital to address the health inequalities seen in this group. Only a minority of people with intellectual impairment currently access screening services, with uptake of smear tests for cervical cancer, and mammography for breast cancer being particularly poor (DH, 2001a). Access to routine screening programmes for people with intellectual impairment is beset with problems. Exclusion from screening may lead to conditions being identified too late for routine treatment to be effective, with a poorer outcome resulting. Read (2005) highlights a number of resources which have been developed to help those with intellectual impairment in relation to health promotion and screening. These include 'Keeping healthy down below' (Hollins and Downer, 2000) and 'Looking after my balls' (Hollins and Wilson, 2004) which encourage carers to explain procedures and tests in a very simplistic and meaningful way.

People with intellectual impairment are known to have higher rates of tooth decay and gum disease than the general population. The fact that their diet is poor, oral hygiene insufficient and oral health promotion inadequate compounds the situation. Dentistry for them is problematic for a variety of reasons including the difficulty getting an NHS dentist to see them in the first instance. Some people with intellectual impairment are seen by the already stretched Community Dental Services and many need sedation for even minor procedures or inspection. Challenging behaviours may also surface with a visit to the dentist and it is essential that good oral hygiene and regular check-ups are encouraged during childhood. The advent of the electric toothbrush has certainly been a positive move in making a 'game' of oral hygiene for many people with intellectual impairment, however, this does not hold true for all people with intellectual impairment, those that have autism in particular. People with Down syndrome have a high rate of oral complications which include gum problems and deformities of the mouth. It is therefore important to think about the individual and their past experience of dental care to find the best way for them to access services which will be acceptable for them.

HEALTH CARE AND HEALTH MAINTENANCE

Although little evidence exists of the most appropriate ways to promote the physical and mental health of those with intellectual impairment, it is reasonable to suggest that the promotion and maintenance of health in childhood and early adult years will promote more positive health outcomes in later life. Training and subsequent support is vital for individuals and their lay or professional carers who have been asked to change current behaviour or lifestyle to improve health.

Consider the case of Nazza in Box 5.2. Nazza's blood sugar is generally poorly controlled and she is experiencing more frequent episodes of both breathlessness and chest pain. Her mother tries to monitor Nazza's blood sugar but is having only limited success. Nazza likes foods that are high in fat and sugar.

- Consider how you might encourage Nazza to eat a more healthy diet and take more exercise.

- How could you support Nazza's mother in maintaining these changes?

- Which health professionals would be supportive to you, Nazza, and her mother in this process?

BOX 5.2   **NAZZA**

Nazza is a 32-year-old Asian woman who has Down syndrome and diabetes. She lives with her family but has expressed a desire to live on her own like her friends from the centre she attends daily. Her parents have explained that it is not their custom for a woman like Nazza to live alone or with others who are not family. Nazza is overweight and her diabetes is not controlled very well as she often snacks and enjoys her food. ■

CHRONIC HEALTH CONDITIONS AND CARE REQUIREMENTS OF ADULTS WITH INTELLECTUAL IMPAIRMENT

As noted elsewhere in this text (especially Chapter 2) there is a higher prevalence of certain chronic conditions amongst people with intellectual impairment. Although they may be linked to the condition causing intellectual impairment, such as Down syndrome, individuals are disadvantaged through membership of a lower socioeconomic group and are less likely to be engaged in health promotion. As Clare and Cox (2003) argue, it is possible that people with learning disabilities who have complex needs (either through impaired communication, challenging behaviour, or chronic physical or mental health conditions) are seen by professionals as being too 'difficult' to involve as users of mainstream services, and thus are excluded and marginalized from treatment and care.

RESPONDING TO NEW OR WORSENING SYMPTOMS

Much of what we know about how people interpret and act on new or worsening symptoms has come from studies of people who are not intellectually impaired. Lay health beliefs are an amalgamation of individual beliefs that are modified through experience of health and care, and medical science and knowledge. There exists great diversity in beliefs across and within individuals, families, communities and cultures. Beliefs about health and illness may change over time, in response to the disease and treatment taken. What individuals believe about their health and the cause of illness has implications for personal risk taking with health; the uptake of preventive healthcare services; and attitudes, behaviours and interactions with healthcare professionals (Ewles and Simnett, 2003). People's views of what has caused their illness may differ from health professionals' views.

Of course, it is probable that people with intellectual impairment experience symptoms that are shared with all members of the population. In one study where women were asked to keep a diary of their health, symptoms were recorded on average on one in every three days, with the most common symptoms being headaches (21% of symptom episodes); tiredness (13%); 'nerves' or depression (9%); aches, pains in joints, muscles or limbs (8%); and 'women's complaints' (8%) (Scambler *et al*, 1981). What is of note, however, is relatively how few times experience of these symptoms resulted in a consultation with healthcare services. This might be influenced by the individual's consideration of the 'normalcy' or commonness of their symptoms resulting in low consultation rates. Only one consultation took place on average for every 60 headaches reported. A reluctance to consult may be due to a feeling that there might not be anything that services could offer. The challenge for those working with people who are intellectually impaired is to recognize or enable the individual to make decisions about how severe or unusual symptoms are, and whether a consultation is necessary.

HEALTH BELIEFS AND ILLNESS BEHAVIOURS

In dealing with the onset of new or worsening particular physical symptoms, for example those of diabetes or heart disease, it is common for individuals without impairment to have informal ongoing dialogue with friends and family members in their social network about the possible causes and significance of their symptoms, and to expect some discussion about recommended actions to be taken. Uncertainty over symptoms is normal, and lay advice is very common, although the relationship between patients, their families and professionals is complex and changes as society changes (Cornford and Cornford, 1999). Indeed in one study of 101 patients consulting in a general practice, around 70% reported having a conversation about their symptoms, most often with their partner, before consulting a doctor (Cornford and Cornford, 1999). Furthermore, those already integrated into the healthcare system are better placed to decide which healthcare provider to alert to their deteriorating health. This raises issues for people who are intellectually impaired as they are often not integrated into the healthcare system.

Social networks can provide support in terms of information, appraisal, emotional and practical support. Such networks generally act in a 'loop' of maintaining or improving the individual's self-esteem, and may encourage use of alternative strategies such as participation in self-help groups, or self-medication (Read, 1998). Social exclusion for people with intellectual impairment can include not being listened to by others, having no friends, experiencing difficulties in completing tasks that others routinely carry out with ease, for example joining in social activities individually or as a group (Read, 2005). They may feel that they are a burden to others, or make little contribution to society, they may also feel physically or emotionally unsafe, and not have personal resources (such as money) to be able to have control over their plans (Morris, 1993). However, social networks may not be as strong for those with intellectual impairment (making it problematic to ask others for help), or the onus may be firmly on family members, carers or friends to take the initiative in health. That involves noticing a problem, interpreting possible causes, and initiating medical help, or navigating the maze of service provision. Changing family networks over the past three or four decades, with smaller family units and wider geographical dispersion, further limits social networks within the family (Scambler and Scambler, 1981).

PERCEPTION AND ASSESSMENT OF NEW OR WORSENING SYMPTOMS

One useful way to illustrate how difficult it might be for people who are intellectually impaired is to consider the complex ways in which the general population assess, evaluate, and act upon their own symptoms. Mechanic (1978) noted many ways that this happens, including consideration and initial interpretation of:

- the visibility or salience of the symptoms;

- the perceived present and future potential seriousness of the symptoms;

- the extent to which symptoms disrupt current social activities;

- the frequency of symptoms;

- the cause of symptoms;

- knowledge and cultural assumptions about the symptoms;

- the availability of information about the symptoms;

- the availability, location and cost (both financial and personal) of treatment.

Most people with intellectual impairment are reliant on those who care for them on a day-to-day basis. In many instances carers may not notice symptoms or be able to evaluate the seriousness of such symptoms. In addition, the client may be unable to communicate the effect the symptom is having on them (Chapter 3). Sometimes they may attempt to communicate their distress through behaviours which may seem challenging. For a further discussion see Chapter 10.

There are many barriers to consultations with health services amongst the general population, including individual, family and social norms of ill health (i.e. what people consider a range of 'normal' health to be). Issues can include normalization of symptoms and diagnostic confusion. Experience of past, present, and expectations of future health may also play a part as may past and current experience of health care (Zola, 1973). A fear of 'overusing' health services, self-blame and fear of chastisement can also come into play in the scenario.

Assessing a new or worsening symptom is particularly challenging for those with intellectual impairment and their carers if the symptom is not visible (e.g. pain). It may be difficult to articulate, or non-specific. Symptoms of chronic illness may be insipid, worsening over time and may not be as noticeable as the onset of new symptoms (Thorpe et al, 2000). Acting on these symptoms later in the disease course is likely to lead to increased morbidity, with a reduction in quality of life experienced, and increased mortality.

Zola (1973) identified a series of triggers to making a healthcare consultation. The usual triggers that lead people to a consultation such as interference with physical activities or social or personal relationships may be relatively easy for carers to recognize under many circumstances. However, they need to be interpreted in this way by the carer and may not be apparent in some people who are severely impaired. However, a potential lack of physical closeness to others displayed by some with intellectual impairment, for example in those who have autism, may mean that some physical symptoms, including those of an intimate nature, will go unnoticed by others. It is also likely that people with intellectual impairment will be unable to make use of other 'triggers' such as the coexistence of an interpersonal crisis, sanctioning by others (i.e. a 'punishment' meted out by a significant other to an individual not seeking medical attention), and temporalizing (deciding to consult after a set period of time with no resolution of symptoms). The centrality both of close friends and family advising in health care, and of lay carers in managing chronic and enduring illness is often not acknowledged by healthcare professionals, or indeed recognized by lay carers themselves.

People with communication deficits may exhibit challenging behaviour, such as violence or aggression, in attempting to demonstrate their need to others. This behaviour might arise from the symptom itself (e.g. pain), or an inability to cope with the symptom. There may be many possible needs for both lay carers and health professionals to address, and challenging behaviour may place a strain on the social support available, leading in a downward spiral to social exclusion. Some helpful areas for further investigating needs, in relation to maintaining health, include a knowledge of the individual's personal characteristics, such as their personal history and discovering whether the need is likely to be physical, mental, emotional (or a combination of these). Diagnostic overshadowing may again feature here in that the assumption is often made that challenging behaviour is due to the intellectual impairment, rather than an underlying physical or mental health problem.

COMPLIANCE WITH TREATMENT AND SELF-CARE

Taking medicines is usually an ongoing decision made with other people (Stimson, 1974). People with intellectual impairment will vary in their ability to negotiate with others their treatment and care plans. Today's health service aims for patients to be concordant; that is, to agree a course of action that is acceptable to both patient and provider. Illness beliefs not only influence patients seeking health care, but also their subsequent concordance with treatment. Compliance is less likely if many changes are recommended, a one step at a time model is more likely to be successful. Poor coping mechanisms and communication problems are also issues here as is the uncertainty of what condition the prescribed medication is for (McCarthy and Millard, 2003). Autonomy and control in treatment decisions is of importance for any patient, however, this is often absent in the person who has an intellectual impairment. Plans for what treatment and care is required currently, and what may be likely for the future, need to be coherent. Not enough effort is put into communicating with individuals with learning disability (DH, 2001a). Provision of accessible information, tailored for the person with intellectual impairment, their carer, and other professional staff is essential and often unavailable.

Consent must also be taken into account with people who have intellectual impairment and this is further discussed in Chapters 8 and 12. It is important that accurate information is given, and that this is understood and remembered by the individual. There needs to be an understanding of the consequences of the decision made, and that the decision is not made under duress. In general, it is essential to make no assumption about the understanding of health issues and symptoms in any patient. The health professional must seek to understand each individual's level of comprehension before imparting information, with constant checking of how much is being understood.

In chronic conditions, regular monitoring of symptoms is necessary in order to maintain health and prevent deterioration of the condition. This is often problematic for those who have intellectual impairment for the reasons that are discussed in other chapters around barriers to health care and a lack of understanding of health issues by untrained carers. There may be difficulties, for example in the case of those with diabetes, for the person who has an intellectual impairment to monitor their own condition by checking and interpreting blood sugar levels, or even in identifying the signs and symptoms that they may be becoming hypo- or hyperglycaemic. Enabling self-care in the management of certain chronic conditions is often not without its issues in the general population, it is essentially much more so in people who have intellectual impairment. Explanation of the condition and its management must be related to both the individual and those that care for them. This can be a lengthy process and a step-by-step approach is vital, often this requires the use of prompts or pictures and constant checking that information has been retained.

EXPERIENCING CONTINUITY OF CARE FOR A CHRONIC HEALTH PROBLEM

The target of 'Valuing People' (DH, 2001a) is to address health inequalities seen for people with intellectual impairment (in this case specifically those with learning disabilities) and for people to use generic health services wherever possible. Health service change has been phenomenal over the last two decades; this may be bewildering for individuals with intellectual impairment, and those who care for them.

In primary care, evidence suggests that when doctors know their patients well, compliance with treatment, accuracy of diagnosis, and patient satisfaction with care are all increased (Cook et al, 2000). Continuity of care is important across primary and secondary care, and also within secondary care services. In thinking about continuity of care in a hospital, Cook et al (2000) note gaps at all levels, between departments, professions, patterns and times of working, as well as differences at an individual level. Furthermore, services may be delivered at different hospital sites which adds to the complexity of access for the person with an intellectual impairment. The multidisciplinary team needs to stay abreast of what information the individual and carers have been given, frequently checking their understanding of that information, and avoid conflicting messages or recommendations.

Fragmentation of services, differing philosophies, priorities, objectives and values adds to the confusion experienced by the person who has an intellectual impairment. A named health professional as a contact or designated health facilitator is the ideal for people with intellectual impairment, especially in complex cases of chronic ill health. The Care Programme Approach (CPA) as described in Chapter 12 which is sometimes used with patients who have more complex mental health problems is an ideal one and a similar model should be considered in the management of people who have intellectual impairment and chronic physical health care problems.

'It is important to recognise that continuity of care when the carer is an institution differs in important aspects from continuity when the carer is a person' (Krogstad *et al*, 2002:36). A particular barrier to supportive and continuing care is the placing of individuals with intellectual impairment and complex needs outside of their own community (Jaydeokar and Piachaud, 2004; Pritchard and Roy, 2006) and away from a supportive social network. Those people who live without carers are often victims of additional social exclusion. Social exclusion only adds to the complexity of managing care for a person with a chronic health problem (Pritchard and Roy, 2006). According to Freeman *et al* (2000), the central element of continuity is the experience of a coordinated and smooth progression of care from the patient's point of view. This requires continuity of information.

THE IMPORTANCE OF MULTIDISCIPLINARY TEAM WORKING

A multi-agency and multidisciplinary approach to chronic health care for people with intellectual impairment is necessary but can be problematic. In order to achieve successful continuity of care the experience of a coordinated and smooth progression of care from the patient's point of view is essential. This requires continuity of information between client, carer, and healthcare teams, cross-boundary and team continuity, both flexible and longitudinal continuity in addition to relational or personal continuity (Freeman *et al*, 2000).

For patients and their families, the *experience* of continuity is the perception that providers know what has happened before, that different providers agree on a management plan, and that a provider who knows them will care for them in the future (Haggerty *et al*, 2003). There is some stability in providing services from a single team with a named individual as coordinator. However, this opposes the plan which is suggested in 'Valuing people' (DH, 2001a) whereby people negotiate mainstream NHS services. Once more this indicates that a Care Programme Approach (CPA) be utilized in chronic and enduring physical conditions, as it is in severe and enduring mental health care – to good effect.

When discussing continuity in secondary care, modern organizations have the need to balance the *division* of tasks with the *coordination* of these tasks (Haggerty *et al*, 2003) which can be problematic and result in a far from seamless service. Issues may also arise due to lack of coordination or communication between different departments or professional disciplines which can have catastrophic consequences for the continuity of patient care. There needs to be an attempt to move towards anticipating needs rather than responding to requests from carers or individuals themselves. One solution offered is patient-held records (Hart, 2002) whereby the patient or carer keeps the information and takes it from one health provider to another.

Sensitivity with personal subjects may cause problems for the person with intellectual impairment and therefore it can be beneficial to arrange for a same-sex professional to talk to them. It is known that there are issues for people who live in households where all other members are of the opposite sex (McCarthy and Millard, 2003).

Let us return to Nazza, who was introduced in Box 5.2.

• Consider what gaps in services Nazza may experience as she receives care from the hospital for complications of her diabetes.

• How can continuity of care be increased for Nazza?

• How can Nazza's carers be helped to navigate the services available to them?

ISSUES ARISING FROM AGEING INTELLECTUALLY IMPAIRED GROUPS

The ageing of populations with many types of intellectual impairment is now mirroring the ageing of the general population. For example, in 1997, the average age at death for people with Down syndrome was 49 years, nearly double the age in 1983 (Yang *et al*, 2002).

Hearing loss, cataracts (refer to Chapter 2) and other bodily degeneration associated with the ageing process are likely to make already problematic communication more difficult. Problems in performing some routine tasks, which are normally taken for granted, often become evident at this stage. However, there is a dearth of research about the ways in which social, economic, behavioural and environmental factors influence the ageing process. Polypharmacy, that is the prescription of multiple medications for both physical and mental health conditions, increases the chance of unwanted drug interactions and side effects. In the current health service configurations it is not usual for this group to be incorporated within generic elderly care services. In any event, these ageing populations are likely to stretch the ability of services to meet their needs (Patja *et al*, 2000).

There are issues of growing old arising from 'normal' ageing and those associated with an underlying syndrome. There is minimal understanding of whether or how people with intellectual impairment perceive themselves as growing older. It may be likely that some challenging behaviour or mental health problems arise from an inability to cope with an ageing body. It is also feasible that reducing social roles as the body ages, together with a limited and possibly shrinking social network, and limited exposure to, or involvement with, social events such as retirement parties, or funerals, will lead to a greater negative health impact when these events are experienced.

Although not strictly a health 'condition', body changes in mid-life will also prove a challenge for those with intellectual impairment. It is important in maintaining a sense of well-being that the social interactions and roles that people are able to fulfil continue for as long as possible. For women, the menopause marks the time of many new bodily sensations including hot flushes (see Chapter 2). Yet women with intellectual impairment, in particular learning disabilities, have seldom been informed of, prepared for, or supported through this time (McCarthy and Millard, 2003); in part, because of the difficulties in understanding age and ageing that exist amongst this group and the negative associations that may be drawn (e.g. dying, bereavement). The need to encourage communication about normal body changes across the lifespan is essential in order to give men and women confidence to speak about their own experiences (McCarthy and Millard, 2003).

Older people with intellectual impairment will also suffer from conditions associated with increasing age amongst the general population, for example falls, incontinence, dementia, stroke, coronary heart disease, rheumatic disease and osteoporosis. Some of these conditions can also be the cause of new intellectual impairments in an ageing population. All these conditions require assessment of the suitability of the individual's living environment, the likely success of adaptations to the environment, and issues surrounding changing locations of care. Little evidence exists to help with understanding the experience or recommendations as to the best ways of responding to these conditions and their effects upon specific intellectually impaired populations. In beginning to address issues inherent in ageing amongst this population, the World Health Organization (Thorpe et al, 2000) has identified 11 broad goals for healthy ageing in intellectually impaired populations:

1. To improve the understanding of normal psychological functioning throughout the lifespan of people with intellectual disabilities.

2. To improve knowledge and awareness of age-related stressors and their impact on older people with intellectual disabilities.

3. To understand and appreciate the social, cultural, environmental and developmental context of behaviours and their functions in older people with intellectual disabilities.

4. To improve the detection and holistic assessment of mental disorders such as depression, anxiety, and dementia in older people with intellectual disabilities.

5. To increase mental health knowledge and skills in professionals, carers and families of older people with intellectual disabilities.

6. To develop living environments that are responsive to the mental health needs of older people with intellectual disabilities.

7. To promote mental health and minimize negative outcomes of mental health problems in older people with intellectual disabilities.

8. To increase mental health services and supports in their own communities for older people with intellectual disabilities.

9. To collaborate with older people with intellectual disabilities and their support system in developing culturally sensitive, humane, and least restrictive mental health interventions with an integrated bio-psychosocial orientation.

10. To improve the quality of life in older people with intellectual disabilities and mental health problems.

11. To develop a research agenda that will provide evidence concerning each goal for all nations.

Return to the case of Nazza whom we met in Box 5.2. You notice that Nazza is taking longer to complete routine tasks than she used to, and seems reluctant to volunteer to do 'jobs' that she once took pleasure in.

• Why do you think this is happening to Nazza?

• Who may be able to advise you on what could be wrong with Nazza?

• How might you encourage Nazza to resume some of the jobs that she used to enjoy?

• What measures might you employ to prevent the situation worsening?

ISSUES ARISING AT END OF LIFE

BEREAVEMENT CARE FOR A PERSON WITH INTELLECTUAL IMPAIRMENT

People with intellectual impairment are more likely than the general population to live with ageing relatives and experience the death of key individuals with whom they have social ties and dependent relationships. Breaking bad news is difficult for health and social care professionals in any situation. Best practice includes checking the individual's desire for the amount of information given, and understanding of the issues under discussion (Bloom, 2005). Being honest, and avoiding such euphemisms as 'lost' and 'gone away' can make communication easier with an individual who is likely to be distressed and less likely to take in information. Sensitively timing the information given, and the place where the news is broken, whilst acknowledging the distress experienced should be taken in to consideration.

Anger, despair and worry are common reactions to the news of the death of a loved one. Professional carers who feel unable to talk to the individual who has an intellectual impairment may inadvertently compound the problems experienced. There exists a host of resources that may be useful in supporting an individual and their carers during a bereavement. In particular is support of staff in order to ease the process. At one time the news of the death of a loved one was often withheld from the person with the view that they would not understand the concept of death, but this can lead to confusion and a feeling of abandonment. Memory boxes, filled with photographs and other memorabilia, are commonly used in bereavement services for children to remember someone close to them who has died. These may be an effective way for the person with intellectual impairment to remember the deceased. In common with the general population many people who have intellectual impairment have religious beliefs and these may be explored and can be very helpful in the grieving process. The area of spirituality and religion is often overlooked in people with intellectual impairment. The process of attending and taking part in the funeral service is also helpful for the individual and may enable them to understand the death.

PALLIATIVE CARE

Palliative care has been defined by the World Health Organization as:

an approach that improves the quality of life of patients and their families facing the problem associated with life-threatening illness, through the prevention and relief of suffering by means of early identification and impeccable assessment and treatment of pain and other problems, physical, psychosocial and spiritual

(WHO, 2005).

Communication is often the key to sensitive, meaningful and caring support for those in need of palliative care (Read, 1998). However, people with intellectual impairment often have difficulties communicating in an effective way as a result of impairment (see Chapter 3) in a number of areas identified by Ambalu (1997). These include:

- *Cognitive skills* – people with intellectual impairment may have a limited attention span, memory problems or experience difficulty retaining information.
- *Hearing* is often a problem and may result in challenging behaviour.

- *Language* – delayed language development may result in a reduced receptive and expressive vocabulary and difficulty understanding abstract concepts such as death and dying.

- *Speech* disorders can range from mild problems such as not being understood by 'new' people to severe problems where the person is unable to be understood at all.

- *Social interaction* – when people with intellectual impairment do not understand a social inter-action they use compensatory strategies to deal with it. Sometimes this can be avoiding the situation, pretending to understand when they do not or withdrawing from communication altogether.

It is important that healthcare professionals have developed their own communication skills and are receptive to hearing the message behind the communication of people with intellectual impairment.

Palliative care is a neglected area in general, with poor communication being a major current problem in its provision. A lack of research exists in palliative care provision for people with intellectual impairment (Read, 2005), despite the holistic, individualized service that it aims to provide. Caring for people with intellectual impairment who require palliative care is extremely problematic and requires expertise and skill.

In terms of end of life care and choice of where to die, people with intellectual impairment may be further disadvantaged. For people living in group homes or residential facilities without on site nursing care a move may be needed because the skills to manage day-to-day needs are not available. Similarly those living with older carers may not have the option of remaining at home. This adds distress at an already traumatic time. The situation is compounded by carers and staff being reluctant to raise the subjects of dying and death, or giving conflicting information to individuals.

People with intellectual impairment are more prone to certain types of cancer, especially gas-trointestinal cancer. This is due to a variety of reasons including a poor diet, lack of exercise, insufficient hydration and the resulting constipation. As with most types of cancer in people with intellectual impairment, diagnosis is made late due to the inability to notice or articulate signs and symptoms of disease. The need for a multidisciplinary and multi-agency approach is more vital than ever when the individual has an intellectual impairment, the involvement of specialist services (e.g. Learning Disability Community Teams) is helpful to this process, although 'Valuing People' (DH, 2001a) would not recognize this as part of their current role. There is also excel-lent material available to help explain some of the procedures that may be carried out in hospital. Donaghey *et al* (2002) have written a superb book which explains 'getting on with cancer' in picture form including relevant investigations, radio- and chemotherapy.

Symptom control

People with intellectual impairment and their carers usually have low expectations of their own health and of services they receive (Koffman and Camps, 2004). Many individuals will tolerate poor health and uncomfortable symptoms unnecessarily (Tuffrey-Wijne, 1997). There is a reluc-tance for people to complain about symptoms and sometimes fear of treatments (needle phobia being common in this group) may encourage the individual to leave symptoms unreported. Failure to diagnose advanced disease and symptoms may mean treatment options are limited. A care coordinator who is known to the family can be of valuable assistance here. By knowing the person with intellectual impairment and being able to communicate in a way which facilitates the person revealing how they feel, healthcare professionals are more likely to be able to find more acceptable treatment modes and ways of managing symptoms.

There is added difficulty in terms of assessment of symptoms. Very little is known about how people with intellectual impairment experience pain (Koffman and Camps, 2004) and evidence suggests they may experience difficulties communicating its presence (Beirsdorff, 1991). Other symptoms, such as dysphagia, nausea or fatigue, are similarly poorly communicated and this may lead to sub-optimal assessment and management (Tuffrey-Wijne, 1997). It is therefore important for healthcare professionals to be person-centred in their approach to symptom assessment. By being mindful of the non-verbal communication of the person with intellectual impairment, listening to their descriptions of symptoms and getting added information from carers, healthcare professionals will be better placed to assess and plan symptom control for people with intellectual impairment.

Psychosocial support

Psychological responses to chronic illness and poor prognosis vary widely in the general population and are influenced by many individual factors. Some of the most important factors include previous coping strategies, emotional stability, social support and symptom distress (Pasacreta *et al*, 2006). All users of the NHS and their families need psychological support within palliative care provision. People with intellectual impairment and their families need it even more so. The key to effective psychosocial support is good communication skills. Healthcare professionals need to be receptive to the non-verbal cues displayed by people with intellectual impairment and acknowledge how difficult it is for them to express their feelings. They may be confused or unable to ask for clarification or help (Read, 1998). It is important for healthcare professionals to actively support the person with intellectual impairment in understanding his/her illness and help him/her to explore feelings arising from impending death. The person needs to be supported in order to enable them to fulfil their last wishes (Read, 1998). Facilitation may include helping to draw up a wish list with creative use of books, pictures, drawings, etc.

Read (1998) has shown a number of ways professionals may help address the challenges posed by communication difficulties with people with intellectual impairment. These include:

- allowing the person more time to digest/inspect new information visually and verbally. Using touch may also prove helpful;
- using visual stimuli such as pictures, books, photographs, together with short simple sentences, may help to improve understanding and recall;
- breaking tasks down into smaller more understandable steps;
- using creative mediums such as drawing, painting music to illicit feelings and emotions;
- using life-story work;
- using drama;
- using language that is simple and concrete and varying the ways in which information is given;
- giving the individual permission to experience difficult feelings such as anger and guilt. Some people may have been taught that anger is a bad feeling and should not be communicated;
- audio taping information so that the person can take it with them and listen to it with relatives or carers;
- involving the individual as much as possible with their treatment.

BOX 5.3   SOPHIA

Sophia is a 58-year-old woman who has uncontrolled schizophrenia and end-stage breast cancer. In addition she has alcohol problems and is homeless. In the last 10 years she has been in and out of different hostels, often being refused entry because of her alcoholism and her aggressive behaviour. Sophia is from the Ukraine and originally came to England in the 1980s. She has a daughter who is 32 years old. Her schizophrenia has meant that she often alienates her family and friends. ■

Understanding the complex concepts around serious ill health, death and dying and recognizing and responding appropriately to spiritual needs may also be difficult for health professionals (Read, 2005). Services need to develop strategies to nurture spiritually sensitive services through client-centred approaches, e.g. person–centred planning, and through practical provisions such as providing quiet spaces for personal reflection and offering appropriate support (Read, 2005). In relation to addressing spiritual issues, although acknowledging spirituality involves more than religion, Read (2005) recommends a guide to good practice by Hatton *et al* (2004) as a useful training resource that explores the meaning of faith in relation to people with intellectual impairment in an interactive way.

Consider the experience of Sophia in Box 5.3. Sophia is at the end stage of her life. Thinking about her gives the opportunity to reflect on the issues outlined above. She is increasingly breathless, spends much of her day sleeping on the street and appears to have increased levels of pain.

- What services are available to provide palliative care to Sophia?

- How might care be provided to Sophia's friends and family?

- Consider how you might support Sophia and her family and friends.

CONCLUSION

This chapter has explained the need for primary, secondary and tertiary mental and physical health promotion for vulnerable populations. It has considered the chronic health problems and care required of adults with intellectual impairment and discussed the transition from paediatric to adult care. In exploring the issues arising from ageing intellectually impaired groups of people, the chapter has stressed the need for collaborative working in order to provide high quality care. Healthcare professionals, social care staff and family members need to work together to address the needs of a diverse population (Read, 2005).

REFERENCES, RESOURCES AND RECOMMENDED READING

Ambalu S. (1997) Communication in: (O'Hara J, Sperlinger A (Eds)) *Adults with Learning Disabilities: A Practical Approach for Health Professionals*. Chichester: John Wiley & Sons.

Biersdorff K. (1991) Pain insensitivity and indifference: alternative explanations for some medical catastrophes. *Mental Retardation* 29(6):359–62.

Bittles AH, Petterson BA, Sullivan SG, Hussain R, Glasson EJ, Montgomery PD. (2002) The influence of intellectual disability on life expectancy. *Journal of Gerontology: Medical Sciences,* 57A(7): M470–2.

Bloom J. Breaking Bad News (Chapter 10), in Grant G, Goward P, Richardson M, Ramcharan P. (2005) *Learning Disability: A Life Cycle Approach to Valuing People.* Berkshire: Open University Press.

Braunschweig CL, Gomez S, Sheean P, Tomey KM, Rimmer J, Heller T. (2004) Nutritional status and risk factors for chronic disease in urban-dwelling adults with Down syndrome. *American Journal on Mental Retardation* 109(2):186–93.

Cardy P. (2005) Learning disability and palliative care. *International Journal of Palliative Nursing* 11(1):14.

Clare L, Cox S. (2003) Improving service approaches and outcomes for people with complex needs through consultation and involvement. *Disability & Society* 18(7):935–53.

Cook RI, Render M, Woods DD. (2000) Gaps in the continuity of care and progress on patient safety. *British Medical Journal* 320:791–4.

Cornford CS, Cornford HM. (1999) I'm only here because of my family: A study of lay referral networks. *British Journal of General Practice* 49:617–20.

Dahlgren G, Whitehead M. (1991) *Policies and Strategies to Promote Social Equity in Health.* Stockholm: Institute for Futures Studies.

Department of Health. (2001a) *Valuing People: A New Strategy for Learning Disability for the 21st Century.* London: DH.

Department of Health. (2001b) *Seeking Consent: Working with People with Learning Disabilities.* London: DH.

Donaghey V, Bernal J, Tuffrey-Wijne I, Hollins S, Webb B. (2002) *Getting on with Cancer.* London: Books Beyond Words. Gaskell/St George's Hospital Medical School.

Ewles L, Simnett I. (2003) *Health Promotion.* Edinburgh: Balliere Tindall.

Freeman G, Sheppard S, Robinson I *et al.* (2000) *Continuity of Care: report of a scoping exercise for the SDO programme* of NHS R&D. London: NHS Service Delivery and Organisation National Research and Development Programmes.

Haggerty JL, Reid RJ, Freeman GK, Starfield BH, Adair CE, McKendry R. (2003) Continuity of care: a multidisciplinary review. *British Medical Journal* 327:1219–21.

Harrison S, Berry L. (2006) Valuing people: health visiting and people with learning disabilities. *Community Practitioner* 79(2):56–9.

Hart JT. (2002) Continuity would be achieved with patient held records. *British Medical Journal* 324: 851.

Hatton C, Turner S, Shah R. (2004) *What About Faith? A Good Practice for Services on Meeting the Needs of People with Learning Disabilities.* London: The Foundation for People with Learning Disabilities.

Hogg J, Lucchino R, Wang K, Janicki M. (2001) Healthy ageing – adults with intellectual disabilities: Ageing and social policy. *Journal of Applied Research in Intellectual Disabilities* 14:229–55.

Hollins S, Downer J. (2000) *Keeping Healthy Down Below.* London: Gaskell and St Georges Medical School.

Hollins S, Wilson J. (2004) *Looking After My Balls.* London: Gaskell and St Georges Medical School.

House of Commons Health Committee (2004) *Palliative Care: Fourth Report of Session 2003–04,* Volume 1. London: The Stationery Office.

Jaydeokar S, Piachaud J. (2004) Out-of-borough placements for people with learning disabilities. *Advances in Psychiatric Treatment* 10:116–23.

Kerr M. (2004) Improving the general health of people with learning disabilities. *Advances in Psychiatric Treatment* 10:200–6.

Koffman J, Camps M. (2004) No way in. In: Payne S, Seymour J, Ingleton C. (eds), *Palliative Care Nursing.* Berkshire: Open University Press.

Krogstad U, Hofoss D, Hjortdahl P. (2002) Continuity of hospital care: beyond the question of personal contact. *British Medical Journal* 324:36–8.

McCarthy M, Millard L. (2003) Discussing the menopause with women with learning disabilities. *British Journal of Learning Disabilities* 31:9–17.

Mechanic D. (1978) Medical Sociology, 2nd edn. New York: Free Press.

Morris J. (1993) *Independent Lives.* London: Macmillan. Cited in Grant G, Goward P, Richardson M, Ramcharan P. (2005). *Learning Disability: A Life Cycle Approach to Valuing People.* Berkshire: Open University Press.

Pasacreta J, Minarik P, Nield-Anderson L. (2006) Anxiety and depression. In: Ferrell B, Coyle N (eds), *Textbook of Palliative Nursing*, 2nd edn. Oxford: Oxford University Press.

Patja K, Iivanainen M, Vesala H, Oksanen H, Ruoppila I. (2000) Life expectancy of people with intellectual disability: 35-year follow-up study. *Journal of Intellectual Disability Research* 46:585–93.

Pritchard A, Roy A. (2006) Reversing the export of people with learning disabilities and complex health needs. *British Journal of Learning Disabilities* 34:88–93.

Read S. (1998) The palliative care needs of people with learning disabilities. *International Journal of Palliative Nursing* 4(5):246–51.

Read S. (2005) Learning disabilities and palliative care: recognizing pitfalls and exploring potential. *International Journal of Palliative Nursing* 11(1):15–20.

Scambler A, Scambler G, Craig D. (1981) Kinship and friendship networks and women's demand for primary care. *Journal of the Royal College of General Practitioners* 26:746–50.

Siegrist J, Marmot M. (2004) Health inequalities and the psychosocial environment – two scientific challenges. *Social Science and Medicine* 58:1463–73.

Stimson GV. (1974) Obeying the doctor's orders: a view from the other side. *Social Science and Medicine* 8:97–104.

The Task Force on the Management of Grown Up Congenital Heart Disease of the European Society of Cardiology (2003) *European Heart Journal* 24:1035–84.

Thorpe L, Davidson P, Janicki MP. (2000) *Healthy ageing – Adults with Intellectual Disabilities: Biobehavioural Issues.* Geneva, Switzerland: World Health Organization. (WHO/MSD/HPS/MDP/00.4)

Tuffrey-Wijne I. (1997) Palliative care and learning disabilities. *Nursing Times* 93(31):50–1.

Yang Q, Rasmussen S, Friedman J. (2002) Mortality associated with Down's syndrome in the USA from 1983–1997: a population based study. *Lancet* 359:1019–25.

World Health Organization. (2005) *Definition of Palliative Care.* www.who.int/cancer/palliative/definition/en/ Accessed 5th September 2005.

Zola K. (1973) Pathways to the doctor: from person to patient. *Social Science and Medicine* 7:677–89.

CHAPTER 6
THE OLDER ADULT, INTELLECTUAL IMPAIRMENT AND THE DEMENTIAS

Emma Ouldred and Catherine Bryant

STUDY AIMS:

1. To understand the prevalence of dementia and the various types of disease.

2. To study the assessment process for dementia and the problems associated with diagnostic overshadowing in people who have intellectual impairment.

3. To study the common medical conditions associated with older adults who have intellectual impairment.

4. To look at some of the therapeutic interventions that are available for dementia clients.

5. To investigate ways that both informal and paid carers of dementia sufferers can be given optimum support.

Dementia is a leading cause of intellectual impairment in older people. As people with pre-existing intellectual impairment grow older they become subject to developing the same medical conditions and problems as the older general population. Dementia is one such age-related condition, the prevalence of which is significantly higher in this group than the general population. The lack of standardized tools for the assessment of dementia in the population with existing intellectual impairment, the lack of awareness of the increased risk of dementia and the way

Learning Disability and other Intellectual Impairments, Edited by L.L. Clark and P. Griffiths
© 2008 John Wiley & Sons, Ltd

dementia might manifest itself differently means that often diagnosis is not made until much later in the disease progression. Alternatively it may be missed altogether and be attributed to the ageing process or the initial intellectual impairment.

In 1929 in England the life expectancy of a person with Down syndrome was only nine years. However, today it is estimated that approximately 80% of people with Down Syndrome live to over 50 years (Kerr, 1997). Overall, the life expectancy of someone with a congenital or acquired intellectual impairment is estimated to be 55 years (Hussein and Manthorpe, 2005) with some people living to 70 years or older (Yang *et al*, 2002). This has been attributed to medical advances and improved living conditions (Janicki *et al*, 1985). However, as with other groups, an extended life span can come with a price in terms of an increased burden of disability.

The White Paper 'Valuing People' (DH, 2001a) aimed to make the lives of people with intellectual impairment and their families better. However, despite recent initiatives, people with intellectual impairment remain marginalized (Bland *et al*, 2003). Certain groups, such as those with Down syndrome, become further disadvantaged as they suffer from premature ageing and become susceptible at an earlier age to the development of Alzheimer's disease. Prasher (2005) refers to this as triple jeopardy.

This chapter outlines the prevalence of dementia and its main forms. The signs and symptoms of dementia are described in addition to the risk factors for the development of the disease. The importance of making an early diagnosis and the difficulties associated with making such a diagnosis are discussed. Diagnostic criteria are outlined in addition to the assessment process. The signs and symptoms of dementia are often mistaken for depression or delirium so a brief description of both conditions is also included. People need to be aware of other medical conditions which might exacerbate cognitive impairment and such conditions are outlined. The management of dementia, including drug therapies, non-pharmacological interventions and carer's needs, is described. The chapter concludes with a discussion regarding service provision and the complexities around this issue and ponders on what the future holds for the care and management of this group of vulnerable people. Guidance on the management of challenging behaviour can be located in Chapter 10.

WHAT IS DEMENTIA?

Dementia is defined as a 'syndrome due to disease of the brain usually of a chronic and progressive nature, in which there is impairment of multiple higher cortical functions including memory, thinking, orientation, comprehension, calculation, learning capacity, language and judgement. Consciousness is not clouded. The cognitive impairments are commonly accompanied and preceded by deterioration in emotional control, social behaviour or motivation' (ICD-10. p. 28). Behavioural and psychiatric symptoms commonly occur with the cognitive symptoms. Cognitive and non-cognitive symptoms will cause a decline in a patient's ability to perform activities of daily living. Before the diagnosis of dementia can be made the decline of memory and other cognitive functions must be present for at least six months (ICD-10 classification of dementia, WHO, 1992).

The commonest form of dementia in people over 65 years is Alzheimer's disease which accounts for 60–70% of all dementias. Vascular dementia (either alone or coexistent with Alzheimer's disease) is probably the second commonest (15–20%) with dementia with Lewy bodies and fronto-temporal dementia also commonly seen. However, there are rarer and potentially treatable causes of dementia including hypothyroidism, vitamin B12 and hypercalcaemia.

Less common causes of dementia include Wenicke-Korsakoff's syndrome, progressive supranuclear palsy, neurosyphilis, Huntington's disease, HIV infection and Creutzfeldt-Jakob disease.

The incidence and prevalence of dementia increases with age. It is estimated that there are over 750 000 people in the United Kingdom suffering from dementia. This number is expected to rise to almost one million by 2026 (Alzheimer's Society, 2003c). However, dementia is not exclusively a disease of older age and there are over 18 000 people under the age of 65 years living with dementia in the UK (Harvey *et al*, 2003) with an estimated prevalence of one per thousand in the 40–65 age group.

There is conflicting evidence available regarding the number of people with Down syndrome who have dementia. It is now thought that it may not be as high as previously stated, mainly due to misdiagnosis. However, a prevalence of over 36% is estimated in the 50–59 age group rising to 54.5% in those aged 60–69 (Prasher, 1995). The prevalence of dementia in people with other forms of intellectual impairment is up to four times higher than in the general population (Alzheimer's Society, 2004).

CLINICAL PRESENTATION OF DEMENTIA

The early stages of dementia may be characterized by personality changes, difficulty with word finding, deterioration in daily performance, disorientation, disturbances of mood and loss of memory. As the individual progresses through the disease difficulty maintaining appropriate conversations, apathy and inactivity, incontinence, loss of self-care skills, delusions, hallucinations and more serious changes in behaviour may emerge. In the final stages of the disease the person will lose basic skills such as eating and drinking, they will have problems in recognizing people, they may develop seizures and become bedridden. As the person becomes more immobile they have an increased risk of other physical complications such as chest and urinary tract infections. The case study in Box 6.1 describes the early presentation of the condition.

Many people like Martha who are in the early stages of dementia may realize that they are more forgetful. Others around them may notice the changes too. However, in Martha's case it may take longer for others to recognize that there is a problem because she lives alone. The early signs and symptoms of dementia may easily be attributed to other mental health conditions.

On the whole, the clinical presentation of dementia in people with intellectual impairment is similar to that in the general population. However, sometimes the sequence of the disease can be different from that shown in the general population. In the general population it is often symptoms of memory loss, loss of judgement and loss of specific cognitive functions that are reported first. However, in individuals with intellectual impairment early signs of dementia may include general slowing, personality changes, apathy and lack of motivation. The symptoms manifested will depend on environmental and genetic factors, the underlying cause of the intellectual impairment, the severity of the impairment and age of onset of the dementia (Prasher, 2005).

ALZHEIMER'S DISEASE

Alzheimer's disease accounts for up to 70% of all dementia cases. It is a neurodegenerative condition. There is a loss of nerve cells in the brain. Alzheimer's disease is characterized by a build-up of abnormal proteins between nerve cells: amyloid plaques, and damaged fibres: tau tangles. There

BOX 6.1   MARTHA

Martha is a 57-year-old woman who is divorced and lives alone now that her children have left home and moved out of the area. She works four days a week as a receptionist at the local group practice. Over the last few months it has been noticed by her work colleagues that she has become a bit forgetful and is certainly not as efficient as she once was. When talking to both colleagues and patients she regularly seems to lose track of the subject that she was talking about and she seems to struggle to find the right word to use on some occasions. A couple of times her apparent frustration has rendered her quite rude to people, this is totally out of character. The practice manager has recently tried to talk to Martha about the situation. She, like her colleagues, believes that Martha is probably suffering from clinical depression. Martha claims that all is well and she is just a bit tired.

Martha herself has actually become aware that she is becoming more forgetful and now has notes pinned up on the inside of her front door reminding her to take her bag and keys with her as she has forgotten them several times. She believes that this is all part of the ageing process.

Matters finally came to a head one morning when Martha appeared to be totally disorientated at work and thought it was time to go home only an hour after she arrived there. ■

is a marked reduction of a number of chemical neurotransmitters such as acetylcholine. The medial temporal lobe dealing with memory is affected first, thus first signs are often forgetfulness and confusion. There is a gradual progression of disease but eventually all areas of the brain are affected leading to full functional dependence. The condition can only be absolutely confirmed by microscopic examination of brain tissue.

In the general population there appears to be a slightly higher risk of developing Alzheimer's disease if a parent or relative has developed the condition. In the general population, familial Alzheimer's disease with an onset under 65 years age is an autosomal dominant disease but is rare (less than 0.1%) (Raber *et al*, 2004). The risk of developing dementia (of the Alzheimer's type) after head injury appears to be greater in people over the age of 50 who have a particular gene profile (ApoE4 gene). It seems deposits formed in the brain as the result of head injury may be linked to Alzheimer's disease. People who have sustained head injury as a result of boxing may go on to develop dementia pugilistica, which is a condition similar to Alzheimer's disease.

Epidemiological studies have shown that multiple vascular risk factors such as diabetes, hyper-cholesterolaemia, hypertension, and high fat intake have been associated with increased incidence of Alzheimer's disease (De La Torre, 2002). Luchsinger *et al* (2005) explored the association of the aggregation of vascular risk factors and Alzheimer's disease. Four risk factors were associated with a higher risk of Alzheimer's disease when analysed separately namely: diabetes, current smoking, hypertension and heart disease. People with Alzheimer's disease who have cerebrovascular disease deteriorate more quickly. The Syst-Eur study also showed treatment of isolated systolic hypertension in people aged over 65 years reduced the incidence of vascular dementia and Alzheimer's disease (Staessen et al, 1997). There is some evidence to suggest that a high intake of vitamins C, E, B6, B12 and folate, unsaturated fatty acids, fish and a modest alcohol intake may be related to a lower risk of Alzheimer's disease but definitive dietary advice in Alzheimer's disease or dietary modifications to prevent Alzheimer's disease cannot be made (Luchsinger and Mayeux, 2004). Research is currently underway to investigate the link between modification of vascular risk factors and rate of disease progression.

Studies have suggested associations of Alzheimer's disease that may be linked to decreased capacity of the brain such as reduced brain size, low educational and occupational attainment, low mental ability in early life and reduced mental and physical activity during later life. However, the greatest risk factor for Alzheimer's disease appears to be advancing age. One in 20 people in the general population over the age of 65 goes on to develop the disease and the risk rises exponentially with age such that one in five people over the age of 80 will develop the condition.

The reason why people with Down syndrome are at an increased risk of Alzheimer's has not been fully confirmed. However, it could be linked to the fact that amyloid protein, associated with genetic susceptibility, is allied to chromosome 21. People with Down syndrome have an extra copy of chromosome 21, which may explain their increased risk (Alzheimer's Society, 2004). The average age of onset is 52.8 years (Janicki and Dalton, 2000). The duration of the disease is highly variable ranging from a few months to 21 years (Prasher and Krishnan, 1993).

The risk of Alzheimer's disease in the intellectual impairment population also increases with age (Prasher, 2005). The clinical link between Down syndrome and Alzheimer's disease was made by Jervis (1948). Jervis and his colleagues observed that many people with Down syndrome who reach the fourth and fifth decade of life undergo dramatic personality changes resulting from intellectual and emotional deterioration. Several researchers (Malamud, 1966; Wisniewski and Hill, 1985; Mann, 1988) have shown that most adults with Down syndrome over the age of 40 show pathological changes of Alzheimer's disease but may not go on to develop the disease. There is little information to establish whether there is an increased risk in the intellectual impairment population if Alzheimer's disease affects a family member. However, there is some evidence to suggest that there is an increased risk (Prasher, 2005).

VASCULAR DEMENTIA

Vascular dementia accounts for up to 20% of all dementia cases. Vascular dementia is caused by problems with the blood supply to or within the brain. The concept of vascular dementia has historically been based on stoke and the multi-infarct model. However, it is now clear that vascular cognitive impairment encompasses a broader clinicopathological range of disorders including post-stroke dementia, multi-infarct dementia, subcortical ischaemic vascular dementia, strategic-infarct dementia, hypoperfusion dementia, haemorrhagic dementia and dementia caused by specific arteriopathies (O'Brien et al, 2003). The uniting feature is that vascular pathology causes or makes a substantial contribution to the cognitive impairment. Post-stroke dementia occurs in up to a third of patients within a year of the stroke and is strongly associated with advancing age. However, more work is needed to define and develop operational criteria for these different subtypes of vascular impairment.

The differentiation between Alzheimer's disease and vascular dementia can be extremely difficult and the two may coexist. Mixed dementia may make up about one-fifth of all dementia. Current criteria for the diagnosis of vascular dementia focus on the presence of dementia and the presence of cerebrovascular disease manifest by the presence of neurological signs on clinical examination and relevant cerebrovascular disease on neuroimaging. There needs to be an association between the two, either that the onset of dementia is within three months of a recognized stroke or there is a stepwise progression in cognitive deficits. The presence of gait disturbances, unsteadiness or falls, urinary symptoms and pseudobulbar palsy are all other features consistent with a diagnosis of vascular dementia. Neuropsychiatric symptoms can occur. Vascular dementia has similar rates of decline to Alzheimer's disease although the development of cerebrovascular disease in an Alzheimer's disease cohort is associated with a more rapid course of illness (O'Brien *et al*, 2003). Each time a person has a stroke it will affect their overall functioning. Sometimes people are unaware they have had a small stroke, but others might feel unwell and confused (Kerr, 1997).

People of Asian descent such as those from India and Bangladesh have an increased risk of coronary heart disease, which therefore increases their risk of developing vascular dementia. Likewise, people from an Afro-Caribbean background are at risk of developing diabetes and hypertension and are thus also at higher risk of developing vascular dementia.

DEMENTIA WITH LEWY BODIES

Lewy body dementia accounts for up to 15% of all forms of dementia. Lewy bodies are microscopic deposits found in damaged nerve cells. It is a progressive condition where there is gradual degeneration and death of nerve cells. Dementia with Lewy Bodies is characterized by fluctuations in cognitive performance (although this can also be seen in other forms of dementia) and, more importantly, consciousness level. Significant variations in attention and alertness are observed. Parkinsonian features such as bradykinesia, limb rigidity and gait disturbance are found. Postural instability increases the risk of falls in this group. People with dementia with Lewy bodies often experience visual hallucinations earlier on in the disease than any other form of dementia. Dementia with Lewy bodies has a similar pathological basis to Parkinson's disease dementia and both are associated with progressive cognitive decline and parkinsonism. Approximately three-quarters of older people with Parkinson's disease develop dementia after 10 years.

Frontotemporal dementia covers a range of conditions including Pick's disease and dementia associated with motor neurone disease. There is frequently a family history of disease (Schott *et al*, 2002). The spectrum of behavioural disorders in frontotemporal dementia reflects frontal lobe dysfunction. They include emotional blunting and apathy, disinhibition and disruption of social conduct and a lack of empathy for others. A spectrum of repetitive and compulsive behaviours can be seen, including wandering, agitation and altered eating habits (Snowden *et al*, 2002). It is caused by damage to the frontal and temporal lobes of the brain, the areas that are responsible for behaviour, emotional response and language skills. Behavioural disturbance occurs much earlier on in the disease.

ALCOHOL-RELATED DEMENTIA

Chronic and heavy alcohol use may lead to a mild or moderate impairment of memory. Other associated problems may be in the learning of new skills, visual–spatial skills and impulse control which is associated with ventricular enlargement and cortical atrophy of the brain. Whether it can be categorically stated that usage of alcohol is a direct cause of dementia is debated by many. Other aspects must also be considered such as multi-organ dysfunction, malnutrition and trauma (e.g. head injury). In many cases withdrawal from alcohol may lead to some improvement in cognitive functioning.

Alcohol-induced amnesia, Korsakoff's syndrome, occurs due to thiamine deficiency and commonly follows on from Wernicke's encephalopathy. Episodes of amnesia can be the result of alcohol intoxication in conjunction with patchy memory loss which does include this condition under the wider term of intellectual impairment.

EARLY DIAGNOSIS

It is imperative that a diagnosis of dementia is made as early as possible. There are several reasons for this. Reversible and medical causes such as depression and thyroid disease can be identified and treated. Giving the correct diagnosis enables carers and families to understand what is causing the changes within an individual and what the disease progression is likely to be. The patient and family are able to come to terms with the diagnosis over time. It allows them to plan for the future and have some control over long-term care management. Early management and treatment strategies may be put in place to maximize the patient's independence and quality of life. Carer support and education can be provided from the early stages of disease throughout the progression of the disease. This enables a rapport to be established between care support agencies and the family.

Making an accurate diagnosis of dementia in a person with existing intellectual impairment is complex and difficult (Oliver, 1999). Assessment of cognitive decline can only be reliably made within the context of previous level of functioning and longitudinal follow-up (Devenny et al, 1996; Visser et al, 1997). There is a high rate of missed diagnosis and inaccurate diagnosis (Prasher, 2005). According to the Foundation of Learning Disabilities, many professionals and carers in specialist intellectual impairment services and generic health and social care are unaware of the increased risk of Alzheimer's in people with Down syndrome in particular.

There are several other reasons why the diagnosis of dementia in people with intellectual impairment is difficult. A lack of understanding and awareness of the symptoms of dementia means that many health and care professionals overlook the possibility of dementia in intellectual impairment. It is dismissed as part of the impairment or it is regarded as part of the normal ageing process. Likewise, family carers may also be unable to differentiate between the underlying intellectual impairment and the insidious onset of dementia.

There is some evidence that dementia may present differently in people with Down syndrome, for example, that personality changes (including apathy and withdrawal) may be the first noticeable signs in comparison with the general population where memory loss tends to occur first (Holland et al, 2000). There is a lack of validated screening tools for the assessment of dementia in the population with intellectual impairment. Scores on dementia tests used within the general population assume that the person's previous level of functioning is within the 'normal' IQ range (Oliver, 1999). Cognitive tests that may be used in other situations are less likely to be successful in people who are non-verbal or have difficulty in following instructions (Whitehouse and Chamberlain, 2000). Due to the lack of objective standardized screening tests there may be an over-reliance put on subjective observations by carers of change in a person's behaviour without being fully aware of how behaviour might change with the onset of dementia (Oliver, 1999).

There is a general assumption that people with intellectual impairment who are cared for by family carers are already known to and supported by professionals. This is often not the case and so people with intellectual impairment may present to the GP or other service in the later stages of dementia, for example, when challenging behaviour occurs. The risk of acquired dementia in adults with Down syndrome is sufficiently high to consider whether screening should be introduced for those who are over the age of 30. Assessments could be made at three or four year intervals whilst the person is in their 30s, with the interval between assessments decreasing as age and consequently risk increase. Wilkinson *et al* (2004) recommend baseline screening, cognitive, health and functional assessments for individuals with Down syndrome over 30. Where periodic screenings are not possible, Janicki *et al* (1995) recommend an alternative method of observing change by keeping a life history record whereby individuals are encouraged to note significant life events, abilities and documentation of other capabilities.

ASSESSMENT FOR DEMENTIA IN INTELLECTUAL IMPAIRMENT

The optimum setting for the initial assessment is normally within an individual's home environment. A person should feel relaxed and comfortable. People examined within the clinic or hospital environment might be more inhibited and be less likely to attempt to respond to questions compared with those assessed at home. It has been postulated that some aspects of neuropsychological function such as orientation to place offer better validity if performed at home. Level of functioning is captured more accurately if conducted in an environment familiar to an individual (Prasher, 2005).

The typical presentation of dementia in people with existing intellectual impairment may not include symptoms of memory loss and cognitive deficit initially. The ICD-10 (WHO, 1992) criteria for diagnosis are advocated in adults with intellectual impairment as there is less emphasis on cognitive ability and more attention on behavioural changes (Aylward *et al*, 1997). ICD-10 criteria are designed to establish a diagnosis of dementia and differentiate between Alzheimer's disease and other forms of dementia.

The Diagnostic Criteria for Learning Disabilities (DC-LD) (Royal College of Psychiatrists, 2001) incorporates the ICD-10 criteria for diagnosis of dementia but is developed for use specifically in the population with intellectual impairment. Aylward *et al* (1997) have published international guidelines on the diagnostic criteria for a diagnosis of dementia in the intellectual impairment population.

Assessment of dementia is multidimensional and incorporates assessment of cognitive level, functional status, clinical screening including physical examination and routine investigations, patient and carer history. There are often several different agencies/professional bodies involved in a person's care. It is therefore important that all members of the multidisciplinary team are involved in the assessment process. This could include carers, GP, community nurse, psychologist, and psychiatrist with special knowledge of intellectual impairment, physiotherapist, occupational therapist and social worker (Kerr, 1997). Hospital workers who have known an individual over time might also be able to provide collaborative history.

Dementia is a disease of exclusion. A decline in adaptive behaviour and performance does not necessarily mean that an individual has developed dementia. Symptoms of dementia and depression often overlap so it is vital that assessment is done comprehensively and diagnosis is made appropriately. There may be underlying medical reasons why an individual is showing signs of deteriorating function. It is therefore important to exclude potentially treatable causes of a decline in cognitive and functional ability. Particular attention should be made to visual and auditory examination as both these can exacerbate a decline in cognition and make communication and therefore assessment of the patient more difficult. Examination will look for comorbid physical disease, risk factors for vascular disease such as hypertension and signs of neurological disease. Sometimes medical problems coexist with dementia. Treatment can improve cognitive impairment in some cases.

THE FORMULATION PROCESS

The Formulation Process is an ongoing assessment involving the mental well-being of the patient. It is undertaken in a variety of ways – through formal and informal observation of a patient, neuropsychological assessment, detailed informant interview, review of case notes and discussion with other disciplines involved in a patient's care. The Mental State Examination is an intrinsic component of the formulation process. It is essentially a 'snap-shot' of that individual at that particular time. Prasher (2005) outlines the components of a standard Mental State Examination:

- **Appearance** – Does the patient look neatly dressed/well groomed? Assess psychomotor behaviour, for example is there evidence of gait/balance disturbance? Does the person have a shuffling gait, which may suggest cerebrovascular disease or Lewy body dementia? Assess posture and level of eye contact. Assess level of consciousness – is the patient fully alert? How well does patient communicate/engage with assessor? What is their attention span?

- **Mood** – Does the patient appear happy? Depressed? Emotional? Anxious? Euphoric?

- **Perceptions** – Are there reports (by the patient or more usually, others) of hallucinations, delusions or illusions?

- **Thought process** – Is the patient able to respond appropriately to questioning? Are their comments logical and appropriate?

- **Insight** – Does the patient exhibit any understanding of their condition/situation?

- **Rituals** – Are there signs of compulsive behaviour or repetitive behaviour?

- **Personality change** – Does the carer report marked change in personality?

- **Cognition** – Orientation to person, time, place, memory, language, recall?

It is important to obtain evidence that the patient's present state represents a decline from prior levels of ability. Many people with intellectual impairment are unable to provide detailed information regarding past medical/psychiatric history, pattern of decline, etc. It is therefore reasonable that an informant is present when assessment is made in order to obtain collateral history. The informant should know the person reasonably well and may be a family member or a care worker. An accurate assessment of the severity of the underlying intellectual impairment is an important factor to consider. The initial consultation between interviewer, patient and carer is the first step in establishing a rapport and a relationship that may last for years. It is important to ask a patient to describe his or her symptoms but, obviously, it is important to check the history with someone else.

It is essential to ask questions relating to current medical problems, past medical history and current drug treatment to determine whether any other medical conditions or drug therapy might have contributed to the current problem (e.g. strokes, myocardial infaction, epilepsy). It is important to obtain history relating to physical features of dementia such as incontinence, seizures and weight loss (Prasher, 2005).

There is an increased prevalence of psychiatric disorders in people with intellectual impairment (Deb, 2001) for example, Cooper and Bailey (2001) estimate the number of people with known learning disabilities and mental disorders to be 40%, higher than the prevalence in the general population. Symptoms of depression are often mistaken for dementia. It is useful to ascertain whether there is a family history of dementia. This should where possible include obtaining information on age of onset, cause of death and type of dementia (Prasher, 2005).

Current and previous drug therapy must be documented whether they are prescribed medications or over-the-counter drug treatments or illegal substances. The use of prescribed, illegal and over-the-counter medication can lead to cognitive impairment and confusion in addition to the use of multiple drugs (polypharmacy). The side effects of some drugs can cause increased confusion and there is evidence to suggest that older people with Down syndrome are particularly susceptible to the adverse effects of certain types or combinations of medication (Kerr, 1997).

It is important to know whether the current problem is impinging on an individual's social life. Has the individual recently given up previously enjoyed hobbies or pastimes? Are work colleagues reporting any changes in a person's ability to perform at work? This all indicates a possible change in prior functioning. If an individual attends a day centre it is useful to question their key worker regarding physical/psychological changes. Many of the scales used to assess cognitive skills (see below) in people with intellectual impairment incorporate functional domains. An assessment of function will be covered as part of the caregiver/informant assessment. NICE (National Institute for Health and Clinical Excellence) (2006) recommends an Assessment of Motor and Process Skills (AMPS) by an occupational therapist at the point of diagnosis.

NEUROPSYCHOLOGICAL ASSESSMENT

Neuropsychological testing formally documents the level of cognitive skills and allows fairly reliable monitoring of change in cognitive function over time. However, it can be very time consuming and tiring for the individual, carer and administrator (Prasher, 2005), which can affect performance and thus may contribute towards a misdiagnosis of dementia.

Ideally testing should be performed at regular periods by the same person who is trained in administering such tests and also familiar with working with people with intellectual impairment. It is important to remember that whilst decline in cognitive function is a significant factor in making a diagnosis of dementia, it can only be considered as diagnostic when coupled with evidence of decline in adaptive function.

Cognitive tests designed for the general population are not appropriate for use within the population with intellectual impairment because they assume a normal level of functioning prior to the onset of impairment. The Mini-Mental State Examination (Folstein *et al*, 1975) is a validated, standardized assessment of cognitive capacities, and is widely used amongst the general population. It has a high degree of specificity and sensitivity for dementia although it cannot be used if an individual suffers from poor hearing, and it is culturally biased. It is a good example of a tool that assumes a certain standard of prior cognitive function. Wisniewski and Hill (1985) developed a version of the Mini-Mental State Examination modified for use in people with intellectual impairment but empirical support for valid classification criteria for the instrument has not been provided.

There are several cognitive assessment tools available for use within the intellectual impairment population. However, it is widely agreed that the population with intellectual impairment and dementia is not as homogeneous as the general population with dementia and thus, no single neuropsychological test will be suitable for all. However, some tools exist which do carry some validity and reliability such as the Down Syndrome Mental State Examination, which assesses a broad range of skills. The Test for Severe Impairment (Albert and Cohen, 1992) is useful for assessing individuals who are functioning at very low intellectual levels. The Dementia Question- naire for Mentally Retarded Persons (DMR) (Evenhuis *et al*, 1990) is an informant-based ques- tionnaire with eight subscales (namely short-term memory, long-term memory, spatial and temporal orientation, speech, practical skills, mood, activity and interests and behavioural disturbances).

The Dementia Scale for Down Syndrome (DSDS) (Gedye, 1995) assesses cognitive decline in individuals with moderate to severe intellectual impairment and comprises 60 questions in an informant-based questionnaire. The Camdex-DS (Holland *et al*, 2000) is a comprehensive assess- ment tool for assessment of dementia in people with Down syndrome and other intellectual impairments. It includes a structured informant questionnaire, and a direct cognitive assessment of the individual. The Camdex-DS focuses on establishing change from best level of functioning. The DMR and DSDS are both recommended as useful assessment tools by NICE (2006) in its guidance on dementia.

The Adaptive Behaviour Dementia Questionnaire (Prasher *et al*, 2004) is a validated assess- ment-screening questionnaire for Alzheimer's disease in adults with Down syndrome. It comprises 15 informant questions and can be used to detect change in adaptive behaviour over time. It can be administered by a clinician via a brief five-minute interview with the caregiver, while in their clinical setting and without the need for special training. It is the first clinical tool to screen specifically for Alzheimer's disease in adults with Down syndrome.

INVESTIGATIONS

The following laboratory tests have been recommended as part of the investigation of the young patient with dementia (Sampson *et al*, 2004).

- Full blood count screen for anaemia, polycythaemia, eosinophilia
- Urea and electrolytes, renal function, liver function, thyroid function, B12 and folate, lipids screen for reversible causes of dementia and vascular risk factors
- Syphilis serology screen for tertiary neurosyphilis
- Erythrocyte sedimentation rate/C-reactive protein screen for inflammatory process
- ANCA, thyroid antimicrosomal, antigastric parietal, antiphospholipid, antineuronal, VGKC, serum electrophoresis screen for vasculitides, atrophic gastritis, Hashimoto's encephalopathy, paraneoplastic syndromes.

CT head scan/MRI scan enables the exclusion of other disorders that cause dementia such as brain tumour and hydrocephalus. Neuroimaging is also helpful to look for medial temporal lobe and hippocampal atrophy suggestive of Alzheimer's disease. Chest radiography is used to screen for pulmonary neoplasm, tuberculosis, some systemic disorders (e.g. sarcoid). Electrocardiogra- phy/echocardiography may reveal cardiac arrythmia or sources of emboli.

Whilst EEG is not recommended in the routine diagnostic assessment of dementia in the general population, Sampson *et al* (2004) recommend its routine use in patients under 65 years with possible dementia. It is also recommended for assessment of dementia in patients with Down syndrome (Prasher, 2005). Although there are genetic links to the development of Alzheimer's disease, routine genetic testing is not recommended.

DEMENTIA AND DEPRESSION

Depressive disorders may coexist with dementia (Mynors-Wallis *et al*, 2002). There is no reliable and valid self-report measure of depressive symptoms for people with intellectual impairment. However, the Glasgow Depression Scale for people with a learning disability (Cuthill *et al*, 2003) was recently developed and showed good correlation with the Beck Depression Inventory (1961) in people aged 26–60. Both these assessments may be useful in investigating possible depression in the population with intellectual impairment.

Depressive symptoms include:

- Mental deterioration

- Emotional deterioration

- Disturbed sleep pattern

- Weight loss

- Motor retardation

- Reduced appetite.

Depression has been referred to as a pseudodementia because the symptoms are very similar to dementia and thus diagnosis is often missed or mistaken. In people with intellectual impairment the prevalence of depression is approximately 1–3.5%, this percentage appears to be higher in people with Down syndrome (Prasher, 1995).

Management of depression in people with intellectual impairment is very similar to that for the general population (Prasher, 2003) and includes antidepressant therapy and psychological approaches. There is limited evidence regarding the use of electroconvulsive therapy in the population with intellectual impairment.

DELIRIUM/ACUTE CONFUSIONAL STATE

It is important to differentiate between symptoms of dementia and delirium (acute confusional state) although it can be quite difficult. Little is known about the occurrence of delirium in intellectual impairment and literature on delirium in this population is scarce. Diagnosis is often missed (Van Waarde and van der Mast, 2004).

The essential feature of a delirium is a disturbance in consciousness that is accompanied by a change in cognition that cannot be better accounted for by a pre-existing or evolving dementia.

(American Psychiatric Association, 1994)

Delirium develops quickly and is treatable. Consciousness fluctuates and hallucinations frequently occur. In contrast the onset of dementia is insidious and the level of consciousness is normal, hallucinations may occur in the latter stages of the disease.

The aetiology of delirium is often multifactorial and will involve an interplay of predisposing factors and acute precipitants. Increasing age and the presence of dementia are important risk factors for delirium.

There are many causes of delirium including:

- Infections – especially chest infection and urinary tract infection
- Metabolic disturbances such as hypothyroidism and diabetes
- Poor diet leading to vitamin B12 deficiency, anaemia, thiamine deficiency
- Constipation
- Dehydration
- Pain (observe for non-verbal signs of pain in people with severe intellectual impairment and people with dementia)
- Bone fractures
- Drugs: toxicity, polypharmacy and psychoactive drug use
- Heart disease
- Renal failure
- Alcohol
- Sensory deprivation – hearing/visual impairment, social isolation
- Dehydration
- Grief reaction
- Environmental, e.g. going into hospital, moving into a care home.

COMMON MEDICAL CONDITIONS EXPERIENCED BY OLDER ADULTS WITH INTELLECTUAL IMPAIRMENT

As people with Down syndrome and other forms of intellectual impairment get older, they become predisposed to the impact of chronic medical disorders which they inherited as part of their condition. Lifestyle and environmental stressors also predispose any individual with intellectual impairment to develop age-related conditions and may result in a different profile of illness compared to the age-matched general population (Wallace and Dalton, 2006). This section addresses a number of common medical problems amongst older people with intellectual impairment:

VISUAL IMPAIRMENT

The prevalence of visual impairment increases with age and level of disability. The prevalence of visual impairments is higher amongst the population with intellectual impairment compared with an age-matched general population. The prevalence of visual impairment is higher in all age groups in people with Down syndrome (Wallace and Dalton, 2006). The commonest forms of visual impairment are cataracts and acute keratoconus. Up to 40% of people with Down syndrome develop cataracts (Hiles *et al*, 1990). There is also a greater percentage of congenital cataracts among people with intellectual impairment than in the general population.

AUDITORY IMPAIRMENT

The prevalence of hearing impairments increases with age and is more common in people with Down syndrome than other aetiologies of intellectual impairment (Wallace and Dalton, 2006). If a person cannot make sense of his world because of a visual or hearing impairment, it can cause frustration, anger and confusion. It can predispose to delirium and exacerbate chronic cognitive problems by hampering communication.

OBSTRUCTIVE SLEEP APNOEA

Up to 63% of people with Down syndrome could suffer from sleep apnoea. It is higher amongst the population with Down syndrome compared with other forms of intellectual impairment; this prevalence increases with age (Telakivi et al, 1987). Obstructive sleep apnoea appears to be linked to cognitive dysfunction (Incalzi et al, 2004), due to hypoxia. This condition is treatable by non-invasive ventilation.

HYPOTHYROIDISM

Adults with Down syndrome are at an increased risk of thyroid dysfunction and this risk increases with age (Rooney and Walsh, 1997). Hypothyroidism occurs in 20–30% of people with Down syndrome (Kerr, 1997). Symptoms of hypothyroidism can mimic symptoms of dementia such as lethargy, functional decline, confusion and depression.

CORONARY ARTERY DISEASE

Coronary artery disease is the second most common cause of death amongst people with intellectual impairment (14–20%) (Hollins et al, 1998). Rates of coronary artery disease are increasing as a result of increased longevity and lifestyle changes (Wells et al, 1997). Up to 50% of people with Down syndrome have some form of congenital heart defect, which may affect their risk of developing hypertension and stroke.

EPILEPSY

People with intellectual impairment appear to be at higher risk of developing epilepsy (Foundation for People with Learning Disabilities, 2002). Drugs used to treat epilepsy can cause side effects such drowsiness and confusion.

DIABETES

The exact prevalence of diabetes mellitus amongst people with intellectual impairment is not known but it is generally assumed that it is more common in people with Down syndrome compared to the age-matched general population (Wallace and Dalton, 2006). Complications associated with diabetes include retinopathy, neuropathy and nephropathy. See Chapters 2 and 5 for a further discussion on the aspects of physical health in people with intellectual impairment.

MANAGEMENT OF DEMENTIA

The care and management of dementia in an individual with intellectual impairment is multi-dimensional and involves multiple agencies, the use of drug treatments, non-pharmacological interventions and provision of support for carers. One of the main aims of management is to promote independence for the individual and maintenance of skills for as long as possible. Quality of life is also an important factor to consider, although it is difficult to measure. Adverse behavioural symptoms associated with the dementia need to be assessed thoroughly and a care plan should be developed with the involvement of the individual and their carer. Significantly, management must also focus on the alleviation of carer burden.

Person-centred care in dementia aims to see the person with dementia as an individual, rather than focusing on their illness and on abilities they may have lost. Instead of treating the person as a collection of symptoms and behaviours to be controlled, person-centred care takes into account each individual's unique qualities, abilities, interests, preferences and needs (Kitwood, 1997). These must be the underlying principles when caring for an individual with a dual diagnosis of dementia and intellectual impairment.

TREATMENTS FOR DEMENTIA

Although there is no known cure for Alzheimer's disease there are drug treatments, which may stabilise the condition or slow down the progression of the disease. Cholinergic deficiency in the brains of Alzheimer's disease patients is well documented and linked to cognitive deficits seen in Alzheimer's disease. Cholinesterase inhibitors (ChEIs) are the mainstay of symptomatic treatment of cognitive symptoms in this disease. The first drug to be licensed for Alzheimer's disease in the UK was donepezil in 1997. There are now three drugs available: donepezil, rivastigmine and galantamine. They all work in a similar way by inhibiting acetylcholinesterase although rivastigmine and galantamine also have additional pharmacological effects.

Cholinesterase inhibitors can slow down the rate of deterioration of Alzheimer's disease in the Down syndrome population (Alzheimer's Society, 2004; Kishnani *et al*, 1999). Positive effects include a reduction in deterioration of cognitive function, improvement in neuropsychiatric symptoms and improvement in adaptive skills (Prasher *et al*, 2004). The National Institute for Health and Clinical Excellence (NICE) recently issued new draft guidance on the prescription of antidementia drugs on the NHS in the general population. It suggested that anticholinesterase inhibitors should only be given to those patients who have Mini-Mental State Examination scores of 20 and below, despite research evidence that suggests these drugs are effective in the early stages of disease. It also stated that memantine, a drug licensed for people in the moderate to severe stages of disease, should no longer be provided on the NHS. Memantine blocks a messenger chemical, known as a neurotransmitter glutamate. Glutamate is released in excessive amounts when brain cells are damaged by Alzheimer's disease, which causes the brain cells to be damaged further. Memantine can protect brain cells by blocking this release of excess glutamate (Alzheimer's Society, 2003b).

This has been strongly opposed by the Alzheimer's Society and allied organizations, health and social care professionals, patients and carers. A further criticism is that the NICE guidelines fail to include people with intellectual impairment in their proposals and although the Mini-Mental State Examination is a validated standardized assessment of cognitive capacity in the general population, it is not a recognized tool for use with people with intellectual impairment. A recent judicial review has found that NICE did breach its duties under the Disability Discrimination Act and the Race Relations Act by not offering specific advice regarding people with learning disabilities and people for whom English is not their first language in guidance. Further guidance specifically addressing this issue will shortly be published.

There are currently no drug treatments available for sufferers of vascular dementia unlike Alzheimer's disease. If the clinical picture suggests a mixed form of dementia then anticholinesterase therapy may be considered. The main aim of treatment for people with vascular dementia is to reduce their risk of further stroke damage through modification of cardiovascular risk factors, namely treatment and prevention of strokes and transient ischaemic attacks. Patients and carers should be encouraged to comply with antihypertensive medication. Management and treatment of elevated cholesterol may be achieved through manipulation of diet alone or in combination with the prescription of a statin.

Patients should be advised to drink in moderation – no more than two units of alcohol per day. Patients should be encouraged to give up smoking. Appropriate guidance regarding smoking cessation clinics and methods to give up smoking should be given. Patients should be advised to exercise regularly such as 30 minutes per day. This does not have to be intensive gym activity but could simply mean a walk in a local park. Patients should be advised to eat a varied low salt, low fat diet. Referral to a dietitian may be required.

Drug therapy is aimed at improving the cognitive symptoms and reducing the parkinsonian features associated with dementia with Lewy bodies. There is evidence to suggest some efficacy with anti-cholinesterase therapy and dopamine replacement therapy. However, this is a relatively new area of research interest and research is currently ongoing into effective treatments for the condition. Neuroleptic sensitivity is a disorder characterized by the acute onset or exacerbation of parkinsonism and impaired consciousness in patients with dementia with Lewy bodies given typical neuroleptic drugs (e.g. haloperidol) and is associated with a high mortality and morbidity (McKeith et al, 1992).

NON-MEDICAL INTERVENTIONS IN DEMENTIA CARE

There are several psychological techniques which have been validated, but there is little research evidence assessing their efficacy within the population with dementia and existing intellectual impairment.

REALITY ORIENTATION AND VALIDATION THERAPY

Reality orientation is a practical tool. Its main aims are to maintain and improve the patient's orientation and awareness of their environment through a variety of prompts and activities: 24 hour reality orientation is intended to be ongoing and involves changes in the environment. The physical environment is important in facilitating orientation by using notices and clear signposting of key locations. Buildings should make finding rooms and directions easy (Kerr, 1997). Staff and carers are encouraged to stress information relating to orientation (e.g. by mentioning the time frequently and referring to an individual by name).

Reality orientation also takes the form of special sessions whereby small groups of people meet with staff/carers on a regular basis for a fixed duration. Questions and comments are raised concerning areas such as weather, day, date, month, history, etc. Reality orientation has been criticized in recent years for devaluing and demeaning individuals (McCarron, 1999). However, Spector et al (2000) undertook a review of orientation therapy amongst adults with dementia in the general population and found that reality orientation has beneficial effects on cognitive function and partial effect on behavioural functions. Prasher (2005) argues that there needs to be further research on the benefits of reality orientation in people with intellectual impairment who may never have been orientated to time. However, McCarron feels that it can help the person with intellectual impairment in a number of ways, for example affixing photographs and pictures on a bedroom door can aid spatial awareness and regularly reminding where the toilet is, ensuring it is well signposted and offering the use of the toilet may help maintain continence.

BOX 6.2   BILLY

Billy is 60 years old and has a moderate learning disability. He wakes up one morning in his care home and is very confused. He gets up, dresses and packs his bag stating that he is going to meet his sister Jenny at Euston Station (Jenny died some years ago).

Reorientating Billy by saying that Jenny has died will cause more upset and confusion, as will blocking his way and locking the door. Validation therapy encourages the care staff to talk to Billy about his sister whilst maintaining the past tense. One could ask Billy what he and Jenny used to do when at Euston Station and did he enjoy travelling by train. By encouraging Billy to talk about Jenny thereby acknowledges his feelings and permits an easier way of introducing diversion, without ignoring or dehumanizing his feelings or emotions. ■

Validation therapy focuses on the importance of an individual's feelings and their attempts to express them. Instead of correcting factual errors in conversation, one seeks to find the true meanings behind verbal and non-verbal communication and attempts to gain a full understanding of a person. The carer is encouraged to utilize validation techniques to acknowledge the feelings expressed while ignoring the content (Feil, 1993). Again, more research needs to be undertaken to explore the benefits of validation therapy amongst people with dementia and intellectual impairment (see Box 6.2).

REMINISCENCE

Reminiscence therapy encourages recollections of details or events in an individual's life. Reminiscence has a positive effect on well-being and personhood, in addition to its effects on autobiographical memory, socialization, long-term memory, communication and social interaction (Rosewarne, 2001). It can be undertaken in different ways:

- **Group activities** – Items such as old photographs, music and everyday objects serve as triggers from the past to be discussed. Participants are encouraged to reminisce and discuss the past in the presence of a group facilitator. This stimulates memory and encourages social interaction.

- **One-to-one work** – This is similar to group work but some individuals with dementia and intellectual impairment might find group work overwhelming and unsatisfactory. They may prefer to work on a one-to-one basis (Kerr, 1997).

- **Life story work** – A 'Life book' is a book compiled by an individual with staff and carers that is a visual and written record of a person's life and contains information about significant people and events in a person's life. The process of collating the materials for the book stimulates memory and the finished piece serves as a visual cue for an individual to remember his or her past.

Reminiscence is interactive and informative. Knowing a little about a person's past and hobbies and interests enables carers to understand an individual better and therefore promote person-centred care. Unfortunately there is little research evidence regarding the cognitive or behavioural effects of reminiscence therapy in any population (Spector *et al*, 2000).

OTHER THERAPEUTIC APPROACHES

Music therapy is a creative use of musical improvisation by an individual and practitioner to create an environment in which healing can take place. A review of music therapy for dementia showed that it might be beneficial in treating the symptoms of dementia and improving quality of life for people with dementia and their carers (Alzheimer's Society, 2003a,b,c). Although research into the benefits of music for people with dementia is focused on the general population, there is some evidence to suggest that older people with intellectual impairment have high affinities to music and rhythm.

Cognitive behavioural therapy works by changing people's attitudes and their behaviour. Therapies focus on thoughts, images and beliefs that are held and how these relate to behaviour. Examples include progressive relaxation techniques, which reduce agitation and anxiety (Prasher, 2005). Cognitive behaviour therapy (CBT) is now a widely accepted and effective form of psychotherapy for many mental health problems and the evidence base is growing on its effectiveness with the intellectual impairment population (Brown and Marshall, 2006). However, Prasher (2005) suggests more research is required before it is initiated in the population with intellectual impairment and dementia.

Guidance on how the environment can play a part in minimizing the symptoms of dementia is increasing. Environments might need to be modified to make them calm, familiar, stimulating and safe (Kerr, 1997). Suggested alterations might include flooring, lighting, access and signposting. There is emerging evidence to suggest aromatherapy is an effective way of alleviating behavioural symptoms in dementia. Ballard and Holmes (2004) showed aromatherapy to be a safe and effective treatment for the management of agitation in severe dementia. However, this research was undertaken in the general population and there is little evidence base for the efficacy of aromatherapy in people with a dual diagnosis of intellectual impairment and dementia.

CARING FOR THE CARERS

There are approximately six million carers in England and Wales. Informal carers provide the vast majority of health and community care and studies have shown their work saves the nation an estimated £57 million per year that would otherwise have had to be spent on services. Nearly two-thirds of carers look after someone with a disability; 7% care for someone with a mental disability; and 15% care for someone with a physical and a mental disability. Half of all adults with intellectual impairment are cared for by relatives in the family home. It is also estimated that one-third of them live with a family carer aged 70 or over (DH, 2001a).

As parents of people with intellectual impairment get older they develop their own health problems and they may have difficulty continuing as full-time carers. This makes them anxious and fearful about the future and they are at an increased risk of developing anxiety, depression and becoming socially isolated (Mencap, 2002). Support networks are likely to diminish with age as friends and relatives move away or die (Hatzidimitriadou and Milne, 2005). It is estimated that 25% of people with intellectual impairment are not known to services until illness or death prevents a parent from continuing to care and there is evidence to suggest that parents are wary of approaching professionals for help (Mencap, 2002).

Research investigating the effects of caring for a person with a dual diagnosis of learning disability and dementia is sparse. However, there is much literature that investigates the effects of caring for somebody with dementia in the general population. We must use this evidence as we imagine what it must be like caring for somebody with a dual diagnosis. There are high levels of stress, distress and psychological illness in family caregivers of individuals with dementia (Mahoney *et al*, 2004). Many studies have shown that the incidence of depression in caregivers is high, ranging from 18 to 47% (Rosenthal *et al*, 1993; Teri and Truaux, 1994) and caregivers who are depressed experience higher degrees of burden (Lawton *et al*, 1991). The degree of behavioural problems in patients with dementia appears to contribute to caregiver burden (Baumgarten *et al*, 1994). When patients with dementia have depression, their caregivers report higher levels of burden (Drinka *et al*, 1987).

CARERS LEGISLATION AND GUIDANCE

Carers often remain unaware of their rights or needs despite increasing stutory requirement for services to consider and provide for them. The Carers (Recognition and Services Act) 1995 gave carers the right to ask for an assessment of their own circumstances and need as part of the assessment for the person they cared for. This was the first legislation that gave specific rights to carers who provide substantial and regular care. In 2002 The Carers and Disabled Children's Act gave carers the additional right to request an assessment of their own circumstances and needs, even when the person they were caring for had been offered but refused an assessment. It also gave councils the power to provide services specifically for carers, as well as the power to make direct payments to carers to meet their own assessed needs.

The National Service Framework for Mental Health (DH, 1999a) focused on people up to the age of 65. Standard 6 (Caring for Carers) highlighted the need for services to recognize the vital role carers play. Extra funding was allocated to provide more support services including carers' grants and funds for carer breaks. A network of local carer support workers was also established. The National Service Framework for Older People (DH, 2001b) focused on people over the age of 65. Standard 7 (Mental Health and Older People) recognized the need for older people to have access to integrated mental health services provided by the NHS and councils to ensure effective diagnosis, treatment and support for them and their carers. The standard emphasized the need to provide information, advice and practical help to support carers.

The National Carers Strategy (DH, 1999b) emphasized three strategic elements:

- **Information** which included advice on long-term care services, introducing the NHS direct careline for carers and providing good health information to carers.

- **Support** involving carers in planning and delivering services and consulting carers' organizations.

- **Care to include** carers' rights to have their own health needs met. Local authorities were empowered to provide more services for carers. Carers' grants and breaks were also introduced.

In Valuing People: A New Strategy for Learning Disability for the 21st Century (DH, 2001a) the government cited carer support as a main objective. This was to be achieved by ensuring carers of people with learning disabilities benefited from all mainstream carer initiatives (including initiatives proposed in the National Carers' Strategy) implementing the recent Carers and Disabled Children Act 2000, funding a National Learning Information Centre and help line in partnership with Mencap and issuing new guidance on exclusion. The government also advised local authorities to pay extra attention to identifying older carers (i.e. those aged over 70) and carers from ethnic minorities.

The Foundation for Learning Disabilities launched a Charter of Rights for Older People with Learning Disabilities and older family carers in 2002 to give the right to flexible health and social care services, assistance in planning for the future and better access to information and support. The Charter stated that older carers (with due consideration paid towards their ethnic, religious and cultural backgrounds) should be offered practical and emotional support, respite breaks, access to support groups and independent advocacy. Carers should be given advice on planning for the future from the age of 60 (rather than 70 as advised by the government). This planning should provide reassurance (in the light of increased life expectancy amongst people with intellectual impairment) that if the carer should cease to care full time or should die, then the person with intellectual impairment will be cared for.

WHAT DO CARERS NEED?

Research has identified lack of communication and information and support as one of the main issues for carers. Two themes identified in a study by Keady and Nolan (1995) were the need for ongoing information on dementia and relevant services and the need for continuing support for the carer. Carers need information about the likely course of the disease and to know how to use the environment to help counteract the impact of the disease. They also require assistance on how to maintain skills and promote independence (Kerr, 1997). A recent survey of over 1100 European caregivers of people with dementia felt that they had received inadequate information at diagnosis: four out of five wanted more information on help and support services (Alzheimer's Europe, 2006).

Older carers of people with a dual diagnosis of intellectual impairment and dementia want help and information on planning for the future should they become unable to care for their loved one. (Morgan and Magill, 2005). Carers have indicated that having somebody to talk to whether it is a friend, relative or professional is beneficial (BMA, 2003). There is evidence to suggest that carers who are linked in to a local support group are better able to continue to provide care (DH, 1999b). The Admiral Nurse Services provide expert advice and support on all aspects of dementia, the service is exclusively for carers. Carers need to be aware of local support groups and should be provided with the contact details of organizations such as the Alzheimer's Society, local carers' organizations, The Down syndrome Association, Mencap and the Foundation for Learning Disability.

Let us consider the case of Stephen and Marion in Box 6.3.

Marion is torn between wanting to care for her husband at home but is now having to cope with being a full time carer. The strain of dealing with Stephen's erratic and sometimes challenging behaviour is taking its toll on both her physical and mental health. Consider what services are available for Marion and Stephen and what is the best course of action the GP should initially take to help the couple.

Carers may want to access social service agencies for extra help or welfare advice. It is important that they are given the right information to achieve this in a timely fashion and with as little inconvenience as possible. Carers have highlighted the need for help carrying out personal care tasks such as using the toilet and bathing and home-based help such as chiropody and physiotherapy. Assistance with household tasks such as cleaning is also appreciated (Carers UK, 2001). Carers also want time off from caring in order to have time to themselves or to carry out other chores (BMA, 2003). Examples include home-based or care-home-based respite, sitting services, befriending services, day centres.

BOX 6.3	MARION AND STEPHEN

Marion and Stephen have been married for 40 years and are both in their middle 60s. Stephen took early retirement on the grounds of ill health four years ago after he was diagnosed with dementia and work became impossible. During the last four years his condition has rapidly worsened, he is often confused for long periods of time, unpredictable, sometimes aggressive and some days needs total support with all his basic daily living needs. He is not known to specialist dementia services and refuses to see anyone bar his own GP.

Marion has always been reluctant to 'put him in a home' and manages with only minimal help at home. Marion and Stephen's children live in other parts of the country and visit for weekends when they can.

Marion's daughter has recently been to visit her parents and has telephoned their GP to express her concerns over her mother's health. She reports that Marion has lost a vast amount of weight, has ceased to care about her appearance and is not getting out of the house at all to see her friends due to Stephen's deterioration. She was also very tearful throughout the visit. ■

The commonest forms of accommodation for people with intellectual impairment in the UK are the family home and small community-based supported housing (Perry *et al*, 2000). People with intellectual impairment are living longer and as a result are at risk of developing age-related illnesses such as dementia. Caregivers in care homes must be provided with the right skills and knowledge to support their ageing residents (Wilkinson *et al*, 2005). Whitehouse and Chamberlain (2000) undertook a study investigating the knowledge and attributions of dementia held by care staff working with older adults who had intellectual impairment. The results suggested that these care workers had limited knowledge about ageing in general and, specifically, dementia. It must also be remembered that people with intellectual impairment are often moved into residential services for older people, where care staff are not used to caring for individuals with intellectual impairment.

Generic care staff require training about the needs of people with intellectual disability and staff working in services for people with intellectual disability need training about the ageing process and age-related ill health.

Hatzidimitriadou and Milne (2005)

SERVICES FOR PEOPLE WITH INTELLECTUAL IMPAIRMENT AND DEMENTIA

There is evidence to suggest that service providers are finding it difficult to find appropriate ways of supporting people with intellectual impairment through the progression of their dementia (Wilkinson and Janicki, 2002) and that there is inadequate provision of appropriate services

(Davidson *et al*, 2004). Research highlights the limited choices that people with intellectual impairment who develop dementia have over their support (Wilkinson and Janicki, 2002). Service providers are unclear and inconsistent about how to provide support for this increasing population (Wilkinson and Janicki, 2002). An important task for care providers is to avoid institutionalization and inappropriate settings for this group of individuals as research has shown that people with intellectual impairment are often moved out of their homes and into nursing care when their needs increase (Thompson and Wright, 2001), a situation deemed unsatisfactory as general settings tend to provide a poorer level of support (Thompson and Wright, 2001).

An International Working Group on Dementia Care Practices met in 2001 to develop universal guidance on the continued community care and support of people with intellectual impairment affected by dementia. This guidance was intended for use by governments, organizations and service providers and became known as The Edinburgh Principles (Wilkinson and Janicki, 2002).

Principle 1: Adopt an operational philosophy that promotes the utmost quality of life of persons with intellectual impairment affected by dementia and where possible bases services and support services on a person-centred approach.

Principle 2: Affirm that individual strengths, capabilities, skills and wishes should be the overriding consideration in decision making for and by the person with intellectual impairment affected by dementia.

Principle 3: Involve the individual, his/her family and other close supports in all phases of assessment and service planning and provision for the individual with intellectual impairment affected by dementia.

Principle 4: Ensure that appropriate diagnostic, assessment and intervention services and resources are available to meet the individual needs and support healthy ageing of persons with intellectual impairment affected by dementia.

Principle 5: Plan and provide supports and services that optimize remaining in the chosen community of adults with intellectual impairment affected by dementia.

Principle 6: Ensure that adults with intellectual impairment affected by dementia have the same access to appropriate services as afforded to other persons within the general population affected by dementia.

Principle 7: Ensure that generic and proactive strategic planning across relevant policy, provider and advocacy groups involves consideration of the current and future needs of adults with intellectual impairment affected by dementia.

SERVICE RECOMMENDATIONS

It is widely recognized that there needs to be a coordinated, needs-led multidisciplinary approach to service provision for people with intellectual impairment and dementia (Watchman, 2003). This entails close collaboration between dementia services and services for people with intellectual impairment. The White Paper 'Valuing People' (DH, 2001a) reviews existing services for people with intellectual impairment and also recognizes the specific needs of older people with intellectual impairment. Valuing People states that mental health services should ensure the needs of people with intellectual impairment who develop dementia or a functional mental illness are met.

It regards partnerships between services for older people with intellectual impairment, mental health services and services for those with intellectual impairment as essential ingredients of service development (Hatzidimitriadou and Milne, 2005).

Younger people with dementia (i.e. those aged under 65) often fall through the net of health and social care services, as they are not old enough to be eligible for generic dementia services. At present there are few designated services for younger people with dementia although organizations such as The Royal College of Psychiatrists (RCP) and The Alzheimer's Society recognize that this group of people have issues quite separate to older people with dementia. The RCP and the Alzheimer's Society have issued guidance on service development for younger people with dementia. This guidance recommends an incremental approach with the appointment at commissioning level (i.e. primary care trusts or their equivalent) of a named person responsible for planning and a consultant clinician (this could be an old age psychiatrist) to act as a focus for referrals (Royal College of Psychiatrists and Alzheimer's Society, 2006).

Evidence suggests that both residential and community-based services are required. The provision of appropriate day and respite care has been identified as particular deficits and the development of supported housing for people with intellectual impairment and dementia is recognised as a new challenge. Specialist long-stay units for elderly people with intellectual impairment must be developed by services for intellectual impairment with the emphasis on environmental modification and highly skilled staff (Prasher, 2005). As mentioned previously care staff need adequate training about the needs of people with intellectual impairment and recognizing age-related changes and diseases such as dementia.

In the UK there are at least 58 memory clinics serving the general population (Lindesay *et al*, 2002). The National Service Framework for Older People recommends that specialist mental health services should provide memory clinics (DH, 2001b). The main aims of a memory clinic are diagnosis, treatment, monitoring of dementia over time, the provision of non-pharmacological interventions, planning for the future, educating carers and professionals and participation in research (Prasher, 2005). Some clinics also have links with the local Alzheimer's Society and advocacy organizations. Memory clinics are multidisciplinary and may consist of psychiatrists, geriatricians, clinical psychologists, dementia support workers, occupational therapists and physiotherapists. There are fewer memory clinics for people with intellectual impairment, but there is an upward trend as the benefits of intensive assessment, regular follow-up and support for this population are slowly becoming recognized.

CONCLUSIONS

This chapter has highlighted the difficulties associated with the diagnosis, care and management of people with intellectual impairment and dementia. However, despite a plethora of guidance and recommendations, the provision of services for this vulnerable group remains patchy and somewhat disjointed. The diagnosis of dementia is still mistaken or made too late in some cases which means that individuals miss out on valuable, quality of life-enhancing drug treatments. There is a distinct lack of research to provide a good evidence base for many of the interventions specified and often people with intellectual impairment are excluded from dementia research studies. There is a need for an ongoing research programme which looks specifically at the needs of this special group. The number of people with intellectual impairment and dementia is increasing, the issues will not go away. 'Triple jeopardy' should not exist. People with intellectual impairment and dementia and their carers have a right to the same standards of care, management and treatment as an individual within the general population. There is a need for greater dementia awareness and access to high quality training for people working with this group if they are to receive equitable care. The care and recognition of people with intellectual impairment has come a long way but there is still a considerable way to go before we can seriously say we have provided the optimal care and service for people with intellectual impairment and dementia and their carers.

REFERENCES AND RECOMMENDED READING

Albert M, Cohen C. (1992) The test for severe impairment: an instrument for the assessment of patients with severe cognitive dysfunction. *Journal of the American Geriatric Society* 40:449–53.

Alzheimer's Europe (2006) *Who Cares? The State of Dementia Care in Europe*. Luxembourg: Alzheimer's Europe.

Alzheimer's Society (2003a) *Information Sheet: Complementary and Alternative Medicine and Dementia*. London: Alzheimer's Society.

Alzheimer's Society (2003b) *Information Sheet: Drug Treatments for Alzheimer's Disease; Information Sheet: Aricept, Exelon, Reminyl and Ebixa*. London: Alzheimer's Society.

Alzheimer's Society (2003c) *Information Sheet: What is Dementia?* London: Alzheimer's Society.

Alzheimer's Society (2004) *Information Sheet: Learning Disabilities and Dementia*. London: Alzheimer's Society.

American Psychiatric Association (1994) *Diagnostic and Statistical Manual of Mental Disorders* (4th edn) DSM IV-TR. American Psychiatric Association.

Aylward EH, Burt DB, Thorpe LU, Dalton A. (1997) Diagnosis of dementia in individuals with intellectual disability. *Journal of Intellectual Disability Research* 41:152–64.

Ball S, Holland T, Huppert FA, Treppner P, Dodd K. (2006) *Camdex DS – The Cambridge Examination for Mental Disorders of Older People with Down's Syndrome and Others with Intellectual Disabilities*. Cambridge University Press.

Ballard C, Holmes C. (2004) *Advances in Psychiatric Treatment*, Volume 10. The Royal College of Psychiatrists: 296–300.

Baumgarten M, Hanley JA, Infante-Ricard C, Battista RN, Becker R, Gauthier S. (1994) Health of family members caring for elderly persons with dementia. *American Journal of Internal Medicine* 120:126–32.

Beck AT, Ward CH, Mendelson M, Mock J, Erbaugh J. (1961) An inventory for measuring depression. *Archives of General Psychiatry* 4:561–71.

Bland R, Hutchinson N, Oakes P, Yates C. (2003) Double jeopardy? Needs and services for older people with learning disabilities. *Journal of Learning Disabilities* 7(4):323–44.

British Medical Association (2003) *Working with Carers: Guidelines for Good Practice*. London: BMA Publishing Group.

Brown M, Marshall K. (2006) Cognitive behavioural therapy and people with learning disabilities: implications for developing nursing practice. *Journal of Psychiatric and Mental Health Nursing* 13:234–41.

Brown J, Hillman J. (2004) *Your Questions Answered: Dementia*. Philadelphia: Churchill Livingstone.

Bullock (2002) Building a Modern Dementia Service. Middlesex: Altman.

Carers UK (2001) *You Can Take Him Home Now*. Carers' Experiences of Hospital Discharge.

Cooke DD, McNally L, Mulligan KT, Harrison MJG. (2001) Psychosocial interventions for caregivers of people with dementia: a systematic review. *Aging and Mental Health* 5(2):120–35.

Cooper SA, Bailey NM. (2001) Psychiatric disorders amongst adults with learning disabilities: prevalence and relationship to ability level. *Irish Journal of Psychological Medicine* 18:45–53.

Cuthill FM, Espie CA, Cooper S. (2003) Development and psychometric properties of the Glasgow Depression Scale for People with a Learning Disability; individual and carer supplement versions. *British Journal of Psychiatry* 182:347–53.

Davidson PW, Heller T, Janicki M, Hyer K. (2004) Defining a national health research and practice agenda for older people with intellectual disabilities. *Journal of Policy and Practice in Intellectual Disabilities* 1(1):2–9.

Deb S, Thomas M, Bright C. (2001) Mental disorders in adults with intellectual disability: 1: prevalence of functional psychiatric illness amongst community-based population aged between 16 and 60. *Journal of Intellectual Disability Research* 45(6):495–505.

De La Torre JC. (2002) Vascular basis of Alzheimer's pathologenesis. *Annals of the New York Academy of Sciences* 977:196–215.

Department of Health (1999a) *National Service Framework for Mental Health*. London: DH.

Department of Health (1999b) *National Carers Strategy*. London: DH.

Department of Health (2001a) *Valuing People: A New Strategy for Learning Disability for the 21ˢᵗ Century*. London: DH.

Department of Health (2001b) *National Service Framework for Older People*. London. DH.

Devenny DA, Silverman WP, Hill AL, Jenkins E, Sersen. (1996) Normal ageing in adults with Down's syndrome, a longitudinal study. *Journal of Intellectual Disability Research* 40(3).

Drinka T, Smith JC, Drinka P. (1987) Correlates of depression and burden for informal caregivers of patients in a geriatrics referral clinic. *Journal of American Geriatrics Society* 35:522–3.

Evenhuis HM. (1990) The natural history of dementia in Down's syndrome. *Archives of Neurology* 50:305–10.

Evenhuis HM, Kengen MMF, Eurlings HAL. (1990) *Dementia Questionnaire for Mentally Retarded Persons* Zwanerdam, The Netherlands: Hooge Burch Institute for Mentally Retarded People.

Feil N. (1993) *The Validation Breakthrough: Simple Techniques for Communicating with People with 'Alzheimer's-Type Dementia'*. Baltimore: Health Professionals Press.

Folstein MF, Folstein SE, McHugh PR. (1975) Mini-Mental State: a practical method for grading the cognitive state of patients for the clinician. *Journal of Psychiatric Research* 12:189–98.

Foundation for People with Learning Disabilities (2002) *Charter of Rights for Older People with Learning Disabilities and Family Carers*.

Gedye A. (1995) *Dementia Scale for Down Syndrome: Manual*. Vancouver: Gedye Research and Consulting.

Harvey RJ, Skelton-Robinson M, Rossor MN. (2003) The prevalence and causes of dementia in people under the age of 65 years. *Journal of Neurosurgical Psychiatry* 74:1206–9.

Hatzidimitriadou E, Milne A. (2005) Planning ahead: meeting the needs of older people with learning disabilities in the United Kingdom. *Dementia* 4(3):341–59.

Hiles *et al.* (1990) Down's Syndrome Group Western Pennsylvanian Newsletter 8:27–30.

Holland AJ, Hon J, Huppert FA *et al.* (2000) Incidence and course of dementia in people with Down's syndrome, findings from a population based study. *Journal of Intellectual Disability Research* 44:138–46.

Hollins S, Attard MT, von Fraunhofer N, Sedgwick P. (1998) Mortality in people with learning disabilities: risks, causes and death certification findings in London. *Developmental Medicine and Child Neurology* 40:50–6.

Holmes C, Ballard C. (2002) Aromatherapy in dementia. *Advances in Psychiatric Treatment* 10:296–300.

Hulse GK, Lautenschlanger NT, Tait RJ, Almeida OP. (2005) Dementia associated with alcohol and other drug use. *International Journal of Psychogeriatrics* 17(Supp 1):S109–27.

Hussein S, Manthorpe J. (2005) Older people with learning disabilities: Workforce issues. *Journal of Integrated Care* 13(1):17–23.

Incalzi RA, Marra C, Salvigni BL, Petrone A, Gemma A, Selvaggio D, Mormile F. (2004) Does cognitive dysfunction conform to a distinctive pattern in obstructive sleep apnea syndrome? *Journal of Sleep Research* 13(1):79.

Janicki M, Dalton AJ. (2000) Prevalence of dementia and impact on intellectual disability services. *Mental Retardation* 38:276–88.

Janicki MP, Ackerman L, Jacobson JW. (1985) State developmental disabilities/ageing plans and day planning for an older developmentally disabled population. *Ment Retard* 23(6):297–301.

Janicki MP, Heller T, Seltzer G, Hogg J. (1995) *Practice Guidelines for the Clinical Assessment and Care Management of Alzheimer's and Other Dementias Among Adults with Mental Retardation.* Washington DC: American Association on Mental Retardation.

Jervis GA. (1948) Early senile dementia mongoloid idiocy. *Am J Psychiatry* 105:102–6.

Jokinen N. (2005) The content of available practice literature in dementia and intellectual disability. *Dementia* 4(3):327–39.

Keady J, Nolan MA. (1995) Stitch in time. Facilitating proactive interventions with caregivers: the role of community practitioners. *Journal of Psychiatric and Mental Health Nursing* 3:163–72.

Kerr D. (1997) *Down's Syndrome and Dementia – Practitioners Guide.* Birmingham: Ventura Press.

Kerr D, Wilson W. (eds) (2001) *Learning Disability and Dementia.* Stirling: University of Stirling, Dementia Services Development Centre.

Kishnani PS, Sullivan JA, Walter BK *et al.* (1999) Cholinergic therapy for Down's syndrome. *Lancet* 353(1064).

Kitwood T. (1997) *Dementia Reconsidered: The Person Comes First.* Buckingham: Open University Press.

Lai F, Williams RS. (1989) A prospective study of Alzheimer's disease in Down syndrome. *Arch Neurology* 46:849–53.

Lawton MP, Moss M, Kleban MH, Glicksman A, Rovine M. (1991) A two-factor model of caregiving appraisal and psychological well-being. *J Gerontol Psychol Sciences* 46:181–9.

Lejeune L, Gautier M, Turpin R. (1959) Les Chromosomes Humaines en Culture de Tissu *Comptes Rendus Acad Sci* 248:602–3.

Lindesay J, Marudkar M, Van Diepen E, Wilcox G. (2002) The second survey of memory clinics in the British Isles. *International Journal of Geriatric Psychiatry* 17:41–7.

Luchsinger JA, Mayeux R. (2004) Dietary factors and Alzheimer's disease. *Lancet Neurol* Oct 3(10):579–87.

Luchsinger JA, Reitz C, Honig S, Tang MX, Shea S. (2005) Aggregation of vascular risk factors and risk of incident Alzheimer's disease. *Neurology* 65:545–51.

Mahoney R, Regan C, Katona C, Livingston G. (2004) Anxiety and depression in family caregivers of people with Alzheimer's disease: the LASER-Alzheimer's disease study. *The American Journal of Geriatric Psychiatry* 13(9).

Malamud N. (1966) The neuropathology of mental retardation. In: I Phillips (ed.), *Prevention and Treatment of Mental Retardation.* New York: Basic Books.

Mann DMA. (1988) The pathological association between Down syndrome and Alzheimer disease. *Mech Ageing Dev* 43:99–136.

McCarron M. (1999) Some issues in caring for people with the dual disability of Down's syndrome and Alzheimer's disease. *Journal of Learning Disabilities for Nursing, Health and Social Care* 3(3):123–9.

McKeith I, Fairbairn A, Perry R, Thompson P, Perry E. (1992) Neuroleptic Sensitivity in patients with senile dementia of Lewy body type. *BMJ* 305:673–8.

Mencap (2002) *The Housing Timebomb.* London.

Morgan H, Magill D. (2005) *Supporting Older Families of People with Learning Disabilities.* London: Mental Health Foundation at The Foundation for People with Learning Disabilities.

Mynors-Wallis L, Moore M, Maguire J, Hollingbery T. (2003) *Shared Care in Mental Health.* Oxford: Oxford University Press.

National Institute for Health and Clinical Excellence and Social Care Institutive for England (2006). *Draft Guidance: Dementia: the Treatment and Care of People with Dementia in Health and Social Care.* London: NICE.

O'Brien JT, Erkinjuntti T, Reisberg B, Roman G, Sawada T, Pantoni L, Bowler JV, Ballard C, DeCarli C, Gorelick PB, Rockwood K, Burns A, Gauthier S, DeKosky ST. (2003) Vascular cognitive impairment. *Lancet Neurol* 2:89–98.

Office for National Statistics (2003) *Census 2001.* London: The Stationery Office.

Oliver C. (1999) Perspectives on assessment and evaluation. In: Janicki M, Dalton AJ (eds), *Dementia, Ageing and Intellectual Disabilities: A Handbook.* Castleton, NY: Hamilton Printing Company; 123–41.

Perry J, Lowe K, Felce D, Jones S. (2000) Characteristics of staffed community housing services for people with learning disabilities: A stratified random sample of statutory, voluntary and private agency provision. *Health and Social Care in the Community* 8(5):301–15.

Prasher V. (1995) Age-specific prevalence, thyroid dysfunction and depressive symptomology in adults with Down syndrome and dementia. *International Geriatric Psychiatry* 10:25–31.

Prasher V. (2003) Psychiatric morbidity in adults with Down's syndrome. *Psychiatry* 2:8.

Prasher V. (2005) *Alzheimer's Disease and Dementia in Down Syndrome and Intellectual Disabilities*. Oxford: Radcliffe.

Prasher VP, Krishnan VHR. (1993) Age of onset and duration of dementia in people with Down syndrome. *International Journal of Geriatric Psychiatry* 8.

Prasher V, Farooq A, Holder R. (2004) The Adaptive Behaviour Dementia Questionnaire (ABDQ): Screening questionnaire for dementia in Alzheimer's Disease in adults with Down's Syndrome. *Res Dev Disb* 25:385–97.

Raber J, Huang Y, Ashford J. (2004) ApoE genotype accounts for the vast majority of Alzheimer's disease risk and Alzheimer's disease. *Pathology Neurobiology of Aging* 25(5):641–50.

Rooney S, Walsh E. (1997) Prevalence of abnormal thyroid function tests in a Down's syndrome population. *Irish Journal of Medical Science* 166(2).

Rosenthal CJ, Sulman J, Marshall VW. (1993) Depressive symptoms in family caregivers of long-stay patients. *Gerontologist* 33:249–56.

Rosewarne M. (2001) Learning disabilities and dementia: a pilot therapy group. *Journal of Dementia Care* July/August:19–20.

Royal College of Psychiatrists (2001) *DC-LD Diagnostic Criteria for Psychiatric Disorders for Use with Adults with Learning Disabilities/Mental Retardation*. Gaskell (Royal College of Psychiatrists).

Royal College of Psychiatrists and Alzheimer's Society (2006) *Services for Younger People with Alzheimer's Disease and Other Dementias*. London: Royal College of Psychiatrists.

Sampson EL, Warren JD, Rossor MN. (2004). Young onset dementia. *Postgraduate Medical Journal* 80:125–39.

Schott JM, Fox NC, Rossor MN. (2002) Genetics of the dementias. *Journal of Neurology, Neurosurgery and Psychiatry* 73(ii):27.

Snowden J, Neary MD, Mann MA. (2002) Frontotemporal dementia. *British Journal of Psychiatry* 180:140–3.

Soininen H, Partanen J, Jousmaki V et al. (1993) Age related cognitive decline and electroencephalogram slowing in Down's syndrome as a model of Alzheimer's Disease. *Neuroscience* 53:57–63.

Spector A, Davies S, Woods B, Orrell M. (2000) *Reality Orientation for Dementia*. Cochrane Database. Systematic Review (4).

Staessen JA et al. (1997) For the Systolic Hypertension in Europe (Syst-Eur) Trial Investigators. Randomised double-blind comparison of placebo and active treatment for older patients with isolated systolic hypertension. *Lancet* 350:757–64.

Telakivi T, Partinen M, Salmi T, Leinonen L, Harkonen T. (1987) Nocturnal periodic breathing in adults with Down's syndrome. *Journal of Mental Deficiency Research* 31:31–9.

Teri L, Truax P. (1994) Assessment of depression in dementia patients: Association of caregiver mood with depression rating. *Gerontologist* 34:231–4.

Thompson D, Wright S. (2001) *Misplaced and Forgotten? People with Learning Disabilities in Residential Services for Older People*. London: The Mental Health Foundation.

Turk V, Dodd K, Christmas M. (2001) *Down's Syndrome and Dementia: Briefing for Commissioners*. Foundation for People with Learning Disabilities.

Van Waarde JA, Van der Mast R. (2004) Delirium in learning disability: Case series and literature review. *British Journal of Learning Disability* 32(September):123.

Visser FE, Aldenkamp AP, van Huffelen AC, Kuilman M, Overweg J and van Wijk J. (1997) Prospective study of the prevalence of Alzheimer-type dementia in institutionalized individuals with Down syndrome. *American Journal on Mental Retardation* 101:400–12.

Visser SL, Stam FC, Van Tilburg W, Op den Velde W, Blom JW, De Rijke W. (1976) Visual evoked response in senile and presenile dementia. *Electroencephalogr Clin Neurophysiol* 40:385–92.

Wallace RA, Dalton AJ. (2006) Clinicians' guide to physical health problems of older adults with Down syndrome. *Journal of Developmental Disabilities* 12(1). Down Syndrome (Supplement 1).

Watchman K. (2003) Critical issues for service planners and providers of care for people with Down syndrome and dementia. *British Journal of Learning Disabilities* 31(2):81–4.

Wells MB, Turner S, Martin DM, Roy A. (1997) Health gains through screening – coronary artery disease and stroke. Developing primary health care services for people with intellectual disability. *Journal of Intellectual and Developmental Disability* 22(4):251–63.

Whitehouse R, Chamberlain P. (2000) Dementia in people with learning disabilities, a preliminary study into care staff knowledge and attributions. *British Journal of Learning Disabilities* 28(4):148–53.

Wilkinson H, Janicki MP. (2002) The Edinburgh principles with accompanying guidelines and recommendations. *Journal of Intellectual Disability Research* 46:279–84.

Wilkinson H, Kerr D, Cunningham C. (2005) Equipping staff to support people with intellectual disability and dementia in care home settings. *Dementia* 4(3):387–400.

Wilkinson H, Kerr D, Cunningham C, Rae C. (2004) *Home for Good? Preparing to support people with learning difficulties in residential settings when they develop dementia.* Joseph Rowntree Foundation/Pavilion Publishing www.jrf.org.uk

Wisniewski KE, Hill AL. (1985) Clinical aspects of dementia in mental retardation and developmental disabilities. In: Janicki MP, Wisniewski HM (eds), *Aging and Developmental Disabilities: Issues and Approaches.* Baltimore: Brookes, 195–210.

World Health Organization (1992) *ICD-10: International Statistical Classification of Diseases and Related Health Problems 10ᵗʰ Revision.* Geneva: WHO.

Yang Q, Rasmussen S, Friedman J. (2002) Mortality associated with Down's syndrome in the USA from 1983–1997: a population based study. *Lancet* 359:1019–25.

CHAPTER 7
EMERGENCY AND URGENT HOSPITAL-BASED CARE

Ian Noonan and Karen Lowton

STUDY AIMS:

1. To explore the type of emergencies that people with intellectual impairment are at increased risk of experiencing.

2. To improve care for people who are intellectually impaired in emergency and admission ward settings.

3. To understand the many ways in which people with intellectual impairment may express physical and psychological pain and distress, and to consider how this might be assessed in an emergency context.

4. To consider how to assess and treat self-harm and self-injury.

This chapter addresses the needs of people with intellectual impairment including learning disability, cognitive impairment, and brain injury, when attending hospital in emergency and unplanned situations. Throughout the focus will be on the client and how healthcare professionals can improve what is potentially a very distressing experience for them. Staff who feel unprepared for working with clients with intellectual impairment can also be distressed by the difficulties in assessing and managing someone who is injured, in pain, and frightened – particularly when the client is expressing this in ways that may appear confused or are problematic to assess. Therefore recommendations will be made at intrapersonal, interpersonal and organizational levels.

Three case studies; Anna, Ken and Angus (all pseudonyms to maintain confidentiality) will be used to illustrate and inform the discussion. In addition Ken has contributed his own comments in

Learning Disability and other Intellectual Impairments, Edited by L.L. Clark and P. Griffiths
© 2008 John Wiley & Sons, Ltd

relation to his experiences in an accident and emergency department and a medical admissions ward. These case studies focus on learning disability and comorbid health problems, self-harm, and anxiety resulting from brain injury. However, the recommendations for practice, which they support, are applicable to a wide range of clients with intellectual impairment. As a framework, steps in the clients' journeys from ambulance, through accident and emergency to admission and discharge, is used to demonstrate the thought and adaptation of practice that is required at each stage.

HEALTH NEEDS AND EMERGENCIES

There are five linked factors, which have led to an increased rate of accident and emergency department attendance for people with intellectual impairment:

- Move from institutionalized to community-based care

- High morbidity and early mortality

- An increasing awareness of the physical healthcare needs of people with intellectual impairment

- An increased life expectancy for people with intellectual impairment, especially learning disabilities

- A change in demographics – more people being born with intellectual impairment or acquiring the condition as neonates.

The development of community provision and the move away from institutionalization for people with intellectual impairment, has seen a change in the way care is organized (Mencap, 1988; Brown, 2005). Many health problems, or episodes of emotional or behavioural disturbance would have been dealt with 'in-house' in older institutions (Iacono and Davis, 2003; Bradley and Lofchy, 2005). Now that people with intellectual impairment are living either in supported homes or with families and carers in the community, there is a need for increased provision in mainstream healthcare settings.

Patja *et al* (2001) and Sherrard *et al* (2002, 2004) have identified specific risk factors for injury, morbidity and mortality in people with intellectual impairment (see Chapter 2). There is an increased risk of death from cardiovascular disease, respiratory disease and neoplasms (Patja *et al*, 2001), and twice the risk of unintentional injury than in the general population. Sherrard *et al* (2002, 2004) consider that there are a number of risk factors for people with intellectual impairment that increase their risk of accidental injury. These include epilepsy, psychopathology, the hyperkinetic disorders (e.g. Attention Deficit Hyperactivity Disorder (ADHD)) an overly sociable temperament, disruptive, self-absorbed and anxious personalities with problems relating to social or communication difficulties, all significantly increase this risk.

An increasing awareness of the physical health needs of people with intellectual impairment is advocated for learning disability nurses (Northway *et al*, 2006) and indeed for all nurses from all branches of the Nursing Register (Barriball and Clark, 2005). This, combined with an increasing political awareness and pressure to improve the inequality in terms of access to health care (DH, 2001), should also contribute to a greater number of physical and psychological needs being identified in people with intellectual impairment, and therefore increased use of primary care services.

Although life expectancy is significantly shorter than that of the general population, increasingly people with intellectual impairment live extended life spans with a growing population of older people who have congenital or acquired intellectual impairment. An increased knowledge, improved interventions and a rise in health promotion activities seem to be contributing to an increasing life expectancy (NHS Health Scotland, 2004; Brown, 2005; Northway *et al*, 2006). Whilst there is an increasing older population with mild to profound intellectual disabilities, there are also more people being born with severe and profound learning disabilities (Sowney and Barr, 2006). The Department of Health estimates that there will be a 1% growth in the number of people with learning disabilities by 2015 (DH, 2001).

Northway *et al* (2006) identify a range of physical and mental health needs which can be acute or enduring, as well as chronic conditions which may underpin these needs (see Chapter 2). Furthermore, people with intellectual impairment have much higher rates of sensory impairment, communication difficulties and offending behaviour, which may further complicate assessment of their presenting complaint. Brown (2005) also identifies sleep disorders, self-harm and self-injury, infections, haematological and musculoskeletal disorders as significant health needs of this population.

It is without question then that people with intellectual impairment will, and should be making use of primary care health services including accident and emergency departments, that their health needs are complex, and that there is therefore an increased likelihood that admission to a hospital ward may be required. However, there is considerable evidence to demonstrate that accident and emergency and general ward healthcare professionals do not feel adequately prepared to work effectively with this client group (Regnard *et al*, 2006; Sowney and Barr, 2006). Bradley and Lofchy (2005) describe accident and emergency departments as confusing and frightening places. These factors combined with the individual patient's fear, pain and possible difficulties in communicating these experiences, result in distressing experiences for both the patient and staff.

THE PATIENT JOURNEY: ARRIVAL

In our first case study (see Box 7.1), Anna's arrival is clearly traumatic. She is in pain, frightened, and two men she has never met before are trying to take her away from her home in an ambulance. Emergency situations generate fast adrenaline-driven responses. The ambulance crew have correctly identified that Anna is having a myocardial infarction (MI), and know that there is very limited time to complete their assessment and begin to treat Anna according to their acute coronary syndrome protocol. No doubt Anna's key worker is also very distressed – finding Anna on the floor, in pain, making an assessment of what is causing Anna's distress and calling the ambulance. This situation will create conflict. The paramedic's need for fast action and Anna's need to feel safe and know the people around her are not at odds. Bradley (2002) and Bradley and Lofchy (2005) advocate a process of 'optimizing the clinical encounter', in which they suggest that it is the clinician's responsibility to adapt to the patient's level of functioning and understanding.

Consider the circumstances around Anna's MI, transfer to and arrival at hospital. She is frightened, in pain, and has difficulty expressing both her fears and her pain, yet assessment and treatment must be carried out expediently in order to save her life.

What could be done to help reassure her?

- Every interaction needs to be adapted to meet individual needs.

- In Anna's case, this adaptation has to happen at an emergency pace.

- Remain calm – Anna will quickly pick up on your anxiety.

- Adopt a warm manner and a calm and caring attitude.

- Anna's carer may be able to offer advice about interpreting and understanding Anna's communication. Routinely, you should address your questions to the client and not the carer,

BOX 7.1   ANNA

Anna is a 50-year-old woman with Down syndrome and type 2 diabetes which is tablet-controlled. She lives in a shared home with 24 hour residential support. Her key worker found her crying on the floor, looking very pale, sweaty, and clutching her left arm. In the ambulance Anna is very frightened, and although she appears in a lot of pain she screams every time the ambulance man tries to touch her. The paramedic thinks she is having an acute coronary event, but is unable to do an ECG on route as Anna repeatedly pushes him away.

In the resuscitation room the physicians decide to go ahead and treat for acute coronary syndrome, and it is not until Anna has been sedated that they are able to complete their assessment. The ECG and Troponin T test reveal that she has had a myocardial infarction. Anna is admitted to the coronary care unit for four days and then transferred to a general medical ward. On the ward Anna is particularly distressed at night and becomes incontinent. She loses weight and spends a lot of her time crying. Anna's name and some other significant details have been changed to protect her anonymity and maintain confidentiality. ■

unless the client has asked you to do so – however, in an emergency situation this may need to be adapted.

- If possible, her carer or someone else with whom Anna is familiar should be present to offer reassurance to Anna.

- Obtain any history and crisis or emergency plans from the carer.

- Anna may already understand certain routines around investigative procedures – ask the carer about these.

- In spite of the adrenaline-fuelled moment, every effort must be made to keep visual and aural stimulation to a minimum.

- Turn off sirens, flashing lights, radios if possible.

- Silence electronic alarms on monitoring equipment.

- Ask any onlookers to leave.

- Only one healthcare professional should speak.

- Try to speak calmly and clearly, explaining what you are doing whether or not you think Anna is able to understand. Her expressive capacity may be reduced by her distress, but she still may be able to understand what is happening and what you are saying.

- Always ask for Anna's consent before touching her or using any equipment to monitor her – although she may not have capacity to give consent, it helps to forewarn her of what is happening.

- Don't correct her if Anna misunderstands that you are a 'doctor' or 'nurse' – she may understand that these are helpful people
- The person leading the assessment should stay with Anna for as long as possible so she can get used to them.

This list includes four points that involve Anna's carer in the assessment process. In an emergency situation the tendency to rely on carers is strong. In their study identifying perceived challenges in caring for people with learning disabilities in accident and emergency departments, Sowney and Barr (2006) considered this to be a complex issue. When asked what would help increase their ability to care for people with learning disabilities, nurses in their study all suggested involvement of the carer, this is of course applicable across the spectra of intellectual impairment. Sowney and Barr (2006) warn that this could become a dependency on the carer. They also highlighted a lack of understanding of the legal rights of an adult with a learning disability and poor understanding of the ethical issues related to obtaining consent, maintaining confidentiality, privacy and dignity. It is also important to consider the needs of the carer. In any emergency setting the carer may have been dealing with either a stressful deterioration of someone's health, or with a shocking accident or sudden change, from which they need to recover. The above list represents a series of suggestions, from which some may prove helpful. However, each situation will have to be taken on its own merits, considering both the client's and carer's needs. The overall aim is to find the optimum way of communicating with and involving the client in their care.

Finding ways to communicate effectively with someone with an intellectual impairment takes time and patience and is difficult to achieve in an emergency context. In addition to seeking advice from the carer and, if appropriate, including them as much as possible, Bradley (2002), Bradley and Lofchy (2005) and Cogher (2005) advocate the use of the following techniques to promote effective communication:

- Use simple words.
- Use short sentences.
- Speak slowly.
- Do not shout.
- Pause – do not overload the individual with words, and give time for a response.
- Wait and listen.
- Repeat questions or instructions if necessary.
- Be sensitive to the individual's non-verbal cues, and adjust your behaviour accordingly.
- Use visuals – for example drawings, faces for pain assessment, etc.
- Respect avoidance of eye contact or test out whether or not the patient prefers direct eye contact.
- Test out how the client likes to be addressed: by name, in the second person – 'you', or in the third person 'she/he'.
- Use gestures or point to support what you say.
- Encourage the use of comforters.
- Be interested in what the patient is holding, touching or saying.

WHY IS IMPROVEMENT IN EMERGENCY AND URGENT HEALTH CARE PROVISION REQUIRED?

Morgan *et al* (2000) have identified that 14% of the general population and 26% of the population with learning disabilities will require hospital-based services in their lifetime. People with learning disabilities have greater health needs and attendances at hospital, but their inpatient admissions are shorter. Rates of admission are likely to be high in other groups with intellectual impairment. Brown (2005) suggests that there are specific risk factors for people with learning disabilities when they are admitted to general hospital: lack of knowledge and understanding of health needs; increased risk of dysphagia and aspiration pneumonia; difficulties with communication and assessing capacity to consent; barriers preventing physical and cognitive access to health care, education and development issues; misdiagnosis or no diagnosis.

Some of the reasons why people with intellectual impairment have poorer health outcomes and shorter admissions may be more to do with our abilities than with any characteristic of the patient. Five different types of barriers to healthcare services for people with learning disabilities have been identified by the Scottish Executive (2002). Such barriers are applicable for all people with intellectual impairment, whatever the cause. They can be divided into organizational and individual subcategories:

1. Organizational barriers include *physical* issues, such as poor wheelchair access to hospitals, and *administrative*, such as unrealistic targets for waiting times, emergency triage systems that fail to acknowledge an individual's capacity to wait as a priority, and longer appointment times for people who need help communicating.

2. The individual barriers identified were *communication* – our inability to understand and adapt to the different communication styles used, *attitudinal* – making negative assumptions about people with learning disabilities and intervening on the basis of these assumptions, for example not giving pain relief to someone who is self-injuring, and *knowledge* barriers – being limited by our lack of experience of working with people who are intellectually impaired.

Sowney and Barr (2006) identified six themes that nurses considered to influence the potential barriers to providing emergency care to people with learning disabilities:

- Existing good practice
- Respect of individuals
- Communication difficulties
- Difficulties gaining consent
- Lack of knowledge
- Dependence on carers.

In their analysis, Sowney and Barr (2005) considered that this would impact on the healthcare professional, carer and patient in a number of ways. These have been summarized in Table 7.1. The lack of knowledge was of both how to care for people with intellectual impairment, and from where and from whom help could be sought in an emergency. There seems to be a strong

TABLE 7.1

Impact of healthcare professionals' lack of knowledge about intellectual impairment in an emergency setting (Sowney and Barr, 2006)

Healthcare professional	Carer	Patient
Over-dependence on carers	Carers' needs not addressed	Risk of needs not being identified and therefore remaining untreated
Passive caring role	Expected to consent on behalf of patient	Reduced communication
	Expected to stay	Lack of involvement in decision making
Fear and vulnerability	Knowledge not being valued	Barrier to a therapeutic relationship
Reduced competence	Expected to provide care	Feeling devalued
	Obligation to remain (to ensure appropriate care is received)	Unmet physical and psychological needs
		Overuse of investigations
		Opportunities for health education/ promotion reduced

relationship between this lack of knowledge and the fear and vulnerability that nurses also reported in Sowney and Barr's (2006) study.

The accident and emergency culture is one of being able to cope with anything. Within departments, hierarchies are delineated not so much by professional role, but by condition-specific knowledge, and insights into the management of certain situations, conditions and clients. This would seem to be at odds with nurses' abilities to look after people with intellectual impairment. Sowney and Barr (2006) raise the concern that a combination of a lack of knowledge and understanding, and a fear of doing (or not doing) something, contributes to the over-identification of all behaviours as part of an individual's intellectual impairment (in this case, learning disability). This means that healthcare professionals run the risk of either misinterpreting behaviours, which are in fact signs and symptoms of something being wrong, or running tests to identify possible pathological causes for all behaviours displayed by a patient, leading to over-investigation and diagnostic overshadowing.

ASSESSMENT

Bradley and Lofchy (2005) describe the phenomenon of diagnostic overshadowing as the attribution of behavioural disturbances to the person's intellectual impairment and the failure to recognize additional mental and physical health disorders when assessing. In order to avoid diagnostic overshadowing in an emergency or urgent hospital care episode it is essential to structure the assessment using a thorough, open-minded approach, whilst also trying to maintain a balance and avoiding the risk of over-investigation.

It is impossible to know on first meeting with someone who has an intellectual impairment how that person is able to communicate and what particular signs and behaviours may mean. Regnard *et al* (2006) found that there is no validated tool for assessing pain or distress in people with severe communication difficulties. In their development and testing of the Disability Distress Assessment Tool (DisDAT) they have attempted to create a tool which can measure for individuals the level of distress – whether the cause be physical, psychological or emotional. Table 7.2 lists the signs and behaviours indicating pain, and those indicating distress identified in Regnard *et al*'s (2006) review of the literature.

Their study concluded that these signs and behaviours varied greatly for different people. However, their results show that there are some signs and behaviours that were common in as many as 80% (for 'content' cues) and 50% (for 'distress' cues) for the 10 patients in their study. Having an indication of the possible cues a patient might give when content and when in distress may help to focus the assessment. 'Common sense' cues such as smiling, spontaneous talking and a relaxed posture were common in contented patients. Lifting hands to head, vocalizations such

TABLE 7.2

Signs and behaviours of pain and of distress (a summary of the literature review in Regnard *et al*, 2006)

Signs and behaviours indicating pain	Signs and behaviours indicating distress
Aggression, wincing, holding head, protecting limb, moaning	Fidgeting, repetitive vocalization, aggression, withdrawal, facial expression, increased body tension, noisy breathing
Quiet withdrawal, rapid blinking, improved vocalization, refusing food, agitation	Reduced locomotor activity (walking and running around)
Facial expression	Autonomic changes (increased BP and PR, sweating and skin colour changes)
Guarding, bracing, rubbing, grimacing, sighing	Body posture
Crying, rigidity, withdrawal, increased body movement	Tone of voice
Changes in quality of non-verbal vocalizations	Changes in facial appearance, skin colour, sweating, eye appearances, body posture, habits, mannerisms, and speech.
Autonomic changes (increased BP, PR, sweating, skin colour changes)	
Noisy breathing, absence of contentment, facial expression, body tension, increased body movement.	

as screaming, wailing and groaning and a quiet withdrawn and tense or restless manner were all signs of distress. As with all assessment processes, a four-stage strategy will help to lead to our initial formulation: history, subjective assessment, objective assessment and measurements, clinical tests and investigations. If this process is followed it should help to reduce both diagnostic over-shadowing and over-investigation.

HISTORY

In an assessment the history is imperative for the practitioner to be able to assess what has led up to the client's presentation, which symptoms have appeared, in what order and over what length of time, but also for the client to be able to tell his or her story and to be able to express what it is that is causing them the most concern. The client's narrative may be difficult to assess when working with people with intellectual impairment, but this makes it no less important. In an emergency or urgent care context, the scope of the history is not to assess the client's complete history, rather their story of changes that have occurred leading up to this presentation; the history of his or her presenting complaint within a medical model.

However, with a client who has intellectual impairment, this assessment process requires the practitioner to be more creative. As identified above, there are communication techniques that can be employed to maximize the clinical encounter. In addition to these it may be necessary to use written or drawn material, or picture boards to help facilitate someone explaining what has happened. If the presenting complaint is not a life-threatening emergency, then one practitioner should spend as much time as possible with the client. The person with an intellectual impairment may take that time to get to know that individual, trust them and to be able to use their communication skills to the optimum.

Although the individual client should be the focus of the assessment process, they may not be able to relate all the information that is needed, so at the earliest opportunity a corroborative history should be sought from the client's carers, family, GP, previous notes, and any other source available. This should of course be done with the client's consent, but it is perfectly possible to ask for information about someone to help with assessment without breaching the client's confidentiality. The assessor should focus their questions on relevant medical and psychiatric history, how this person usually appears, whether the carers/family or health professionals have noticed any recent changes that they are concerned about, and whether there is anything they could recommend to make the assessment process easier for the client.

SUBJECTIVE

The signs and behaviours described by Regnard et al (2006) and cited in Table 7.2 are of most use in making the initial subjective assessment. Even if a client is refusing or unable to speak, and is not allowing anyone to touch them in order to assess them further, there is a great deal that can be observed, even if at this stage the exact meaning of what is observed is unclear. A 'sensory' model could be employed to structure this initial, subjective assessment.

Consider Regnard et al's (2006) signs of pain and distress in Table 7.2. Which of those signs and behaviours can be seen, heard, smelt, or touched? How could the practitioner notice if a client's taste, appetite, or nutritional status were affected?

The signs and symptoms that can be easily observed help to focus our attention on those symptoms that need more thorough investigation. They can be compared with the history obtained from the client and other sources in order to establish whether or not there is a marked change. If during a subjective assessment it is noted that someone appears in pain – this should be considered, even if the informant history suggests that someone often behaves in this manner. It could be the case that something has become a chronic complaint and the symptoms have been incorporated into other people's view of how this person usually presents.

Furthermore, if there was a suggestion that someone is in pain, it would be unethical not to give analgesia. If the pain is relieved, it will make the rest of the assessment easier and help to establish trust and rapport with the client. The subjective assessment indicates those aspects of a client which need further objective assessment and measurement.

OBJECTIVE

In Anna's case the paramedics were disappointed by the fact that they had been unable to perform an electrocardiogram (ECG) in the ambulance. In fact, they had correctly identified the history from the story of how Anna's carer had found her, and were able to make a subjective assessment based on what they had observed: her fear, pain, clutching her arm, appearing sweaty and very pale. This was enough for them to correctly diagnose acute coronary syndrome (ACS) and rush her to hospital. Usual practice would be to identify the exact rhythm in which her heart was beating – however, it would not have made any difference to their management plan at this stage. Any further attempt to obtain the ECG may have been perceived by Anna as an assault, and would likely have given equivocal results because of her distress and agitated movements. In fact, it was not until after she had been mildly sedated in the resuscitation room, that the objective assessment of her pulse, blood pressure, temperature, ECG, etc., could be made.

It is not being suggested that people with intellectual impairment should not have standard tests done, but rather that we must consider the number, timing and necessity of them. Over-investigation sits at the opposite end of a continuum with diagnostic overshadowing, with a number of competing driving forces shifting the ultimate aim of a balanced, thorough, and holistic assessment, towards one end or the other, as illustrated in Figure 7.1.

The objective assessment should therefore involve those assessments indicated by the history and our subjective assessment. Iacono and Davis (2003) and Bradley and Lofchy (2005) note that hospital procedures can be distressing for clients who are intellectually impaired. However, it is

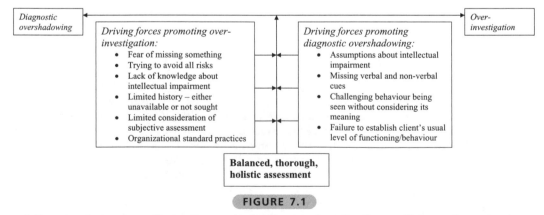

FIGURE 7.1

Influencing factors on a diagnostic overshadowing–over-investigating continuum when assessing people with intellectual impairment in general hospital settings

essential that signs and symptoms are properly investigated – and this can only be achieved on a case-by-case basis. Using Anna's example once more, if she had been held down in the ambulance in order to take an ECG – what else would we have learnt? If her situation had deteriorated or there was a sudden or unexpected change, then this could have been noticed through observation, or using minimally invasive equipment such as pulse oximetry.

CLINICAL TESTS AND INVESTIGATIONS

There is in essence a funnel leading from history of presenting complaint, through subjective and objective observations to clinical tests and investigations. If further clinical tests or investigations are required:

- Employ the same communication techniques outlined above.
- Take time to find out from the client what they understand about the procedure.
- Explain using pictures or showing the equipment if appropriate.
- Demonstrate on someone else if it is a non-invasive and risk-free procedure.
- Find out from carers whether there is a rehearsed protocol for this particular investigation.
- Allow the client to have anyone or anything they find comforting with them.
- If possible ensure the same healthcare professional remains with them.
- Consider what can be brought to the client rather than moving them around the hospital.

It is also possible to 'multitask' in this context. For example, if you need to take a blood sample for a liver function test, and we know that this client may also be at risk of type 2 diabetes, blood can be drawn for HbA1c at the same time. This may read as though it is contrary to the cautions of over-investigating, but it essentially reduces the number of occasions on which the client will need to have a blood sample taken and can identify conditions in addition to those currently being investigated – providing health protection and promotion opportunities.

This will only reduce the number of investigations if results are shared with, or are accessible to, the client's GP and other healthcare professionals. Rigorous systems of reporting or shared access to databases of results are essential.

THE PATIENT JOURNEY – ASSESSMENT

Box 7.2 gives Ken's story. On a number of occasions the history of his presenting complaint has been overlooked. Ken has been assessed at triage and then treated according to the department's protocol for overdoses. He has certainly taken an overdose of paracetamol, he complies with having his paracetamol levels taken at four-hours post-ingestion, and to some degree he allows treatment with acetylcysteine (Parvolex). However, two assumptions are frequently made: (i) that Ken has taken the paracetamol in order to harm or kill himself; and (ii) that he speeds up the intravenous infusion with some manipulating intent. Assessment is always made of whether or not he intended to kill himself, and Ken sometimes answers that he 'wants to die' when he is subsequently referred to the psychiatric liaison team.

BOX 7.2   KEN

Ken is a 21-year-old man who regularly attends the emergency department complaining of lower back pain, and having taken excessive amounts of paracetamol. Ken doesn't view his behaviour as self-harm, but takes the tablets to stop his back from hurting. He regularly requires treatment with parvolex, but doesn't like staying in hospital, so he speeds up the intravenous infusion and then tries to self-discharge. Ken has an IQ of 68 and has been described as having 'impulsive behaviour' and 'poor problem-solving skills'. He lives at home with his mum. Ken experiences low mood and occasionally says he wants to die. However, the local Community Mental Health Team have discharged him. He used to have a key worker from the local learning disability team, but he no longer meets the criteria for support from the adult service. Ken has given his permission for his story and experiences to be used here. His name has been changed to protect his anonymity. ■

Ken is not self-harming, nor is it clear that this is self-injurious behaviour from a challenging behaviour perspective. Ken has very poor problem-solving skills and often behaves impulsively. He agreed that his case could be used for this textbook and agreed to contribute by talking about his experiences of being assessed in the emergency department and treated on a medical admissions ward. The following are excerpts from a tape-recorded interview:

Nurse: Why do you take the paracetamol, Ken?
Ken: My back hurts, and mum is fed-up of me going on you know . . . I take two at a time though . . . when they don't work I take two more.

Ken continues to take two at a time, sometimes taking 24 in less than an hour, expecting that the pain will go away. His understanding of how paracetamol works is poor, but in eight attendances at the hospital, he had neither had his pain assessed further, nor had he been referred for assessment and treatment of his back. If Ken was listened to in detail at the history-taking stage, his reasons for the overdose are clear, and subjectively – he is smiling, chatting to staff, looks well kempt, well fed and seems to enjoy the company on the ward. Not the appearance of a depressed and suicidal man.

Nurse: What's it like on the ward, Ken?
Ken: They don't like me (said urgently and conspiratorially) . . . They tell me off all the time, and I'm scared of [name of doctor omitted]. I know I'm wrong . . . They tell me off for the paramol and to come back when I do it again . . .

Nurse: Do you speed up the drip?
Ken: I can't lie down all day. I'm not ill . . . (said defensively), I want to go home. I feel OK. I have to go and see mum. I'm not allowed to go until it's finished.

Ken's assessment by his previous learning disability team states that he has poor problem-solving skills. However, if the problem is not being allowed to go home, he solves it rather deftly. When the 'rules' of the hospital are explained to Ken, he feels as though he is in trouble. He wants to go home quickly so that he won't be in trouble for long. He also finds the advice he has been given confusing. His experiential learning that if he takes too many tablets, he can come to hospital and will be all right, is more powerful than the information he has been given about the risks. Moreover, he seems to have picked up that in their discharge/crisis planning, Ken thinks the staff expect him to take more tablets and come back. He clearly does not understand the subjunctive tense and it would seem imperative that Ken's discharge instructions are given clearly and simply. Furthermore, his understanding of a plan needs to be assessed.

Consider the diagnostic overshadowing – over-investigation continuum in Figure 7.1. What factors do you think have influenced Ken's assessment in the past?

SELF-HARM AND SELF-INJURY – PRIMARY CARE ASSESSMENT AND TREATMENT

The language used to describe how and why people harm or injure themselves can reflect the judgements that are often made about this client group: 'self-abuse' and 'self-mutilation' assume emotive aspects such as guilt or self-loathing, whereas purely descriptive terms such as 'cutting' or 'blood letting' convey neither the choice that the client has made nor the fact that the act is harmful. Weber (2002) cites several terms that have been used to describe such behaviour: self-injury, self-abuse, indirect self-destructive behaviour, parasuicide, self-inflicted injury, self-injurious behaviour, self-mutilation, as well as deliberate self-harm. The terms used often reflect the theoretical standpoint of the clinician using them rather than the client who harms him or herself. Self-abuse, self-destructive behaviour or self-mutilation suggest a psychodynamic understanding of the motivation for the behaviour. Whereas deliberate self-harm conveys some sense that the person has chosen to act in this way and that it is a behaviour rather than an illness per se. Self-injurious behaviour implies a medical model understanding that the challenging behaviour is an involuntary part of someone's intellectual behaviour and may be a maladaptive form of communicating distress.

Deliberate self-harm can include a wide range of behaviours which damage an individual's body, either externally or internally, with a meaning or purpose that can vary for any one client on each occasion that they self-harm, and from person to person. The act might be impulsive or planned, with immediate or long-term effect. The term only describes the behaviour and is not an illness (Noonan, 2004). Harker-Longton and Fish (2002), Wisely *et al* (2002) and Lovell (2004) identify a development in the definition of self-injurious behaviour from focusing on the repetitive or compulsive nature of the behaviour, to including a consideration of the harm done by the act. Lovell (2004) considers the most common self-injurious behaviours to include:

- Head-banging
- Banging other body parts
- Biting
- Scratching
- Picking at the skin
- Hair pulling
- Placing inedible objects into the mouth or other body cavities.

A further distinction is drawn with self-harm syndrome, which includes:

- Cutting

- Burning

- Carving behaviours (Lovell, 2004).

Noonan (2004) proposes a three-stage model for assessing self-harm including assessment of mechanism, meaning and motivation.

1 MECHANISM

Assessment of the mechanism of injury reveals any urgent risk issues to the individual's health and gives an indication of what emergency action may need to be taken. The mechanism can also suggest where on a continuum of self-injury to self-harm syndrome to deliberate self-harm, the behaviour fits.

2 MEANING

The meaning of the behaviour is what, for example, distinguishes Ken's paracetamol overdoses from self-harm. With clients who self-injure, the learning disability is more likely to be profound, making the meaning of the act for them almost impossible to illicit, whereas self-harm is more common in clients with a primary diagnosis of personality disorder or mental illness, who may be able to communicate what the self-harm means to them quite clearly (Lovell, 2004). However, we still may be able to attribute meaning to someone's self-injurious behaviour. It may be that the part of the body they are banging is causing them pain, or that they are distressed for some other reason, and further assessment is indicated. Attempting to understand the meaning may suggest behavioural interventions that could be employed to help reduce the frequency or the harm done by someone's self-injurious behaviour.

Behavioural phenotype research has demonstrated the link between a number of syndromes and self-injurious behaviour:

- Lesch-Nyhan syndrome

- Smith-Magenis syndrome

- Cornelia de Lange syndrome

- Cri-du-chat syndrome

- Smith-Lemli-Opitz syndrome.

All of these syndromes include signs and behaviours that could be described as self-injurious. However, Oliver and Petty (2002) provide a critique of the studies connecting the self-injurious behaviour and the phenotype for the syndrome. Studies may have been skewed by not considering features of the syndromes such as opisthokinesis, other environmental factors, or by biases in sampling. They propose that a combination of commonality of behaviours, in particular syndromes revealed by identifying the phenotype, learning and neurotransmitter dysfunction, may contribute to the theoretical understanding of self-injurious behaviour.

Although the evidence to support the effects of learning on self-injurious behaviour is limited, it does suggest that it may be possible to understand the meaning of a behaviour for an individual who is quite severely disabled by their intellectual impairment, albeit by relying on history from carers or family. Therefore, we could consider meaning in choosing psychopharmacological and/or behavioural treatments of the self-injurious behaviour.

3 MOTIVATION

Within a self-harm context, an assessment of motivation is undertaken in order to identify whether or not someone is suicidal – how they see their future, whether or not they want to live, what goals they have in the short, medium and long term, and whether or not they feel hopeless. There is also a second stage to the assessment that identifies an individual's readiness to change. By listening to the client and identifying any motivational statements they make, it is possible to identify at what stage of change they might be, and to use techniques to see if this can be moved forward through the cycle of change (Prochaska *et al*, 1993). It is of course still possible to elicit motivational statements from someone with an intellectual impairment who is self-harming.

With self-injurious behaviour it is more complex, but none the less important. With both the cases of Ken (Box 7.2) and Angus (Box 7.3) there are times when they do feel like they want to die. Ken's occasional ambivalence about whether or not he lives is not related to his self-injurious behaviour, or self-poisoning in order to treat his back pain. However, he is at risk of killing himself by continuing to take large doses of paracetamol. His motivational thoughts are revealed in this ambivalence. Angus does not self-harm, but monitoring of his mood and motivational cues in his speech content would ensure that we were able to screen for depression, and suicidal plans should they occur.

Although the evidence is inconsistent, it is largely agreed that a number of theories explain self-injurious behaviour: behavioural phenotypes, neurotransmitters and dependence on opiates released in response to pain, learned patterns of behaviour where responses to self-injury are reinforced, communication difficulties and environmental factors (Harker-Longton and Fish, 2002; Oliver and Petty, 2002; Wisely *et al*, 2002; McClintock *et al*, 2003; Lovell, 2004). The management of challenging behaviour is considered in detail in Chapter 10, but we cannot choose an appropriate protection or restraint, psychopharmacological or behavioural treatment for a client without an understanding of what motivates his or her self-injury.

PRIMARY CARE RESPONSIBILITIES

Guidelines for the primary care assessment and management of self-harm have been provided by the National Institute for Clinical Excellence (NICE, 2004). The guidelines emphasize the need for respect and kindness from health professionals and the recommendations are focused on primary care (non-mental health) professionals' response to patients who self-harm. The guidelines are clear that they include people with 'learning disabilities' who self-harm, but not people with repetitive self-injurious behaviour. Nevertheless the recommendations are equally applicable.

In summary the guidelines suggest that an urgent assessment of risk and emotional, mental and physical health should take place. Everyone who self-harms should be referred for further psychosocial assessment. Assessment needs to take place in an atmosphere of respect and understanding. Account must be taken of emotional distress as well as physical injury when prioritizing care. Psychosocial assessment should not be delayed until after someone has been physically treated. If someone does have to wait for treatment a safe, supportive environment must be provided. If someone who has diminished capacity wants to leave before they have had a psychosocial assessment, provision should be made to prevent them from leaving.

Further guidance has been provided based on the findings of the National Inquiry into Self-Harm and Young People (Brophy, 2005), which identified that young people with learning disabilities, and young people in residential settings were at an increased risk of self-harm compared to the general public. McClintock *et al* (2003), in their meta-analysis of the risk markers associated with challenging behaviour in people with 'intellectual disabilities', also identified that there were specific high-risk groups. People with a severe/profound degree of 'disability' were more likely to self-injure and show stereotyped behaviours; those with a diagnosis of autism and those with deficits in receptive and expressive communication were also at an increased risk of self-injurious behaviour.

Although it may not be possible for each primary care setting to establish an intellectual impairment liaison service like the models proposed by Dinsdale (2001) and Glasby (2002), what is clear from the recommendations is that we need to be prepared. One of the knowledge deficits identified by Sowney and Barr (2006), was from where and from whom help could be obtained. In an emergency context, when assessing someone with either self-injurious behaviour or self-harm, it will be difficult to track down this information. Departments and wards must identify their sources of support from liaison psychiatry and/or learning disability community teams in advance, so that they are accessible when clients attend.

ADMISSION AND DISCHARGE PLANNING

ADMISSION

As already noted, people with intellectual impairment have an increased morbidity and more complex needs than the general population. Their admissions are, however, often shorter. Furthermore, people with intellectual impairment can lose skills and abilities whilst in hospital. For example, someone who is usually able to feed themselves might not eat whilst in hospital because they have not been 'given permission' to do so, or had it explained to them that the food placed on a tray in front of them is theirs. A client, who can normally achieve continence with prompting or reminders, may become incontinent whilst in hospital if their routine is not maintained.

In a survey of people with 'developmental disabilities', Iacono and Davis (2003) explored the extent to which these basic needs were met for people admitted to general wards. They found that in relation to getting to the toilet, receiving the right medication on time and getting enough to eat or drink, that 39%, 22% and 18% of their sample respectively, did not have their needs met whilst in hospital. In the group that did have its needs met, this seemed to be largely attributed to having a carer or support worker with the person all the time. Communication difficulties, nurses' lack of patience, and an underestimation of the person's intellectual abilities, all contributed to these basic needs being unmet. Also the provision of equipment made an impact. Patients needing mobility equipment such as wheelchairs tended to bring their own. However, if someone used specialist or adapted utensils for eating, these were often left at home and no alternative supplied by the hospital – the result being that they went without food.

Bradley (2002) emphasizes the importance of gathering information on the patient's baseline level of function and supports required before the onset of this particular illness, and prior to admission. This includes:

- Cognitive functioning
- Adaptive functioning
- Communication
- Social functioning
- Residential circumstances
- Daily activity.

Cognitive functioning refers to more that just an individual's IQ; assessment includes their usual verbal and non-verbal functioning, problem-solving ability, ability to read and write and any longstanding cognitive deficits. The level of independence in activities of daily living can describe an individual's adaptive functioning. What help or support do they usually have around personal hygiene, dressing, eating, and using the toilet? Hospital staff need to take special care to note the routines that someone has associated with these activities and make every effort to ensure they are maintained whilst they are in hospital.

When assessing someone's baseline communication abilities, ensure that consideration is taken of both their receptive and expressive capacity, and find out what techniques or equipment they use to help this. For example if someone uses gestures or Makaton (a more basic version of British Sign Language) to communicate, most healthcare professionals could learn their key signs for basic needs such as toilet, food or pain, in a few minutes.

Individuals with intellectual impairment may have a number of idiosyncrasies or abnormalities in their social responses. Their ability to tolerate eye contact, and direct gaze, their ability to understand and interpret facial expression, acceptance of physical proximity and contact may all be affected. Establishing the usual boundaries from family, carers and other healthcare professionals will enable us to make the experience less distressing for the client, other patients and staff members.

Whether a patient with an intellectual impairment lives on their own, in a shared home, with family or other full-time carers, or in fully supported residential accommodation, admission is likely to represent a severe disruption in the routine enshrined in their usual residential circumstances. Assessing the level of support the person usually requires will give an indication of the support needed, and importantly of the level of independence that should be promoted whilst in hospital.

As soon as possible, features of the person's daily activity should be reintroduced. If someone is in hospital for investigations, they could be allowed to attend other organized activities that form part of their regular daily activity. The longer these routines are disrupted, the harder it will be to reintroduce them.

Although primarily concerned with psychiatric admissions, Bradley (2002) identifies four key factors that result in a poor outcome associated with hospitalization, and four factors which contribute to a successful admission. These are summarized in Table 7.3.

TABLE 7.3

Factors associated with poor outcomes and successful hospital admissions

Poor outcomes	Successful admissions
Premature discharge	Attention to routines – trying to match those in the hospital to those in the patient's usual accommodation
Over-medication (over-sedation)	Physical environment – using a bed space that considers the patient's level of distress, ensuring space for carers
The patient regresses whilst on the ward	Staff – providing consistency and continuity of care, and clearly allocating responsibility for liaison with the community
Poor communication between the hospital and community care providers	Communication – with the patient, carers, other healthcare professionals

PATIENT JOURNEY

ADMISSION

Ken, the patient introduced earlier (Box 7.2) clearly finds the admissions ward distressing:

> **Ken**: They all tell me what I've done wrong. It feels bad . . . and I don't like being in trouble.

It would seem that there is some degree of 'over-communicating'. The structure on the admissions ward involves assessment by a medical team, a nursing team, a toxicology ward round, a psychiatric liaison team, and changes of nursing shifts three times within a 24-hour period. If each person thinks it is their responsibility to explain to Ken the risks involved in his overdoses, it is no surprise that he perceives it to be telling him off. The communication problem is not with Ken's expressive ability, he may, however, have some difficulty understanding the paternalistic, well-meaning overtones of being warned of how dangerous his behaviour is. However, the primary problem is with no one individual being identified as having primary responsibility for working with him whilst he is in hospital. With one person, Ken could establish a relationship, and there would be the opportunity to explore more thoroughly Ken's understanding of what has happened and what needs to happen.

> **Ken**: I can't lie down all day. I'm not ill . . . (said defensively) I want to go home. I feel OK. I have to go and see mum. I'm not allowed to go until it's finished.

Assessment of Ken's adaptive and social function, and the importance of his residential circumstances and daily activities have been overlooked. Ken is a healthy young man and does not think he should lie down in bed. In fact there is no reason for him to do so. Although intravenous access is required to administer medication in a infusion, Ken could walk around, watch the television in the day room or go to the canteen. Whilst he is dependent on his mum and wants to see her, he also wants to express his independence and does not like being 'mothered' by the nursing staff who tell him to stay in bed. There is a risk that Ken will leave the hospital, but being made to stay in his bed all day increases this. Allowing Ken to maintain his optimal level of functioning and independence whilst in hospital will help to build a trusting relationship between him and the staff, and may decrease his feeling of being punished or reprimanded.

DISCHARGE PLANNING

The process of planning for someone's discharge should start from the moment they are admitted. For nearly all assessments, investigations and procedures, there is an approximate timescale of how long someone will be in hospital. In addition to someone with an intellectual impairment having increased and complex needs, there is the additional risk that changes, both admission and discharge, may cause distress. Many of the recommendations and guidelines around discharge planning are focused on the organizational needs of the hospital. However, as with planning the discharge for any patient, these principles have to be adapted in their application to the individual for discharge planning to be successful.

One of the major aims of Valuing People (DH, 2001) is to focus on the need for person-centred care planning. Priest and Gibbs (2004) identify five key principles that underpin person-centred planning. The person is central to all aspects of their life, and person-centred planning is founded firmly on rights, independence and choice. Family members, other carers and friends are full partners in the planning of care. Person-centred planning reflects the person's capabilities and what is important to that person, and specifies the support each individual requires to make a valued contribution to the community. Planning builds upon a shared commitment that will uphold the individual's rights and must involve continual listening, learning and action.

In other populations, the effect of quality discharge planning and community liaison has resulted in reduced hospital admissions and reduced re-admissions. It has lengthened the time to first re-admission and decreased the cost of care (Naylor *et al*, 1999). These improvements can be mirrored when caring for people with intellectual impairment when educational initiatives are provided by specialist staff (Dinsdale, 2001; Glasby, 2002). The principles outlined in the Department of Health guidelines on discharge planning (DH, 2003) should be applied to all inpatients:

- Understand your local community and balance the range of services to meet health, housing and social care needs.

- Ensure individuals and their carers are actively engaged in the planning and delivery of their care.

- Recognize the important role carers play and their own right for assessment and support.

- Ensure effective communication between primary, secondary and social care to ensure that prior to admission and on admission each individual receives the care and treatment they need.

- Agree, operate and performance manage a joint discharge policy that facilitates effective multidisciplinary working at ward level and between organizations.

- On admission, identify those individuals who may have additional health, social and/or housing needs to be met before they can leave hospital and target them for extra support.

- At ward level, identify and train individuals who can take on the role of care coordination in support of the multidisciplinary team and individual patients and their carers.

- Consider how an integrated discharge planning team can be developed to provide specialist discharge planning support to the patient and multidisciplinary team.

- Ensure all patients are assessed for a period of rehabilitation before any permanent decisions on care options are made.

- Ensure that the funding decisions for NHS continuing care and care home placement are made in a way that does not delay someone's discharge.

Many of the recommendations have a political and organizational frame of reference, but there are also specific guidelines for working with people with a learning disability. These include using the patient's Health Action Plan (HAP), arranging pre-admission visits, and making the links with the community teams prior to admission, in order to facilitate smooth and effective. It is also noted that:

During recovery, health professionals need to take into account that a person with a learning disability may require longer time and additional encouragement to make a full recovery. It is important to gain the co-operation of the patient at their own pace.

(DH, 2003 p. 83)

This suggests that whilst the discharge planning needs to be commenced at the earliest opportunity, it will also have to be flexible. Furthermore, the home care and primary care teams must be jointly involved in coordinating the discharge plan. In addition, HAPs should also be recommended for all people with intellectual impairment and not just those who have a known learning disability.

DISCHARGE

Box 7.3 describes the experiences of Angus who has recently been discharged from hospital. Since he has left hospital, he has been experiencing panic attacks and when neither able to decide nor to remember what to do, he returns to the hospital as he sees it as a safe place. The emergency department staff reinforce the plan that has been agreed with Angus's community team, and it is possible that there is some frustration that he is not following the agreed plan. However, Angus cannot remember the agreed plans, and when he is anxious this further reduces his cognitive ability to concentrate on problem-solving techniques. None the less, at each stage that he has been discharged – from ICU to neurology, to neuropsychiatry, and subsequently to a community mental health team – there have been agreed plans.

Two things are missing however, which might improve the success of his discharge plan, and lessen the distress Angus experiences. First, although he has been involved in the construction of his discharge plan, he does not own a copy of it. The problem-solving and cognitive–behavioural techniques could be incorporated into his HAP, and he could keep this as a resource of how to manage his anxiety and where to seek help. If he were able to bring this with him when he returned to the emergency department, it might promote greater continuity of care, and reduce Angus's frustration that he cannot remember what he is supposed to do.

Second, his discharge plan focuses on long-term aims, and does not include a crisis plan. Angus could be provided with a plan or crisis card, listing the phone numbers he could use for help, one or two basic techniques to manage his anxiety, and the trigger factors or experiences that indicate he should seek help immediately. He could use this to assess for himself the intensity and urgency of the problem when he feels distressed and anxious at night.

BOX 7.3   ANGUS

At the age of 31, Angus sustained a severe head injury in an aggravated assault. Following treatment in an intensive care unit (ICU), neurological and neuropsychiatry units, he has been discharged home. Angus experiences acute panic attacks and chronic anxiety. He is aware that he has lost his job, girlfriend and home since the accident, and becomes overwhelmed when thinking about who he used to be. When Angus has a panic attack, he comes to the accident and emergency department as he cannot think what else to do. He describes symptoms of panic, and occasionally thoughts about ending his life, but he has no specific suicidal plan. His community mental health nurse has attempted some problem solving and cognitive–behavioural interventions to help Angus manage his anxiety, but he cannot remember what he has been taught and feels angry and guilty about not knowing what to do. Angus has given permission for his case to be used here, and his name has been changed to protect his anonymity. ∎

CONCLUSION

This chapter has looked at how people with intellectual impairment who generally have more complex health needs than those of the general population now utilize mainstream hospital services to a greater degree. Evidence suggests that such mainstream NHS services are ill equipped to care for this client group and the patient journey from arrival to discharge has been discussed in some detail and suggestions have been made for improvement.

Healthcare professionals require creativity and flexibility when working with people who have intellectual impairments within mainstream services. They are the chameleons who need to adapt as individuals and organizations in order to meet the needs of this patient group when they utilize our services.

REFERENCES AND RECOMMENDED READING

Barriball KL, Clark LL. (2005) All pre-registration students should develop skills in learning disabilities. *British Journal of Nursing* 14(3):166–9.

Bradley E. (2002) *Guidelines for Managing the Patient with Intellectual Disability in Accident and Emergency.* http://www.intellectualdisability.info/how_to/P_AandE_eb.html

Bradley E, Lofchy J. (2005) Learning disability in the accident and emergency department. *Advances in Psychiatric Treatment* 11:45–57.

Brophy M. (2005) *Truth Hurts: Report of the National Inquiry into Self-Harm among Young People.* London: Camelot Foundation and The Mental Health Foundation.

Brown M. (2005) Emergency care for people with learning disabilities: what all nurses and midwives need to know. *Accident and Emergency Nursing* 13(4):224 31.

Brylewski J, Duggan L. (2006) Antipsychotic medication for challenging behaviour in people with learning disability. *Cochrane Database of Systematic Reviews.*

Cambridge P, Carpenter P, Forrester-Jones R, Tate A, Knapp M, Beecham J, Hallam A. (2005) The state of care management in learning disability and mental health services 12 years into community care. *British Journal of Social Work* 35:1039–62.

Cogher L. (2005) Communication and people with learning disabilities. In: Grant G, Goward P, Richardson M, Ramcharan P. (eds), *Learning Disability: A Life Cycle Approach to Valuing People.* Maidenhead: Open University Press, 260–84.

Department of Health (2001) *Valuing People: A New Strategy for Learning Disability for the 21st Century.* London: The Stationery Office.

Department of Health (2003) *Discharge from Hospital: Pathway, Process and Practice.* London: The Stationery Office.

Dinsdale P. (2001) Learning disability nurses start liaison service in local hospital. *Learning Disability Practice* 4(4):5.

Glasby AM. (2002) Meeting the needs of people with learning disabilities in acute care. *British Journal of Nursing* 11(21):1389–92.

Halliday S, Mackrell K. (1998) Psychological interventions in self-injurious behaviour. Working with people with a learning disability. *British Journal of Psychiatry* 172:395–400.

Harker-Longton W, Fish R. (2002) 'Cutting doesn't make you die': one woman's view on the treatment of her self-injurious behaviour. *Journal of Learning Disabilities* (now *Journal of Intellectual Disabilities*) 6(2):137–51.

Hassiotis A, Hall I. (2006) Behavioural and cognitive–behavioural interventions for outwardly-directed aggressive behaviour in people with learning disabilities. *Cochrane Database of Systematic Reviews.*

Iacono T, Davis R. (2003) The experiences of people with developmental disability in emergency departments and hospital wards. *Research in Developmental Disabilities* 24:247–64.

Lovell A. (2004) Learning disabilities: people with learning disabilities who engage in self-injury. *British Journal of Nursing* 13(14):839–44.

McClintock K, Hall S, Oliver C. (2003) Risk markers associated with challenging behaviours in people with intellectual disabilities: a meta-analytic study. *Journal of Intellectual Disability Research* 47(6):405–16.

Mencap (1998) *The NHS – Health for All? People with Learning Disabilities and Health Care.* London: Mencap.

Merrick J, Kandel I, Birnbaum L, Hyam E, Press J, Morad M. (2004) Adolescent injury risk behaviour. *International Journal of Adolescent Medicine and Health* 16(3):207–13.

Morgan C, Ahmed Z, Kerr M. (2000) Health care provision for people with learning disability: record-linkage study of epidemiology and factors contributing to hospital care uptake. *British Journal of Psychiatry* 176:37–41.

NHS Health Scotland (2004) *People with Learning Disabilities in Scotland: The Health Needs Assessment Report.* Glasgow: NHS Health Scotland.

National Institute for Clinical Excellence (2004) *Self-harm: The Short-term Physical and Psychological Management and Secondary Prevention of Self-harm in Primary Care.* London: NICE.

National Patient Safety Agency (2004) *Understanding the Patient Safety Issues for People with Learning Disabilities.* London: NPSA.

Naylor MD, Brooten D, Campbell R, Jacobsen BS, Mezey MD, Pauly MV, Swartz JS. (1999) Comprehensive discharge planning and home follow-up of hospitalised elders. *Journal of the American Medical Association* 281(7):613–20.

Noonan I. (2004) Therapeutic management of attempted suicide and self-harm. In: Norman I, Ryrie I (eds), *The Art and Science of Mental Health Nursing: A Textbook of Principles and Practice.* Maidenhead: Open University Press, 747–70.

Northway R, Hutchinson C, Kingdon A. (2006) *Shaping the Future: A Vision for Learning Disability Nursing.* London: UK Learning Disability Consultant Nurse Network.

Oliver C, Petty J. (2002) Self-injurious behaviour in people with intellectual disability. *Current Opinion in Psychiatry* 15(5):477–81.

Patja K, Molsa P, Iivanainen M. (2001) Cause-specific mortality of people with intellectual disability in a population-based, 35-year follow-up study. *Journal of Intellectual Disability Research* 45(1):30–40.

Phillips J. (2004) Risk assessment and management of suicide and self-harm: within a forensic learning disability setting. *Learning Disability Practice* 7(2):12–18.

Priest H, Gibbs M. (2004) *Mental Health Care for People with Learning Disabilities.* Edinburgh: Churchill Livingstone.

Prochaska JO, DiClemente CC, Norcross JC. (1993) In search of how people change: applications to addictive behaviours. *Addiction Nursing Network* 5(1):2–16.

Regnard C, Reynolds J, Watson B, Matthews D, Gibson L, Clarke C. (2006) Understanding distress in people with severe communication difficulties: developing and assessing the Disability Distress Assessment Tool (DisDAT). *Journal of Intellectual Disability Research.* doi: 10.111/j.1365-2788.2006.00875.x

Riemsma RP, Forbes CA, Glanville JM, Eastwood AJ, Kleijnen J. (2001) General health status measures for people with cognitive impairment, learning disability and acquired brain injury. *Health Technology Assessment* 5(6):1–100.

Scottish Executive (2002) *Promoting Health, Supporting Inclusion: The National Review of the Contribution of all Nurses and Midwives to the Care and Support of People with Learning Disabilities.* Edinburgh: Scottish Executive.

Sherrard J, Tonge BJ, Ozanne-Smith J. (2002) Injury risk in young people with intellectual disability. *Journal of Intellectual Disability Research* 46(1):6–16.

Sherrard J, Ozanne-Smith J, Staines C. (2004) Prevention of unintentional injury to people with intellectual disability: a review of the evidence. *Journal of Intellectual Disability Research* 48(7):639–45.

Sowney M, Barr OG. (2006) Caring for adults with intellectual disabilities: perceived challenges for nurses in accident and emergency units. *Journal of Advanced Nursing* 55(1):36–45.

Weber MT. (2002) Triggers for self-abuse: a qualitative study. *Archives of Psychiatric Nursing* 16(3):118–24.

Wisely J, Hare DJ, Fernandez-Ford L. (2002) A study of the topography and nature of self-injurious behaviour in people with learning disabilities. *Journal of Learning Disabilities* (now *Journal of Intellectual Disabilities*) 6(1):61–71.

CHAPTER 8
ADMISSION TO ACUTE MENTAL HEALTH SERVICES

Mary O'Toole, Mike Reid and Rob Winterhalder

STUDY AIMS:

1. To learn about ways of assessing people who have intellectual impairments on acute mental health wards.

2. To consider some of the psychosocial interventions that can be used with people who have intellectual impairments on acute mental health wards.

3. To understand the legal issues and the interface between capacity and mental health legislation.

4. To explore different care issues for people with intellectual impairments in acute mental health care, including service issues and training.

The care of people with intellectual impairment is part of the everyday work of any acute mental health ward. In addition to those with known learning disabilities, acquired brain injury or dementia, acute mental illness of any form can have a negative impact on cognitive functioning. Depressed, hypomanic, anxious or psychotic people all have difficulties with a range of cognitive activities including attention, recall and processing. People who suffer the long-term consequences of schizophrenia are well known to be at greater risk of chronic cognitive impairment and there is increasing evidence that cognitive deficits precede the symptoms of schizophrenia in many individuals (Fearon

Learning Disability and other Intellectual Impairments, Edited by L.L. Clark and P. Griffiths
© 2008 John Wiley & Sons, Ltd

and Murray, 2002). Severe bipolar disorder may also be associated with long-term cognitive deficits (Osuji and Cullum, 2005). The teams working on mental health units are therefore used to working with individuals who have intellectual impairment in the broad sense used in this book.

However, it is not just those people whose intellectual impairment is related to their mental illness who are admitted to acute mental health units. People with mild or moderate learning disabilities are frequently admitted for assessment and/or treatment of mental health problems. Occasionally, people with more severe learning disabilities or with neuropsychiatric and neurodegenerative illnesses are admitted. Whilst the presence of people admitted to generic mental health units with cognitive impairment related to mental illness is uncontroversial, that of people with even mild learning disability or other types of intellectual impairment is often contested. Perceptions that these people are different, perhaps 'difficult' and that they belong elsewhere (in 'specialist' units) can undermine effective care. Along with genuine differences in the way people with intellectual impairment present, these perceptions leave ward staff feeling unskilled and unsupported. The effect on the service user is worse – they may feel unwanted, misunderstood and marginalized.

In this chapter we concentrate on how to help teams work with people with mild to moderate intellectual impairment. We believe that the teams working on acute mental health units already possess many of the skills required to work effectively with all people who have intellectual impairment, because they are currently working with those who have cognitive deficits, and such skills are transferable. In addition, insights can be applied from research within the field of learning or intellectual disability. This chapter is therefore intended to outline and apply some of those insights to the assessment and treatment of someone with intellectual impairment admitted to a mental health ward and to suggest ways that care can be organized to ensure it is both effective and inclusive.

People are admitted to acute mental health wards for a variety of reasons. In all cases some form of mental health problem is either already identified or at least suspected. But it is unusual for the main driver for an admission to be solely the assessment or treatment of mental illness. There is usually a breakdown in social functioning and some form of risk to self or to others, which necessitates admission to hospital. Consequently, two fundamental aims of the assessment process are the assessment of the mental illness itself and of the social and/or risk factors.

In some cases it may turn out that there is no mental illness and that the admission is related to the individual's intellectual impairment alone, or to other factors, such as difficult social circumstances, cultural misunderstanding or malingering. Sometimes assessment and treatment of the mental illness alone is enough to alleviate the social difficulties that precipitated the admission. However, in many cases changes have to take place in a variety of aspects of the individual's life in order to discharge the service user back into some form of normal living in the community. Changes might include adressing problem behaviours, physical health problems or difficulties in relationships. Some may be central to the reason for admission and some may be incidental. Moreover, rather than just identifying *problems* it is important to establish areas of strength in the individual's life. These can be built into resources to help the person enjoy a more productive or enjoyable life.

THE ASSESSMENT PROCESS

An assessment of someone with intellectual impairment admitted to an inpatient mental health unit includes identification of:

- The extent of any intellectual impairment
- Underlying mental health problems (Mental State Examination – MSE)
- Physical health problems

- Behavioural problems which pose difficulties for the individual or for those they are in contact with

- Risk of harm to the individual or to others

- The individual's social circumstances and their relationships with others, including work and leisure activities

- The individual's quality of life, including their subjective expression of satisfaction with their life (or happiness).

When someone is admitted to an acute mental health ward, it may or may not be known whether they have some form of intellectual impairment. They may come in with a well documented history of developmental disorder, or acquired brain injury, or a clear cut case of cognitive impairment owing to chronic mental illness. Equally, they may have never been assessed for intellectual impairment, they may be new to the country or have navigated the first few years of their life without their intellectual impairment being identified. They may have a chronic mental illness which only now is beginning to significantly affect their cognitive functioning. This intellectual impairment may be readily apparent on first contact, or may take some time to unravel, perhaps being confused with mental illness.

It is not intended that this chapter should include a large amount of coverage in the assessment of specific intellectual impairment per se. The assessments of learning disability, neuro-psychiatric deficits or dementias form their own psychiatric specialties and there are large literatures for each. The assessment of borderline learning disability or cognitive impairment related to chronic mental illness is more contentious. Nevertheless, there are established neuro-psychological tests which psychologists can carry out to aid assessment, in addition to the well known, but limited, Mini-Mental State Examination. Brain scans such as MRI (Magnetic Resonance Imaging) may also be able to detect changes in the brain's structure giving clues that there are changes in cognitive functioning. Nevertheless, determining such changes may do little to inform which interventions can help the individual who is experiencing the results of such alterations. Therefore this chapter contents itself with addressing two main areas: the assessment of mental illness in someone with concomitant intellectual impairment; and the assessment of the broader needs of that person.

Identifying the biological, psychological and sociocultural factors which make up each individual is often a complex task. Adding intellectual impairment into the mix brings not only any primary deficit, but also, and often even more significantly, differences in life history, relationships and social inclusion. This adds another level of complexity that can leave the care team feeling overwhelmed and deskilled in its attempts to understand the service user. Some of the challenges affecting this process include:

- Disentangling intellectual impairment from mental illness, often confused due to 'diagnostic overshadowing'

- Differences in ways of communicating, leading to symptoms of mental illness (and also physical ill health) being expressed by changes in behaviour

- Differences in behaviour being misunderstood as symptoms of mental illness

- Differing effects of life events

- The effect of the setting itself.

DIAGNOSTIC OVERSHADOWING

'Diagnostic overshadowing' was first described by Reiss in the 1980s who was considering the way that the diagnosis of 'learning disability' affects the diagnosis of mental illness (Reiss *et al*, 1982). It can be thought of as having dual aspects; primarily it is the idea that professionals may attribute behaviour in individuals with learning disability as being due to that learning disability, rather than to a symptom of mental illness. Hence they fail to recognize a mental illness in the individual. For example, someone who becomes more talkative, sleeps less, and becomes sexually disinhibited is described as having a behavioural disturbance related to their learning disability, rather than being assessed as hypomanic. This can help explain why, historically, the existence of affective disorders in people with learning disability was denied. The second aspect of diagnostic overshadowing is that professionals may recognize a symptom as being caused by mental illness (e.g. depression manifested as increasing social isolation) but downplay its significance compared to the person's learning disability (Mason and Scior, 2004). This translates in very real terms into denial of treatment for someone or the refusal to accept someone affected by learning disability into a generic service for mental illness.

Some authors have doubted the generalisability of these studies to real clinical settings as they have generally been demonstrated via analogue studies in which clinicians are asked to make diagnoses on the basis of vignettes. Studies have appeared to demonstrate that the effect is only applied when assessing people with an IQ of less than 70 (Mason and Scior, 2004). It is possible that greater awareness of the issues involved in diagnostic overshadowing may have improved the accuracy of diagnosis. A study by Hurley *et al.* (2003) examining real clinical situations (the diagnosis of depression in a US outpatients department) failed to find evidence of diagnostic overshadowing affecting diagnosis, but they did find that caregivers who accompanied people with learning disabilities to clinics tended to describe the symptoms of their relative or client as behavioural problems (such as aggression or somatic complaints), whilst the subsequent diagnosis was of depression or anxiety. This suggests that whilst diagnostic overshadowing may not always operate in the consulting room or ward round, it may be more prevalent to the broader care team. Individual behaviours may still be attributed to learning disability rather than as an expression of a mental illness. Moreover, Jopp and Keys (2001) reviewed a number of studies of diagnostic overshadowing and concluded that the concept did exert a robust influence on diagnosis.

THE ROLE OF COMMUNICATION

Traditionally mental health assessment relies heavily on the verbal expression of symptoms by the person assessed. This is either at the level of accepting at face value the problem expressed by the service user, or by using verbal communication as a clue to indicate what is happening with someone, for example, through their expression of delusional ideas. For people with communication difficulties who cannot express themselves well as a result of intellectual impairment this may compound the assessment process – Sovner's *intellectual distortion*.

Sovner (1986) suggested four ways in which assessment might be compromised when working with those with learning disability:

1. **Intellectual distortion**: due to deficits relating to the intellectual impairment, individuals cannot communicate their emotions or thoughts. Symptoms are less likely to be elicited verbally, particularly using conventional interviews.

2. **Psychosocial masking**: because of reduced social skills or reduced exposure to social interaction symptoms may present as less detailed or 'rich' as for those without intellectual impairment.

3. **Cognitive disintegration**: the process whereby anxiety becomes overwhelming and thus bizarre, and apparently 'psychotic' behaviours, may arise. People with intellectual impairment are likely to have a lower threshold for this to happen.

4. **Baseline exaggeration**: occurs when existing behaviours or deficits increase due to another pathology such as depression, potentially leading to diagnostic overshadowing.

For people with Asperger's syndrome or other autistic spectrum disorder there may be relatively specific difficulties with understanding or expression. They can cause problems in comprehending non-verbal cues from assessors, or in a lack of understanding of the metaphorical or idiomatic usage of words, the avoidance of eye contact is also problematic in these service users. They may have difficulties in addressing the issues questioned on, and instead discuss apparently unconnected topics.

EXERCISE

Consider some of the issues that may be problematic in the assessment process in a patient who has autism or Asperger's syndrome. How can the assessor overcome some of these barriers? ■

Hints for successful assessment of people with autism:

1. Ensure a quiet, undisturbed environment, without interruption.

2. Keep your voice modulated and not high-pitched.

3. Do not make sudden movements.

4. Avoid metaphors and idiomatic use of language, people with autism will always make 'literal interpretations'.

5. Avoid touch as many people with autism feel extremely uncomfortable with this.

6. Eye contact may be problematic and many of these patients will wish to avoid it.

7. Do not rely on cues generated by body language as people with autism find difficulty in interpretation.

8. Attempt to 'steer' the conversation back to the subject in hand if the patient discusses other interests (which is a common problem).

9. Speak to carers first and discover any rituals or routines that the patient may have and do not try to prevent the patient carrying them out during the interview as they often provide comfort in unfamiliar surroundings.

For further reading see Shellenbarger (2004) who gives a simple discussion of this which can aid the assessing professional.

For others with less clear-cut differences in functioning and communication, assessment may accordingly be more complex. In the absence of effective verbal communication distress or illness are often communicated by behaviour. It is increasingly being understood that people with intellectual impairment may change their behaviour as a result of a mental illness. For example, depression may manifest itself in agitated behaviour, perhaps with an increase in someone's normal pattern of self-injurious behaviour (**baseline exaggeration**).

For teams used to working with predominantly verbal expressions of symptoms this may appear challenging; making the service user's internal world inaccessible, and subsequently, the patient becomes more problematic to help. But at times, most of us communicate our distress behaviourally rather than verbally. For example, we shout at those close to us when we ourselves are upset, or withdraw into ourselves if we are angry at what is going on around us. This is the phenomenon of 'acting out', often regarded as complex behaviour manifested by those with intact cognitive functioning. Teams working on acute mental health units are used to interpreting behaviour as signs of underlying distress, even though it is easy to get entangled in the behaviour by responding to it rather than to the underlying problem. The fundamental approach of 'thinking' about what is going on rather than accepting it at face value is equally applicable to those with intellectual impairment.

In an attempt to interpret such behaviour, one can look for altered behaviours which may indicate underlying depression. These might include losing one's temper, increased or altered self-injurious behaviour, changes in seeking social contact, an alteration in patterns of drug or alcohol misuse and so on. These might occur alongside more traditional symptoms such as loss of appetite, early morning wakening, feelings of worthlessness and so on. Assessment of someone with intellectual impairment therefore requires teams to actively consider whether what they are seeing is a behaviour that is related to someone's intellectual impairment directly, or to the circumstances in which they have found themselves, or alternatively to an underlying and unnoticed depressive illness. Robert's case study (Box 8.1) helps to understand this phenomenon.

Diagnostic overshadowing may occur when those behaviours are displayed on an acute mental health unit. The staff who are undertaking the assessment process may attribute these behaviours to the normal presentation of the person, and fail to spot that these are symptoms of an underlying episode of mental illness. Clearly it is difficult to attribute these behaviours to depression based on a 'one-off' assessment. What is vital here is to get a history of what has been happening over a period of weeks or months, in order to establish changes that have taken place during that time, which may indicate the onset of an illness. Such a history can be difficult for the service user themselves to give and often only a 'collateral history' involving carers can give that with accuracy.

In Robert's case (Box 8.1) imagine how much harder it would be to make a diagnosis without the crucial history of change which staff were able to provide. For people with intellectual impairment, a significant amount of diagnosable illness may be missed if a collateral history is not obtained. Changes in behaviour within all settings should be noted, as well as more long-term changes, and, as stated above, events which may play a part in triggering illness or behaviour can be investigated. Carers' accounts may need to be interpreted with caution, however. For those living with family carers external circumstances in a carer's own life may affect their ability to care for someone, and they may (perhaps without even realizing what they are doing) describe this as a worsening condition in the service user rather than in their capacity to provide care. Cooper *et al* (2003, p.5) note that imperfect communication within teams as well as inexperience or lack of observation skills of professional carers may affect the ability to give reliable histories. Additionally, Chaplin and Flynn (2000) point out that listening to parents may exclude some vital information – for example, 'illicit' sexual encounters.

Hamilton *et al* (2005) confirmed previous associations between life events and emotional or behavioural disturbances. They also found differences between different groups with regard to the strength of this effect – people with mild learning disability appeared to be more affected by

BOX 8.1   **ROBERT**

Robert is a 35-year-old man, living in a residential home, housing 12 clients, all with moderate to severe intellectual impairment. Robert is an easy-going person, popular with both staff and residents, recently, however, he has appeared to be irritable and has frequently lost his temper over relatively minor events such as television and mealtime choices. Staff have also become concerned as they have started to notice superficial cuts on Robert's arms. He will not talk about the cuts when asked and has become even more irritable if pushed, resulting in some minor damage to property on two occasions. He seems to have lost his appetite, merely picking at his food at meal times and consequently has lost weight.

Following a client review meeting, Robert is referred to the local mental health team for an assessment, they conclude that he has a depressive illness which requires treatment. He is prescribed an antidepressant and referred for cognitive behavioural therapy. After two months Robert has become a lot less irritable and more like his former, easy-going self. His appetite has improved and he is now interacting more with staff and fellow residents. Staff notice that there are no new cuts on Robert's arms. ◼

events than people with autism. It seems reasonable to suspect that people with other cognitive impairments (such as those with chronic schizophrenia) may react in a similar way. One key difference between people with intellectual impairment and others is their ability to link what is happening in their lives to how they feel. For example, a care worker leaving the care establishment in which someone lives may be a significant loss to that individual. This can impact on the individual's behaviour or even trigger an episode of mental illness such as depression or even psychosis. However, they may be unable to make the link between the loss and how they are feeling, forcing the assessors to discover the link for them.

One of the most significant life events that someone can face is bereavement. Dodd *et al* (2005) reviewed evidence that grief can bring up a range of behavioural and emotional disturbances for people with learning disabilities. They found that conventional scales were not effective in assessing this and suggested other methods such as using drawing or other non-verbal methods. What is unclear is whether this 'traumatic grief' forms a distinct condition or whether it triggers 'depression', and this requires more research in order to inform treatment options.

When working with someone who is of a different cultural background to one's own collateral history-taking becomes even more important. There is very little literature in working cross-culturally with people with intellectual impairment. In any circumstances speaking to families or friends from the same culture, or to other agencies who might support individuals outside the dominant culture with mental health problems, is important, but it may be doubly so when working with someone with intellectual impairment.

Other communication difficulties may have a psychosocial or cultural origin, and reflect the different life history of the service users compared with a professional. A history of abuse, in an institutional context, for example, is likely to negatively influence communication with other health or social care professionals. Indeed the setting in which assessment takes place may significantly affect the assessment. Acute mental health wards are often chaotic places with high numbers of distressed and sometimes aroused service users. They are often poorly decorated environments clearly identifiable as hospitals rather than homes.

The lack of the usual structure and of familiar faces may be difficult for those with even a mild or moderate intellectual impairment who live in care or family homes. The dramatically different environment may result in a disturbance of behaviour which can compound the assessment process further still. Additionally there is a concern that some people with intellectual impairment may repeat what others say (echolalia) and therefore may seem to present with symptoms such as 'hearing voices'. Nevertheless, if someone is admitted to an acute mental health unit, the assessment is necessarily going to be in that environment and so teams there must develop the skills in determining an accurate diagnoses whatever the setting.

ASSESSMENT TOOLS AND TECHNIQUES

So far two ways have been discussed in order to improve the accuracy and validity of assessment: an emphasis on taking a careful history and the bilateral use of a collateral history provided by family or others, albeit used with care is recommended. Whilst history is important, face-to-face assessment is, of course, equally so and the Mental State Examination (MSE) forms a key part of that process.

The Royal College of Psychiatrists (2001) has produced a classification of mental health diagnoses for people with 'learning disabilities/mental retardation' the 'DC-LD'. This typology was found in a study by Cooper *et al* (2003, p.3) to have a 96.3% concordance rate with clinical opinion. The DC-LD also suggests ways in which the standard interview can be adapted to aid accurate assessment of those with learning disability and some of these principles can be applied to those with other forms of intellectual impairment.

Usual good practice, such as allowing sufficient time, in a quiet area with no interruptions or noise is especially important when assessing people with intellectual impairment. Questioning should use straightforward language, avoiding multiple questions and overly abstract concepts. Interviews must take into account the nature of the impairment: is there a problem with hearing impairment, or understanding? Is the person using a word they have heard without a full understanding of it? Are social cues being misunderstood? Is the person saying 'yes' because of the need to agree with someone whom they feel is in 'authority'?

Both 'open' and 'closed' questioning should be adopted, rephrased from time to time to check understanding. Questions should be short and address one concept only (no multiple questioning). Open questions such as 'Is anyone against you?' allow the person space to reveal a possible delusional content, and the question is straightforward and easy to understand. Closed questions can be used to check against this, with either/or questions being effective whilst yes/no questions may lead to acquiescence rather than information. The use of other non-verbal methods such as drawing or pictures is also helpful in certain circumstances. For a more detailed discussion see Chaplin and Flynn (2000, p.132) and Raghavan and Patel (2005, pp.47–87).

Other ways of improving assessment for many groups of people with intellectual impairment include the use of rating scales or other tools, either generic or specially designed for those with learning disability. An excellent overview is given in Priest and Gibbs (2004). Examples include the Psychiatric Assessment Schedule for Adults with Developmental Disabilities (PAS-ADD), which aids diagnosis by asking questions in broad areas such as mood, anxiety symptoms and psychosis (Moss *et al* 1998 and other papers cited in Priest and Gibbs, 2004, p.95). This particular tool is composed of three parts, the first two use the clinicians' input to screen service users for mental health problems and then elucidate symptoms and possible triggers. The third part is a semi-structured clinical interview with the service user and clinician which then produces an ICD-10 diagnosis (Priest and Gibbs, 2004, p.98). Whilst total reliance on these tools is not recommended, they can aid accurate assessment in many circumstances. It is important that they are performed by people who have had specific training in their use. Their interpretation (and that of the rest of the assessment process) should, however, be placed in the broader context – that of the 'whole person'.

RISK ASSESSMENT

Risk assessment for mental health service users has received a huge amount of attention in both the academic and lay literature in the past few years. A number of tools to systematically assess risk to self or more particularly to others have been developed both locally and in the wider context. Less attention has been given to the application of those tools to people with intellectual impairment. Whilst there is an oft cited link between low IQ and an increased risk of offending, only a few empirical studies have addressed this. In particular, there is no specialist tool for assessing risk of violence in people with learning disability or intellectual impairment. Factors such as a perceived increase in impulsivity, poor impulse control, and limited ability to learn from the environment or to absorb normative morals have been cited as reasons why people with intellectual impairment are more likely to harm others.

Yet a review by Johnston (2002) of risk assessment in people with 'intellectual disability' found few studies to provide an evidence base to quantify this. No major studies or random control trials were found. Thus the question of whether tools designed for the general adult population can be applied to people with intellectual impairment remains unanswered. Within the wider literature of risk assessment the use of actuarial versus clinical measures of risk is debated: that is, methods based on a range of objective demographic and clinical data as opposed to specific assessment methods based on current clinical presentation. The lack of any validated 'actuarial' tools suggested to Johnston that much risk assessment of people with intellectual impairment was done using clinical models (Johnston, 2002, p.50). A number of conflicting and confounding factors that might affect assessment were outlined. Some issues suggested underestimation of risk: a resistance to prosecute 'vulnerable people'; 'under-diagnosis, minimization of offence level and use of unfitness to plead'; and a belief that therapy will be effective. Other factors suggested overestimation: personal prejudice against those with intellectual impairment; and a variety of professionals' ideas about people with intellectual impairment including the concepts that inevitable deterioration of those with mental illness/intellectual impairment will occur (Johnston, 2002, pp.50–1).

The implications for the person with intellectual impairment admitted to an acute mental health unit are that it might be difficult to develop an objective appreciation of risk. Whilst there are a number of validated risk assessment tools for the general adult population – the 'HCR-20' (Webster et al, 1997) being one widely used tool – their validity for those with intellectual impairment is not confirmed. Less systematic approaches may be used, which pay closer attention to the individual and less to broader demographic data, but clinicians must be aware of the confounding variables described that may affect their assessment. Taylor (2002) adds a summary of research that indicated that the best way of establishing potential for aggression related to anger was (perhaps not surprisingly) to ask the service user to rate their own anger. Not only did this prove reliable and valid, but also opens up the potential for effective and collaborative interventions for that anger.

Risk plays a large part in modern discussion around mental health services, with services either criticized for not doing enough to reduce risk or to being preoccupied with risk and consequently failing in their duty to provide care rather than control. The received ideas or prejudices that teams or others have around people with intellectual impairment may amplify concerns over risk. Well meaning but ultimately regressive ideas that people with intellectual impairment need protecting from themselves may paralyse teams and prevent them from giving the freedom to make mistakes they would allow someone without intellectual impairment. The notion that someone has a 'mental age' below 16 can suggest that staff or carers are 'in loco parentis' of a child, acting (literally) paternalistically and reinforcing dependence.

Although this is not a fully validated *tool*, Boulter and Pointu (2006, pp.112–13) provide a more 'person-centred' *framework* for assessing and managing risk for people with intellectual disability. The framework looks at issues such as: who should be involved in assessing and managing the risk? What is the nature and extent of the risks involved? What could be the consequences of the risk; what would the individual miss out on if the risk were eliminated? How can the person be supported adequately in order to perform the issue concerned? How should the issue be documented and communicated? By using such a framework, involving relevant others in decision making and thinking about the pros and cons of the issue concerned, a more balanced and robust assessment and plan can develop. In order to do this, all aspects of the person must be considered – and critically, their emotional and social needs.

ASSESSMENT OF SPECIFIC DIAGNOSES

For many people with intellectual impairment, and in particular those with the ability to verbalize their feelings reasonably well, assessment of mood disorders follows a similar pattern as with the general population. Negative cognitions, psychomotor retardation, early morning wakening, social withdrawal, anhedonia, loss of appetite indicate depression, although being mindful of the occasional agitated depression in which the person is active rather than slowed down. Equally, mania follows similar lines as in the general population, such as an increase in activity, poor sleep and grandiose cognitions, although Priest and Gibbs (2004, p.56) state that often irritability rather than euphoria is a key sign. However, for some individuals the signs that someone is depressed are more likely to be read in their behaviour, and this may require careful consideration of their past history, which has been discussed above.

The assessment of psychosis or schizophrenia in people with intellectual impairment has some distinctive features. Assessing typical symptoms of schizophrenia such as hallucinations, delusions, formal thought disorder and the negative symptoms of apathy and withdrawal pose challenges for the clinician. It may be difficult to conclude that someone is definitely hallucinating if they are not able to communicate fluently, and equally, it may be difficult to establish thought disorder in someone whose thinking is already different.

EXERCISE

Consider how the presentation of hallucinations and delusions may differ in people who have intellectual impairment compared with the general population.

To what extent is diagnostic overshadowing problematic when assessing the possible presence of hallucinations and delusions? ■

As Levitas *et al* (2001, p.9) point out, people with learning disability are particularly prone to the 'auditorisation of thought', where one's own thoughts are interpreted as a voice. They state that these are reasonably easily distinguishable from true hallucinations because the former is experienced as inside rather than outside the head, and because the content is usually beneficial in the former and detrimental in the latter. In practice, however, it is often rather more difficult to make these distinctions and the question of whether a hallucination is 'real' or 'pseudo' often remains unanswerable.

Delusional thinking is another symptom which differs in people with learning disability. The historical position defines delusions as fixed false beliefs unavailable to reasoning and often bizarre. This position has been moderated to some extent by the discovery that techniques such as cognitive behavioural therapy (CBT) can not only render the belief rationally understandable, albeit in a unusual way, but also amenable to change. Delusional thinking has been reported to be particularly plastic in people with intellectual impairment. It is reported that people with some forms of intellectual impairment can be quite easily 'talked out' of a delusional belief, perhaps in order to acquiesce with authority.

The delusional beliefs of people with intellectual impairment may have different content to that of the general population, it may be particularly 'simple' due to limited verbal expression or differing life history. This may lead to it being dismissed as 'childish or manipulative behaviour' rather than as a delusion – Sovner's *psychosocial masking*. Paranoia may be manifested as social withdrawal and general behaviour change, rather than as symptom of psychosis if not verbalized. As Levitas *et al* (2001) point out, persecutory ideas may take the form of someone saying that others are 'bothering him'; whether or not that is a delusional belief may take careful investigation and may represent a genuine case of bullying.

Equally, differences in expression may mean that someone with an intellectual impairment may describe something in an unusual way, and incorrectly be interpreted as being deluded. Cooper *et al* (2003, p.6) note that people with intellectual impairment may well talk to themselves. It is common for this to be misinterpreted as 'responding to voices' by staff on acute mental health wards.

The negative symptoms of schizophrenia may be very difficult to distinguish from other behavioural changes, or of a depressive illness, particularly in the absence of positive symptoms such as hallucinations or delusions. A trial of treatment may be necessary in some circumstances in order to make an accurate diagnosis.

If the assessment of functional psychoses or mood disorders in people with intellectual impairment is complex, then even more so is that of personality disorder. As Raghavan and Patel point out (2005, p.73) the broad description of personality disorder is similar in many ways to the description of 'mental retardation' as discussed by DSM-IV-TR (American Psychiatric Association, 2000). Both represent a stable pattern of altered and socially abnormal behaviour which began prior to adulthood. In principle the two are usually distinguished by differences in aetiology. Learning disability is likely to be apparent at an earlier age than personality disorder. Other acquired forms of intellectual impairment occur later in life.

However, in practice, it may be difficult to establish whether an altered pattern of behaviour may by related to a primary intellectual impairment or to personality disorder. The diagnosis of 'organic personality disorder' may well be applied to many with intellectual impairment, in particular those with acquired brain injury. The use of other diagnoses such as emotionally unstable/ schizoid/dependent and so on are more contentious. Gagnon *et al* (2006) discuss at length the differential diagnosis of organic personality disorder and 'borderline personality disorder' for someone with acquired brain injury, a distinction that may well be useful for teams embroiled in the complex business of establishing how to help someone who has a change in behaviour after a brain injury, in addition to pre-existing disturbances.

Alexander and Cooray (2003) reviewed the literature addressing the diagnosis of personality disorder and extracted a number of themes. Some have questioned that people with intellectual impairment can be diagnosed fully as having a personality disorder, due to their difficulties with cognition and delayed development. Others point out that in the absence of clear cut verbalizations to aid diagnosis it is difficult to make a diagnosis based on behaviour alone, as altered behaviour may be described as a 'behavioural disorder' rather than a personality disorder – an example of diagnostic overshadowing. Equally there is a concern that some symptoms of personality disorder may be interpreted as a psychotic or affective illness thus misinforming treatment options, leading to treatment with psychotropic drugs when talking therapies may be more appropriate. Of course, as in the general population treatment of personality disorder may well include the pragmatic use of psychotropic drugs, but misdiagnosis may adversely affect treatment particularly in the face of a professional presumption against the benefits of talking therapies in people with intellectual impairment.

Flynn *et al* (2002) studied inpatients with intellectual impairment and challenging behaviour using a tool called the Standardized Assessment of Personality (SAP), a tool devised to measure personality disorder in those with 'learning disability'. They found that a significant proportion of their sample (39%) met the criteria for 'severe personality disorder' and found an association with childhood trauma a well known causative factor. This suggested to them that clinicians may need to think differently about treatment options for people with these diagnoses. In particular, they suggested that further evidence needed to be gathered to inform the most effective treatment, discussing the possibilities that psychotherapeutic, behavioural or pharmacological approaches to personality disorder could be applied to work with people with concomitant intellectual impairment .

HOLISTIC ASSESSMENT OF NEEDS

It is often not illness but 'behaviour' that brings people to acute mental health wards. Behaviour is likely to be a response by the individual to a range of factors. These would include the person's intellectual impairment, their mental health problems, their personality, thoughts and feelings; their physical health and their social situation. By viewing the behaviour as embedded within that environment, it can be seen as a response which makes sense given the circumstances around it. By changing those circumstances, it may be possible to change the behaviour. One way, of course, is to treat the mental illness and the behaviour may change. But another way to address the problem is through the technique of 'Functional Analysis'.

Assessment of the *physical health* of any person who is admitted to a mental health unit is a key priority both in its own right, but also as a potential cause of mental disorder. Infections, epilepsy and endocrine disorders often have a greater or idiosyncratic effect on people with intellectual impairment, and may be less likely to be identified by the person suffering them. The side effects of prescribed medication may also differ in people with intellectual impairment as Rob Winterhalder discusses in Chapter 9. In addition the reader is strongly advised to refer to Chapter 2, where physical health is addressed in detail.

Mental health units assess service users' needs as part of their local 'Care Programme Approach' and/or assessing them against their local authority's eligibility criteria for access to services. These assessments are likely to be generic, aimed at picking up the broad spectrum of health and social needs, so will not be focused specifically on the needs of people with intellectual impairment.

Raghavan and Patel (2005, p.100) describe a number of more rigid attempts to systematize the needs assessment of people with intellectual disability. The familiar Camberwell Assessment of Need (Phelan *et al*, 1995) has been adapted by Xenitidis *et al* (2000) for people with learning disabilities. Raghavan and Patel further describe Marshall *et al*'s (1995) four-stage model of a needs assessment which can be applied to those with intellectual impairment. This uses various assessment tools to identify needs in either the clinical domain (anxiety, sensory impairment, socially embarrassing behaviour being three such categories) or the social domain (domestic skills, social life and safety, for example). These 'cardinal needs' can then be used to inform subsequent interventions.

Systematic tools such as these provide excellent ways to measure needs of populations, to measure the effects on individuals of psychosocial intervention or on which to base decisions about eligibility for services. They can be studied across many individuals and their validity and reliability determined. What they are not so good at is helping to make sense of the individual's social and emotional needs or addressesing their own feelings about those needs. For example, high scores on some social criteria might suggest that someone requires high level of supported accommodation whilst a fiercely independent person may wish to continue to live alone despite the risks or problems that that entails. Needs assessments must be balanced with the service user's wishes, along with the wishes of any carers they may have and any identified risks.

Assessment of the holistic needs of the service user is intended to inform the use of interventions by mental health staff. Whilst it is often assumed that interventions start when assessment stops, in fact there is a much more dynamic relationship between the two. Intervention may begin the moment someone walks into a ward, depending on the level of distress experienced by the service user, or the interactions they have with others. The effects of interventions are monitored and this feeds back into the assessment process which should always be an ongoing process.

PSYCHOSOCIAL INTERVENTIONS

This section will briefly address some of the psychosocial and psychotherapeutic interventions aimed at helping those who are experiencing specific symptoms of mental ill health, in addition to their intellectual impairment, which might be used in the context of an acute mental health inpatient setting. In Chapter 9, Rob Winterhalder discusses the use of biological treatments more widely, whilst in Chapter 10, Michael Kelly examines physical restraint and de-escalation in relation to challenging behaviour.

Individuals with an intellectual impairment often have difficulties communicating their needs clearly, resulting in the individual experiencing feelings of disempowerment with the potentially negative consequences of anger, violence and other challenging behaviours. It is likely that this situation could very easily be exacerbated within the chaotic and often highly charged atmosphere of an acute mental health ward. Indeed, a review by Chaplin (2004) concluded that people with intellectual impairment appear to be inadequately catered for in general mental health services. Patients with intellectual impairment admitted to general mental health wards were more likely to be restrained, secluded or given emergency medication. They were also at higher risk of being assaultive than those without an intellectual impairment.

Just as assessment is compromised when working with those with learning disability through intellectual distortion, psychosocial masking, cognitive disintegration and baseline exaggeration these same factors, compounded by communication difficulties, will also affect a person's ability to engage in psychosocial interventions and consequently may limit the effectiveness of those interventions. Indeed, clinicians will make choices in terms of the type of treatment intervention depending on the way the client is presenting and expressing their problems. A challenge for mental health clinicians working in acute inpatient settings, therefore, is to work with a range of therapeutic intervention strategies and explore how these might be adapted to meet the needs of people with intellectual impairments.

COGNITIVE BEHAVIOURAL THERAPY

Historically, clinicians have been reluctant to engage in cognitive behavioural therapy (CBT) with clients who have intellectual impairment due to beliefs that these individuals are unable to recognize or express mental distress in a meaningful way. More recently, however, attitudes are beginning to change and there is emerging support and acceptance for the use of CBT in people with intellectual impairment and a variety of concurrent mental health problems.

Cognitive behavioural therapists recommend that a person with an intellectual impairment is assessed in a number of areas including communication skills, cognitive aptitude and capacity to identify emotions, before engagement in CBT can take place (Hatton, 2002). For example, the person engaging in therapy will need both receptive and expressive language skills (Black *et al*, 1997). They will need to be able to monitor their own emotions, thoughts and behaviours and recognize when symptoms get better or worse and they will also require sufficient memory skills in order to carry out 'homework' tasks. Other clinicians (Dagnan and Chadwick, 1997) have argued that people with intellectual impairment may have difficulty in both identifying and labelling their emotions and may oversimplify them by labelling feelings as either 'happy' or 'sad'. In these cases simple line drawings might be used whereby emotions are represented by happy and sad faces along a continuum. Hollins *et al* (1995) describe the use of picture books for patients with limited verbal skills (for example, *Feeling Blue*, which is a story about a man recovering from depression).

A small number of case studies have demonstrated the efficacy of modified CBT for adults with mild/moderate intellectual impairment and a diagnosis of depression. Improvements were noted in daily monitoring of depressive feelings and there were improvements in crying behaviour and behavioural signs of depression (Lindsay *et al*, 1993; Dagnan and Chadwick, 1997).

Cognitive behavioural interventions can also be effective in treating the hallucinations and delusions associated with schizophrenia. Clients are encouraged to view auditory hallucinations as their own thoughts and then challenge them in order to reduce the stress that they cause. There is, to date, however, only minimal evidence examining the use of CBT for people with intellectual impairment and psychosis (Hatton, 2002). CBT has also been shown to be effective for anger management of clients with intellectual impairment (Rose *et al*, 2000; Lindsay *et al*, 1989). Howells *et al* (2000) describe a CBT approach where clients were taught skills around recognizing feelings in others, recognizing signs of anger in themselves, possible triggers and exploring the consequences of anger. Through the use of role-play and videos, clients were taught to employ alternatives to anger and aggression such as assertiveness, negotiation and problem solving. A number of case studies have also been reported that demonstrate a reduction in anger and aggressive behaviour after cognitive behavioural interventions had been used (Black and Novaco, 1993; Murphy and Clare, 1991).

Despite the promising evidence from case studies there remains a paucity of large-scale controlled trials examining the effectiveness in the use of CBT with people who have mental health problems and intellectual impairment and further research is indicated.

PSYCHOTHERAPY

In contrast to CBT, psychodynamic interventions aim to address a person's underlying problems rather than their actual symptoms and behaviour. They are typically used to help treat depression and anxiety problems. Clients are encouraged to develop insight into their problems and work at changing their feelings and behaviours through the therapeutic relationship. Historically, therapists have been reluctant to engage in psychotherapeutic interventions with people with intellectual impairment owing to the erroneous belief that these individuals lack the intelligence to express their emotions and develop the necessary insight. Individuals with intellectual impairment were often seen to express their emotions through aggression.

As with CBT, this view is now being challenged as it is recognized that people with intellectual impairment do experience emotional distress and suffer difficulty in talking about emotions as do the general population. Moreover, Gravestock (1995) argues that people with intellectual impairment may well be more willing to share their feelings and 'open up' than those without impairment as they lack the usual defence mechanisms. Again, there is little research into the effectiveness of psychosocial interventions (Oliver *et al*, 2003; Hatton, 2002) and what is available is limited to case studies and small uncontrolled trials.

LEGAL ISSUES

Central to any therapeutic relationship between a clinician and a patient is the tension between the autonomy of the patient and a clinician's duty of care. The moral dilemmas which can occur can usually be resolved by adhering to professional codes of practice which are underpinned by a common set of ethical principles. Ultimately, a clinician must respect a patient's decision to, for instance, not accept treatment as long as the patient has the capacity to make an informed decision on this point.

People with intellectual impairment are at risk of developing additional mental illnesses or behaviour disorders which may require further assessment and treatment under the Mental Health Act. In addition, either as a result of the intellectual impairment per se or because of additional mental illness, they may temporarily or permanently develop cognitive impairments which are severe enough to interfere with their capacity to make certain informed decisions. In the field of intellectual impairment the two acts which are most relevant are the 1983 Mental Health Act and the Mental Capacity Act 2005 (Chapter 11 considers the Mental Capacity Act in more detail, especially as it relates to the definition of capacity and consent to physical care.)

MENTAL HEALTH ACT (1983)

This act is the legislation concerning the formal detention into hospital care of mentally disordered people. The act is split into ten parts covering various aspects of detention and care, and each part is further split into numbered paragraphs which have become known as 'sections', hence the term to 'section' someone into hospital.

The Mental Health Act (1983) specified four categories for mental disorder: mental illness, mental impairment, severe mental impairment and psychopathic disorder. The 2007 act has done away with these categories in favour of a generic definition of mental disorder as 'any disorder or disability of the mind'. Drug or alcohol dependence are explicitly excluded as mental disorders so that no one may be detained solely to treat their dependence on alcohol or other substances.

The intention in removing the categories was to prevent arbitrary exclusion of mental disorders which did not fit into the previous categories and so is very relevant to the detention and treatment of people with intellectual impairment. In particular, people suffering acquired brain injury are likely now to be covered by this definition, alongside learning disability and mental illness. However, the act is not intended to be used to detain those who suffer disorders of the brain, unless they 'affect the mind'. In addition there is a restriction of certain powers under the act (for example, treatment under 'Section 3') when considered for people with 'learning disability', reserving these powers for individuals whose 'disability is associated with abnormally aggressive or seriously irresponsible conduct on his part'. This restriction derives from the previous definitions of mental impairment and severe mental impairment.

The 2007 act will continue, of course, to be used to detain people suffering from mental illness. Neither act defines mental illness and leaves this as a matter for clinical judgment. The Department of Health has provided a guide to the symptoms associated with mental illness, which includes: significant impairment of intellectual functions, shown by failure of memory, orientation, comprehension and learning; significant alterations of mood; delusions; hallucinations and illusions; and disordered thought. The mental illness (now disorder) should be of a nature or degree to warrant the detention of a patient in the interest of his health or safety, or for the protection of others. From a clinical perspective, disorders such as schizophrenia, bipolar affective disorder, dementia, etc., come within the remit of this definition.

The term mental disorder will continue to include the 'personality disorders'. There are numerous personality disorders, for example dis-social (anti-social), borderline, or paranoid personality disorder. Individuals with a significant impairment of intelligence may of course have, in addition, a personality disorder which, if severe enough and requiring detention, may lead to detention under this category.

The act allows for the involuntary admission, detention, assessment and treatment of people under closely prescribed circumstances. The following covers some of the 'civil sections' most frequently used in the community or in hospital. It does not address the 'forensic' sections which apply to patients in the judicial system.

1. Admission for assessment (Section 2)

Section 2 of the act allows compulsory admission from the community and detention for assessment, or assessment followed by treatment for mental disorder for up to 28 days. This period of detention is not renewable and if continued detention is required, it may be followed by Section 3. Patients may be detained under Section 2, if they have no previous history of admission to hospital and the diagnosis/prognosis is unclear, or if it is uncertain if the patient would accept medication voluntarily. Grounds for detention include suffering from a mental disorder of a nature or degree which warrants such detention for a limited period, and the detention is for the patient's own health or safety or for the protection of others.

Two doctors, one of whom must be approved for this purpose under Section 12 (II) of the Mental Health Act are required to make the medical recommendations. It is the duty of the Approved Social Worker (ASW), or very rarely the nearest relative, to make an application to the hospital, once they are in possession of the two medical recommendations and they are satisfied that detention in hospital is the most appropriate way of providing the care and medical treatment which the patient requires.

Although this section is called 'Admission for Assessment', doctors may treat mentally disordered patients, with medication with or without their consent. The patient may be discharged from detention by the responsible medical officer (or consultant), the nearest relative, hospital managers or the Mental Health Review Tribunal, although certain restrictions and statutory requirements may apply.

2. Admission for treatment (Section 3)

Section 3 allows compulsory detention for treatment for up to six months. This is renewable for a further six months in the first instance and thereafter yearly. The patient must be shown to be suffering from mental disorder as defined above, severe enough to warrant such treatment in hospital. Detention must be necessary in the interests of the patient's health or safety, or the protection of others and such treatment cannot be provided unless they are detained. Finally, the treatment must be regarded as appropriate, taking into account the nature and degree of the mental disorder and all of the circumstances of the case.

Similar to Section 2, two medical recommendations are required, and the application is made by an approved social worker (or nearest relative). Discharge options are also similar to Section 2. It is important to highlight that treatment refers not only to the use of psychotropic medication, but also includes nursing care, psychological therapies, rehabilitation etc.

3. Other powers of admission/detention

Occasionally, use of Section 4 (Emergency Admission for Assessment) is necessary. It allows compulsory admission and detention for assessment for up to 72 hours in emergency situations, where in the community those involved cannot cope with the person's mental state and the person needs to be forcibly admitted to hospital. This should only be used when the delay in waiting for a second opinion for a Section 2 would be undesirable due to the serious nature of the patient's current illness and the ability to cope within a community setting. There should be a clear intention that an assessment under Section 2 will be arranged once the patient is in hospital. One medical recommendation is required and the application is made by an approved social worker (or nearest relative).

For a patient who has already been admitted to a psychiatric unit on an informal basis and is wishing to leave the unit a Section 5 (2) (Report on Hospital Inpatient) may be necessary as an emergency Holding Order in order to give time to complete a Section 2 or 3. One medical recommendation is required and arrangements should be made for a Section 12 doctor and approved social worker to then assess the patient. A registered nurse (Mental Health or Learning Disability parts of the Register) can detain an informal patient who has already been treated for a mental disorder for up to six hours under Section 5 (4) (Nurses Holding Power). Grounds for detention are that the patient is suffering from a mental disorder to a degree that makes it necessary for their health and safety, or the protection of others, for them to be immediately restrained from leaving hospital. It can only be used if the patient is indicating that they wish to leave the hospital and it is not practicable to obtain a doctor for the purpose of completing a Section 5 (2).

For patients detained under Sections 4, 5 (2) and 5 (4) treatment can only be given with the patient's consent or in an emergency under common law, that is, although the patient is detained under the Mental Health Act, this in itself does not allow treatment without their consent.

4. Guardianship (Section 7)

The purpose of guardianship is to enable patients to receive community care where it cannot be provided without the use of compulsory powers. It enables the establishment of an authoritative framework for working with the patient with the minimum of constraint to achieve as independent a life as possible within the community. The patient must be over the age of 16 years, be suffering from a mental disorder (as defined by the act) and require guardianship in the interests of the welfare of that person or for the protection of others.

Initially, the guardianship is for six months. Two medical recommendations are required; following this the approved social worker (or nearest relative) may make the application for guardianship. The application has no effect until it is accepted by the local social services authority. It is then renewable for a further six months and then for a year at a time – the Responsible Medical Officer (RMO) is responsible for renewing the Order. The guardian who may be an individual or a social services authority, has the power to require the person to:

- Reside at a specified place

- Attend at places and at specified times for the purpose of medical treatment, occupation, education or training

- Give access to the place where the person subject to the Order is living, to any medical practitioner, approved social worker or other person specified by the guardian.

The powers given to the guardian cannot be directly enforced, but rely on the cooperation of the patient. If the patient moves away from the specified residence without the guardian's consent, they can be taken into custody and returned but the order does not allow for force to be used to secure attendance at specified places or for medical treatment to be administered without the person's consent.

Guardianship orders are of limited use in day-to-day practice. They seem to work more often in elderly mental health services, especially for people with mild dementia and in learning disability services for people with a mild level of the condition. In such cases the guardianship works because the patient acknowledges the authority of the guardian – they often seem to have a need to be contained within such a legal 'framework' and respond positively to these powers. Occasionally, guardianships are successful when applied in adult mental health services but this is fairly rare. There is no place for a guardianship order if the patient does not recognize the authority of the guardian and is not willing to comply with the powers of the order.

THE MENTAL CAPACITY ACT (DH, 2005)

This act provides the statutory framework for assessing whether a person has the capacity to make decisions for the first time. It only applies in England and Wales although there is similar legislation in Scotland. In Northern Ireland this area remains subject to common law. The act defines how others can make decisions on behalf of someone who lacks such capacity. Not only does it relate to financial affairs but it also includes care and treatment (personal welfare). This section will focus primarily on capacity issues applied to assessment and treatment of medical and psychiatric disorders. For further discussion of the act including determination of 'capacity' and issues of consent that arise see Chapter 11.

The act defines a lack of capacity as 'a person lacks capacity in relation to a matter if, at the material time, he is unable to make a decision for himself in relation to the matter because of an impairment or a disturbance in the functioning of the mind or brain'. The act provides protection for people whose capacity is called into question. It asserts the fundamental right that no matter what a person's diagnosis or behaviour may indicate they must be assumed to have capacity unless proven otherwise even if they already have a diagnosis of dementia or learning disability. It legally recognizes the principle of 'best interest decisions' and provides an independent support service for the most vulnerable people in the form of advocacy. The act also provides legal protection for carers working with people who have impaired capacity.

The act allows for people who currently have capacity to plan ahead for a time when they may lack capacity by assigning another person to make treatment decisions on their behalf if they lose capacity to do so themselves (lasting Power of Attorney). They will also be able to record their wishes for future treatment, especially the refusal of treatment through an 'advanced decision'. The act also empowers staff working with people who lack capacity to make decisions on their behalf and for these decisions to be acted upon.

For people who have been assessed as not having the capacity to make a specific decision the act allows another person involved in the matter to make a 'best interests' decision on their behalf. The decision maker must consider all the relevant circumstances, the person's past and present wishes and feelings, the beliefs and values that would be likely to influence the person's decision, for example religious, cultural and lifestyle choices, and also consult and take into account the views of other key people such as family, friends, health professionals, any lasting Power of Attorney or any deputy appointed by the Court of Protection, etc. The act covers financial and personal welfare decisions which can include care, such as washing, dressing, etc., provision of services, such as occupational therapy, physiotherapy, nursing care (in the community and in hospitals), medical treatments and diagnostic investigations.

The Mental Capacity Act (2005) does now provide a means to admit a person lacking capacity to hospital through a 'best interests decision'; and through the amendments made to the Mental Health Act (MHA) there may be ongoing detention of an individual who lacks capacity. The act allows lawful restraint of a person lacking capacity and defines restraint as 'the use or threat of force to make a person do something they are resisting or the restriction of liberty of movement, whether or not the person resists'. Restraint therefore includes verbal or physical actions, threatening a person with such an action, holding them down or locking them in a room, and sedation with psychotropic medication.

In addition to lacking capacity on a certain decision, it must be demonstrated that it is in the person's best interests for the act of restraint to be performed, that the individual authorizing the restraint believes reasonably that it is necessary to restrain a person to prevent harm to them, and that the intention is to employ the minimum force necessary for the shortest possible time. The person carrying out the restraint (or authorizing it) must justify it. A lasting Power of Attorney may authorize someone else to restrain the person, in particular circumstances, if the criteria are met. A court appointed deputy cannot authorize the restraint of a person unless the criteria above are met and they have the authority for a restraint conferred on them by the Court of Protection.

The act provides for 'Independent Mental Capacity Advocates' to provide an independent review of important best interest decisions made by health and social services. This represents two fundamental changes to existing advocacy services – advocates will have legal powers and there will be a legal duty placed on NHS and local authorities to refer to advocates in specific circumstances. Advocates will have the legal powers to interview a person they represent in private, examine records (NHS, local authority, private/voluntary sector) which the record holder considers may be relevant to the advocate's role. They may make submissions to the NHS or local authority that must be taken into account, obtain further medical opinions if considered necessary for treatment decisions and challenge proposed decisions by the NHS or local authority via the Court of Protection. Relevant NHS bodies have a legal duty to instruct an advocate in certain circumstances when a person concerned lacks capacity. Situations include when an NHS body is proposing serious medical treatment or provision of accommodation in hospital for a period of more than 28 days (or in a care home for more than eight weeks). There are exceptions to this, however, including when treatment is required under part 4 of the 1983 Mental Health Act or when accommodation is provided as a result of an obligation imposed by the 1983 Mental Health Act. If the treatment or move to a hospital, care home or residential home needs to be provided as a matter of urgency, then this may be done without consulting an advocate.

In general, the Mental Health Act (1983, 2007) overrides or 'trumps' the Mental Capacity Act regarding decisions about the treatment of mental disorders. The patient detained under an appropriate section of the Mental Health Act can be treated for their mental disorder with or without their consent. Even if the patient does have the capacity to make an informed decision regarding treatment, the Mental Capacity Act does not apply. However, if the decision pertains to treatment of a general medical disorder and the patient is assessed as not having the capacity to make an informed decision, it will be necessary to refer to the Mental Capacity Act. This would apply to people with severe dementia or moderate to profound learning disability. It might also apply to people experiencing florid psychotic symptoms, for example during an acute episode of schizophrenia if the mental illness interferes sufficiently with their capacity to make informed decisions regarding their own general medical care. (See also section of act on Advanced Decisions to Refuse Treatment.)

DEVELOPING AN EFFECTIVE SERVICE

Perhaps the biggest challenge facing the person with intellectual impairment admitted to an acute mental health unit is the issue of inclusion. Whilst the person with a primary diagnosis of mental illness is likely to be expected and even welcomed to acute units, those with learning disability, acquired brain injury or dementia may well meet with a different response. The reasons for this are manifold. Pressure on beds in many areas leads to attempts to deflect admission if at all possible – if there is any other service which may possibly be thought to be responsible for those people, referral is directed there instead, sometimes regardless of its appropriateness. Priest and Gibbs (2004, p.163) maintain that staff are sometimes afraid that offering a service to someone with intellectual impairment may set a precedent, so that decisions are not made on the basis of individual need.

Staff on acute wards, which often have a low status within mental health services, may feel unskilled or overwhelmed by the complexity of the presentations of people with intellectual impairment. In more high-functioning units there may be concern that people with intellectual impairment are likely to be disruptive to other people's care, and may also be unable to engage with others (in the use of group activities for example). Concerns about the difficulties experienced in placing people with intellectual impairment in supported accommodation may also affect their welcome.

Boundary 'disputes', in which teams attempt to deflect people with intellectual impairment, need to be addressed early on in any admission. Areas differ markedly in their provision for different conditions, some with good levels of specialist provision for neuropsychiatry to treat people with acquired brain injury, for example, and some where such people would be admitted to a general acute ward. People with intellectual impairment may have access to specialist community provision from a learning disability or other specialist team, such as one dealing with pre-senile dementias, for example (see Chapter 6); many will not, either because no such teams exist, or because of exclusion criteria. Certainly those people with a borderline learning disability or other cognitive impairment are unlikely to have such access.

There has been an extensive debate around whether people with learning disability should be admitted to generic mental health provision or to specialist services. In the UK, the white paper, 'Valuing People' (DH 2001) advocates that all mainstream hospital and community health services are made available to people with learning disabilities. Thus in the case of learning disability there is a significant challenge for learning disability community teams in supporting people in accessing these services (Chaplin, 2004). A direct result of this is that clients with learning disabilities are often admitted to acute mental health wards for treatment of their mental health problems. This has not always met with approval from those working in learning disability services or indeed from those within generic services. Day (1994), for example, is clear that generic mental health wards 'cannot satisfactorily meet the needs of people with mental retardation and psychiatric and behaviour problems'. He states that 'people with mental retardation are disadvantaged and vulnerable in generic treatment settings: they do not on the whole mix well with other mentally disordered patients, the pace of life is usually too fast for them and it is difficult to gear therapeutic interventions to meet their needs' (Day, 1994, p.277).

Whilst there are many opinions favouring one or the other approach, the evidence that people with learning disability are better off in either specialist or generic services is inconclusive. Xenitidis et al (2004) describe a comparison of outcomes between people with 'intellectual disability' admitted to a specialist unit and generic services and found that the service was beneficial and patients there were 'less likely to be discharged to out-of-area placements' (Xenitidis et al, 2004, p.11). However, Chaplin, (2004) reviewed a number of studies comparing specialist and generic provision and found few robust studies able to identify differences in outcomes, except in cases of 'severe intellectual disability'. Nevertheless, he did opine that care in generic units may be 'sub optimal due to lack of specialist training, resources and unhelpful attitudes' (Chaplin, 2004, p.1). Supporting this view is one study by LePage et al (2005), who found that mixing young people with mental illness and people with 'mental retardation' led to an increase in violent incidents. They related this to an inability to engage in groups and lack of staff training in behavioural techniques.

Chaplin and Flynn (2000) highlight some of the potential problems when people with learning disability require acute psychiatric hospitalization under the care of general adult psychiatrists, many of whom have had little training in the assessment and treatment of mental illness in this group. For example, people with learning disability will often have come from relatively protected environments such as family homes or residential care. They will be particularly vulnerable on an acute ward where they may be exposed to smoking, alcohol, drugs and exploitation such as sexual abuse and violence from other patients. It is possible that the client will have no access to learning disabilities trained staff and the quality of care may be compromised as a result.

TRAINING AND EDUCATION

Regardless of evidence either way, people with intellectual impairment, whether mild or more pronounced, will be admitted to generic mental health services which must be prepared to offer quality care. Whilst much attention is given in the training of specific learning disability health professionals there has been little emphasis placed on the needs of generic mental health staff in terms of caring for clients with both mental health problems and learning disabilities. Naylor and Clifton (1994) argue that staff working in generic mental health settings generally perceive themselves to lack the expertise and skills to care for learning disability clients. As the current drive is to develop and improve services to meet the mental health needs of people with learning disabilities, training of generic mental health workers should form an integral part of this.

Current nurse training programmes include a limited amount of teaching in the field of intellectual impairment theory (usually amounting to two weeks as part of the Learning Disability Insight placement) but clinical placements are not mandatory and relatively uncommon. Student nurses training in mental health may have no further opportunity to gain any experience in either learning disability or the broader area of intellectual impairment, before qualifying. Specialist post-registration courses in learning disability are rare.

However, there are models for improvement. Barriball and Clark (2005) describe a teaching and learning strategy aimed at non-learning disability preregistration nurse education which addresses this deficit. The aim of the strategy is for nurses on adult, mental health and child programmes to be given opportunities to develop their confidence and skills in the care of this patient group. Since April 2000, psychiatrists are required to have six months' experience in either learning disability or child and adolescent psychiatry at senior house officer level. There are also specialist registrar training schemes in learning disability although some are struggling to fill their posts (Chaplin and Flynn, 2000).

CONCLUSION

In order to best help people with intellectual impairment admitted to acute wards staff may well have to be creative. For people suffering from a particular disorder such as Asperger's or Down syndrome help can be found from a range of sources. Literature is available in trust libraries or online to provide background information as well as evidence for interventions. Local groups focusing on specific conditions can provide information. Whilst specialist learning disability teams may not accept individuals as clients they may be willing to provide advice or training.

Most of all, unhelpful attitudes must be challenged. People with intellectual impairment will continue to be admitted to acute mental health wards, and must be made to feel included into the ward atmosphere. Addressing boundary issues early on and deciding whether the person is best helped in the acute setting will help to ensure that staff are aware of their responsibilities, even if they feel unprepared to execute them. If such boundary issues continue, as often happens around the issue of placements, the team will have to work hard not to communicate that issue to the service user.

Taylor (2002) is damning about the commitment of healthcare professionals to engage at an emotional level with people who have intellectual impairment. He states that there is little interest in their internal worlds and that this may well be mediated by a reluctance to engage with people seen as unattractive because of their disability. Applying the principles of empowerment to acute mental health care for people with intellectual impairment needs sustained and conscious effort. Practically speaking it requires the multidisciplinary team to make significant efforts to increase the choices available to and the power of the service users on the ward. It is hoped that with careful and thoughtful assessment and the application of both creative and evidence-based interventions underpinned by the values of equality and respect, that care on acute mental health wards can be both effective and humane.

REFERENCES AND RECOMMENDED READING

Alexander S, Cooray S. (2003) Diagnosis *of* personality disorders in learning disabilities. *British Journal of Psychiatry* 182(44):28–31.

American Psychiatric Association (2000) *Diagnostic and Statistical Manual of Mental Disorders (DSM-IV-TR)* Washington DC: APA.

Barriball KL, Clark LL. (2005) All preregistration students should develop skills in learning disabilities. *British Journal of Nursing* 14(3):166–9.

Bethlem and Maudsley NHS Trust (1997) *The Maze. Mental Health Act. (1983) Guidelines.*

Black L, Novaco RW. (1993) Treatment of anger with a developmentally handicapped man. In: Hatton C. (2002) Psychosocial interventions for adults with intellectual disabilities and mental health problems: A review. *Journal of Mental Health* 11(4):357–73.

Black L, Cullen C, Novaco R. (1997) Anger assessment for people with mild learning disabilities in secure settings. In: Stenfert Kroese B, Dagnan D, Loumidis K (eds), *Cognitive Behavioural Therapy for People with Learning Disabilities*. London: Routledge.

Boulter P, Pointu A. (2006) Risk and care planning and delivery in intellectual disability nursing. In: Gates B (ed.), *Care Planning and Delivery in Intellectual Disability Nursing*. Oxford: Blackwell Publishing, Ch. 6.

Chaplin R. (2004) General psychiatric services for adults with intellectual disability and mental illness. *Journal of Intellectual Disability Research* 48(1):1–10.

Chaplin R, Flynn A. (2000) Adults with learning disability admitted to psychiatric wards. *Advances in Psychiatric Treatment* 6:128–34.

Code of Practice: Mental Health Act 1983 (Revised 1999). London: The Stationery Office.

Cooper SA, Melville CM, Einfeld S. (2003) Psychiatric diagnosis, intellectual disabilities and Diagnostic Criteria for Psychiatric Disorders for Use with Adults with Learning Disabilities/Mental Retardation (DC/LD). *Journal of Intellectual Disability Research* 47(Supp 1):3–15.

Dagnan D, Chadwick P. (1997) Cognitive-behavioural therapy for people with learning disabilities: assessment and intervention. In: Stenfert Kroese B, Dagnan D, Loumidis K (eds), *Cognitive Behavioural Therapy for People with Learning Disabilities*. London: Routledge.

Day K. (1994) Psychiatric services in mental retardation: generic or specialised provision? In: Bouras N (ed.), *Mental Health in Mental Retardation: Recent Advances and Practices*. Cambridge: Cambridge University Press.

Department of Health (1983) Mental Health Act. London: DH.

Department of Health (2001) *Valuing People: A New Strategy for Learning Disability for the 21st Century*. London: The Stationery Office.

Department of Health (2005) Mental Capacity Act. London: DH.

Dodd R, Dowling S, Hollins S. (2005) A review of the emotional, psychiatric and behavioural responses into bereavement in people with learning disabilities. *Journal of Intellectual Disability Research* 49(7):537–43.

Fearon P, Murray R. (2002) Intellectual function and schizophrenia. *British Journal of Psychiatry* 181:276–7.

Flynn A, Matthews H, Hollins S. (2002) Validity of the diagnosis of personality disorder in adults with learning disability and severe behavioural problems. *British Journal of Psychiatry* 180:543–6.

Gagnon J, Bouchard M, Rainville C. (2006) Differential diagnosis between borderline personality disorder and organic personality disorder following traumatic brain injury. *Bulletin of the Menninger Clinic* 70(1):1–28.

Gilbert T, Todd M, Jackson J. (1998) People with learning disabilities who also have mental health problems: practice issues and directions for learning disability nursing. *Journal of Advanced Nursing*, 27:1151–7.

Gravestock S. (1995) Individual family and social adjustment. In: Priest H and Gibbs M. (2004) *Mental Health Care for People with Learning Disabilities*. Edinburgh: Churchill Livingstone.

Hamilton D, Sutherland G, Iacono T. (2005) Further examination of relationships between life events and psychiatric symptoms in adults with intellectual disability. *Journal of Intellectual Disability Research* 49(11):839–44.

Hatton C. (2002) Psychosocial interventions for adults with intellectual disabilities and mental health problems: A review. *Journal of Mental Health* 11(4):357–73.

Hollins S, Esterhuyzen A. (1997) Bereavement and grief in adults with learning disabilities. *British Journal of Psychiatry* 170:479–501.

Hollins S, Curran J, Webb B. (1995) *Feeling Blue*. London: St George's Mental Health Library.

Howells P, Rogers C, Wilcock S. (2000) Evaluating a cognitive behavioural approach to teaching anger management skills to adults with learning disabilities. *British Journal of Learning Disabilities* 28:137–42.

Hurley AD, Folstein M, Lan N. (2003) Patients with and without intellectual disability seeking outpatient psychiatric services: diagnosis and prescribing patterns. *Journal of Intellectual Disability Research* 47(1): 31–50.

Johnston SJ. (2002) Risk assessment in offenders with intellectual disability: the evidence base. *Journal of Intellectual Disability Research* 46(Supp1): 47–56.

Jopp DA, Keys CB. (2001) Diagnostic overshadowing reviewed and reconsidered. *American Journal on Mental Retardation* 106:416–33.

Jukes M, O'Shea K. (1998) Transcultural therapy 1: Mental health and learning disability. *British Journal of Nursing* 7(15):901–6.

LePage J, Mcghee M, Aboraya A, Murphy J, VanHorn L, Pollard S. (2005) Evaluating risk factors for violence at the inpatient unit level: combining young adult patients and those with mental retardation. *Applied Nursing Research* 18:117–21.

Levitas A, Desnoyers, Hurley A, Pary R. (2001) The Mental Status examination in patients with mental retardation and developmental disabilities. *Mental Health Aspects of Developmental Disabilities* 4(1):2–16.

Lindsay W, Baty F, Mitchie A *et al.* (1989) A comparison of anxiety treatments with adults who have moderate and severe mental retardation. *Research in Developmental Disabilities* 10:129–40.

Lindsay W, Howells L, Pitcaithly D. (1993) Cognitive therapy for depression with individuals with intellectual disabilities. In: Priest H, Gibbs M. (2004) *Mental Health Care for People with Learning Disabilities*. Edinburgh: Churchill Livingstone.

Marshall M, Hogg LI, Gath DH, Lockwood A. (1995) The Cardinal Needs Schedule – a modified version of the MRC Needs for Care Assessment Schedule. *Psychological Medicine* 25(3):605–17.

Mason J, Scior K. (2004) 'Diagnostic Overshadowing' amongst clinicians working with people with intellectual disabilities in the UK. *Journal of Applied Research in Intellectual Disabilities* 17:85–90.

Moss S. Prosser H, Costello H, Simpson N, Patel P, Rowe S, Turner S, Hatton C. (1998) Reliability and validity of the PAS-ADD checklist for detecting psychiatric disorders in adults with intellectual disability. *Journal of Intellectual Disability Research* 42(Pt 2):173–83.

Murphy GH, Clare ICH. (1991) MIETS: a service option for people with mild mental handicaps and challenging behaviour or psychiatric problems 2: Assessment, treatment and outcomes for service users and service effectiveness. *Mental Handicap Research* 4:180–206.

Naylor V, Clifton M. (1994) People with learning disabilities: meeting complex needs. *Health and Social Care* 1:343–53.

Oliver P, Piachaud J, Regan A. (2003) Difficulties developing evidence-based approaches in learning disabilities. *Evidence-Based Mental Health* 6:37–9.

Osuji IJ, Cullum CM. (2005) Cognition in bipolar disorder. *Psychiatric Clinics of North America* 28(2):427–41.

Phelan M, Slade M, Thornicroft G, Dunn G, Holloway F, Wykes T, Strathdee G, Loftus L, McCrone P, Hayward P. (1995) The Camberwell Assessment of Need: the validity and reliability of an instrument to assess the needs of people with severe mental illness. *British Journal of Psychiatry* 167(5):589–95.

Priest H, Gibbs M. (2004) *Mental Health Care for People with Learning Disabilities*. Edinburgh: Churchill Livingstone.

Raghavan R, Patel P. (2005) *Learning Disabilities and Mental Health: A Nursing Perspective.* Oxford: Blackwell Publishing.

Reiss S, Levitan GW, Szyzsko J. (1982) Emotional disturbance and mental retardation: diagnostic overshadowing. *American Journal of Mental Deficiency* 86:567–74.

Richards S, Mugal AF. (2006) *Working with the Mental Capacity Act 2005.* Matrix Training Associates Ltd.

Rose J, West C, Clifford D. (2000) Group interventions for anger in people with intellectual disabilities. *Research in Developmental Disabilities* 21:171–81.

Royal College of Psychiatrists (2001) *DC/LD Diagnostic Criteria for Psychiatric Disorders for Use with Adults with Learning Disabilities/Mental Retardation.* London: Gaskell Press.

Shellenbarger T. (2004) Overview and helpful hints for caring for the ED patient with Asperger's syndrome. *Journal of Emergency Nursing* 30:278–80.

Sovner R. (1986) Limiting factors in the use of DSM-III criteria with mentally ill/mentally retarded people. *Psychopharmacology Bulletin* 22(4): 1055–9.

Taylor JL. (2002) A review of the assessment and treatment of anger and aggression in offenders with ID. *Journal of Intellectual Disability Research* 46(Supp1):57–73.

Webster CD, Douglas KS, Eaves D, Hart SD. (1997) *HCR-20: Assessing Risk for Violence.* Vancouver: Mental Health, Law and Policy Institute: Simon Fraser University.

Xenitidis K, Thornicroft G, Leese M, Slade M, Fotiadou M, Philp H, Sayer J, Harris E, McGee D, Murphy DG. (2000) Reliability and validity of the CANDID – a needs assessment instrument for adults with learning disabilities and mental health problems. *British Journal of Psychiatry* 176:473–8.

Xenitidis K, Gratsa A, Bouras N, Hammond R, Ditchfield H, Holt G, Martin J, Brooks D. (2004) Psychiatric inpatient care for adults with intellectual disabilities: Generic or specialist units? *Journal of Intellectual Disability Research* 48(Part 1):11–18.

CHAPTER 9
PSYCHOPHARMACOLOGICAL ISSUES

Rob Winterhalder

STUDY AIMS:

1. To understand the development of the normal brain and how such development may differ in people with intellectual impairment.

2. To study the links between abnormalities in the brain and mental illness.

3. To investigate the specific types of medication used in the treatment of mental illness and behavioural disorders and their suitability for certain patient groups within the spectrum of intellectual impairment.

4. To comprehend other issues which are involved in psychopharmacology, including compliance.

This chapter addresses clinical issues surrounding the pharmacological treatment of mental illness and/or behaviour disorders in people with comorbid intellectual impairment which includes learning disability, developmental disorders (including autism and attention deficit hyperkinetic disorder), dementia and acquired brain injury. The focus is primarily on principles that can be applied in a community setting within both primary and secondary care. Whilst the management of mental health and behavioural problems in this group of patients can be difficult, there is no room for therapeutic nihilism in patients with dementia, acquired brain injury or learning disabilities who develop additional psychiatric disorders such as psychosis or depression, or behavioural disorders. By using a rational approach to the selection of psychotropic drugs, significant therapeutic responses and remission can be achieved.

Some psychiatric disorders are significantly more prevalent in the learning disabled population than in the general population – these include disorders such as schizophrenia, bipolar affective disorder and other types of affective disorder. Behaviours such as aggression, over-activity, pica, self-injurious behaviour (SIB) which can be conceptualized as a habit disorder, and other stereotypies

Learning Disability and other Intellectual Impairments, Edited by L.L. Clark and P. Griffiths
© 2008 John Wiley & Sons, Ltd

are also particularly prevalent in the learning disability and pervasive developmental disorder groups. These behaviours are sometimes referred to as 'challenging behaviour' (see Chapter 10), which is not a clinical diagnosis but instead a service construct, or organic behaviour disorder.

Acquired brain injury, dementia, and epilepsy and other causes of intellectual impairment are also considered risk factors for a variety of psychiatric disorders, including depression and some types of psychotic disorder. A variety of behavioural problems including aggression, destructive behaviours, over-activity, etc., are also associated with dementia, acquired brain damage, etc. Of course, whilst acquired brain injury may be a causal aetiological factor in the development of mental illness (or personality disorder/change), it may be purely coincidental especially if the mental illness or personality problems pre-date the acquired brain injury.

It is axiomatic that brain damage underpins all of the conditions encompassed within the term intellectual impairment. Patients with intellectual impairment have significant abnormalities not only in brain structure but also in functioning. This in turn may modify their response to psychotropic medication.

BRAIN DEVELOPMENT

Most neurones are formed by the end of the second trimester of prenatal life – neuronal migration starts within weeks of conception and is essentially complete by birth. Human brain development is more dynamic before birth than during adulthood, and brain volume is 95% of its adult age by the age of five. However, several processes affecting brain structure persist throughout life – myelination of axon fibres and branching continues at least throughout adolescence, whilst synaptogenesis occurs throughout the life span.

Both the neurone and its synapses are 'plastic', changeable and malleable. It is possible that some neurones may even divide after birth in human brains. Interestingly, up to 90% of the neurones that the brain makes during foetal development die between conception and birth in a process called *apoptosis*. Apoptosis is programmed into the genome of various cells, including neurones, and when activated, causes a cell to self-destruct. This is a different process to necrotic cell death, which is characterized by a severe and sudden injury associated with an inflammatory response. Apoptosis is a natural mechanism to eliminate unwanted neurones and ensures that the healthiest neurones survive. The selected neurones must then migrate to the correct part of the brain which occurs during the foetal stage. Later only axons can move, and the fact that axonal grown is retained in the mature brain suggests that neurones continue to alter their targets of communication, perhaps by repairing, regenerating and reconstructing synapses.

More synapses are present in the brain by the age of six than at any other time in the lifecycle. During the next five to ten years and into adolescence, the brain systematically removes half of all synaptic connections present at the age of six. Neurodevelopmental experiences and genetic programming lead the brain to select which connections to keep and which to destroy – if done appropriately, the brain matures normally into adulthood. Impairments in this process can lead to a variety of neurodevelopmental disorders.

Epilepsy and many learning disabilities are disorders that in part may result from neurones migrating to the wrong places during foetal development. Abnormal neuronal migration may also contribute to schizophrenia, attention deficit hyperactivity disorder, dyslexia and other developmental disorders. With particular reference to schizophrenia, subtle abnormalities in the cytoarchitecture of the hippocampus, frontal cortex, etc., have been observed. These abnormalities are not associated with gliosis and are likely to be due to disturbances in the late migration or in the final differentiation of neurones during brain development. Post-mortem studies have shown that the lateral ventricles, particularly in the anterior and temporal horns, are enlarged and that this is associated with a reduction in the volume of medial temporal structures such as the hippocampus and parahippocampal gyrus. There is a tendency for the pathological changes in schizophrenia to be more apparent on the left side of the brain. The left hemisphere matures later than the right and may be more vulnerable to disruption by pathological processes such as viral infections.

As part of normal ageing, cell loss and a reduction in dendritic processes occurs – there is a relative decrease in cortical grey matter compared with white matter. There is an accumulation of pigment within the nerve cells, and production of neurofibrillary tangles which can destroy some nerve cells. These tangles are confined to a small number of cells, for example in the hippocampus. In addition, senile plaques which consist of groupings of neuronal processes with extracellular amyloid within the central core can occur both in the cortex and amygdala, as well as in the hippocampus. The brains of some older adults also contain inclusion bodies called Lewy bodies (see Chapter 6).

Not only can psychiatric and associated neurodevelopmental disorders result if synapses are malformed early in life, but brain disorders can also occur if normal healthy synapses are disrupted later in life. In Alzheimer's disease, there is an increase in senile plaques and neurofibrillary tangles throughout the cortical and subcortical grey matter, particularly in the limbic regions. Ultimately, this results in a subtle loss of neurones as a result of apoptosis. More catastrophic loss of neuronal tissue and synapses may occur in disorders such as encephalitis, traumatic brain injury, stroke, etc.

Whilst schizophrenia has often been considered a neurodevelopmental disorder, there is evidence to suggest that, in addition, subtle neurodegenerative processes including apoptosis, may explain the progressive course of schizophrenia into the so called 'negative' or residual phase. In cognitive terms the full scale intelligence quotient of patients with schizophrenia may be reduced by up to 15–20 points. Neuroimaging has consistently demonstrated structural and functional abnormalities affecting particularly the temporal and frontal lobes with reduced volumes, impaired blood flow in the frontal and prefrontal cortex (known as hypofrontality), etc. All these abnormalities have been observed also in neuroleptic-naïve patients, therefore medication side effects cannot explain these findings. Whilst some of the structural abnormalities are clearly developmental in origin, research evidence suggests that progressive degenerative changes may also occur in adulthood. Cognitive dysfunction in schizophrenia seems to result from impaired thalamic gaiting and dopamine deficits in the mesocortical pathways. It is of note that atypical neuroleptics, because of their relative serotonin receptor selectivity (in comparison to dopamine receptors) lead to high levels of dopamine release in the mesocortical pathways.

Neurodegenerative phenomena may also play a role in the 'kindling' phenomena of various affective disorders, including the development of rapid cycling bipolar disorder, and treatment resistance in depression, panic disorder and other psychiatric illnesses. Finally, the kindling model has been used extensively to help explain the progression of a variety of epilepsy syndromes.

SUBSTRATE FOR ACTION

The clinical benefits (and side effects) of psychotropic medication result from its interaction with receptors in the central nervous system, and more specifically the brain. Within the large spectrum encompassed by the term intellectual impairment, there are at least four ways in which the brains of this patient group can differ from the general population, depending in part on which type of disorder the patient has. In intellectual impairment the brain may differ in terms of:

1. **Quantity** With regard to people with mental retardation, dementia, acquired brain injury, etc., there may be less brain substrate, and therefore fewer receptors, on which the drug can act.

2. **Quality** It has become increasingly recognized that the brains of people suffering from schizophrenia, some epilepsy syndromes, various types of learning disability, pervasive developmental disorders, etc., are qualitatively different from those of people with normal intelligence. This can relate to differences in anatomy, histology, neurochemistry or function. Examples can include enzyme deficits, anatomical dislocations or abnormal growth/development of cells, pathways or systems, imbalance in the relative sizes or distribution of competing pathways, etc.

3. **Developmental stage** Hyperactive patients with IQs below 45 or a mental age of 4½ fail to benefit from methylphenidate, while patients with higher mental ages and IQs do benefit – the relationship with mental age is stronger than with IQ. There is also evidence that children with depression respond less favourably than adults to tricyclic antidepressants, although there may be other confounding factors involved.

4. **Degeneration** Dementia is essentially a degenerative condition – of course this process may in itself lead to abnormalities in quantity (of brain substrate), quality (in terms of functioning) due to neuronal loss, dendrictic 'pruning', neurofibrillary tangles and so on. Some patients with learning disability may show premature ageing or degeneration associated with the underlying learning disability itself – the most well-known example being Alzheimer's disease in Down syndrome. (It is important to note that even if one excludes the Down syndrome population from epidemiological studies, dementia is more common in the learning disability population compared with the general population.)

EXERCISE

Consider how the differences in brain structure and function in people with intellectual impairment may have an impact on pharmacokinetics. ■

PHARMACOKINETICS

Pharmacokinetics refers to how the body handles drugs and includes drug absorption, distribution, metabolism and excretion. In individuals with a learning disability or pervasive developmental disorder due to, for instance, a genetic syndrome, there may be additional congenital conditions such as duodenal atresia, renal abnormalities, etc., which may affect aspects of pharmacokinetics such as absorption and excretion. In the older adult a range of age-related changes including reduced liver mass and renal blood flow, relative increase in body fat, reduced body weight and total water, and reduced gastrointestinal function may lead to changes in all aspects of pharmacokinetics. This is particularly relevant in the management of mental illness and behaviour problems in people with dementia.

SIDE EFFECTS AND SENSITIVITY

Clinical experience repeatedly illustrates that people within the intellectual impairment group in general tend to be more sensitive to psychotropic medication compared with the general population. Several of the factors mentioned in the previous sections contribute to this increased sensitivity, for example reduced quantity of neuronal tissue (and receptors), qualitative differences, abnormalities in developmental and/or degenerative terms and pharmacokinetic abnormalities. These concepts help explain why lower doses of psychotropic medication are often sufficient to bring about a therapeutic response and why this particular group may be more sensitive to side effects compared with the general population.

Quantitative and qualitative differences may occasionally explain why some patients paradoxically require much higher doses than generally used in order to obtain a therapeutic response. There may be insufficient receptors available or they are less sensitive to the usual doses employed in the general population. Qualitative factors may also explain why some psychotropic agents such as naltrexone may be more effective in people with a learning disability and self-injurious behaviour than in the general population.

However, the research literature is conflicting on the issue of whether this client group is in fact more prone to side effects than the general population. There are three main groups of side effects which have attracted the attention of clinicians and researchers. Many psychotropic drugs have adverse cognitive side effects, which is clearly a significant issue in this group, which already tends to be intellectually compromised. Similarly, most psychotropic drugs lower seizure threshold, and in view of the fact that brain integrity has already been breached in this patient group, the risks of iatrogenic seizures are significant. Finally, there has been significant debate, particularly in the learning disability field, as to whether neuroleptic medication is more likely to lead to parkinsonian side effects or tardive dyskinesia, compared with the general population. Many clinicians believe that this is in fact the case and that brain damage is a significant risk factor.

MANAGEMENT

The decision to commence psychotropic medication is influenced by several factors including the diagnosis and its associated course and prognosis, the severity of the signs and symptoms, the risk to the patient and/or the environment, the failure (in relative or absolute terms) of psychosocial interventions, compliance and the wishes of the patient (if they have capacity to make informed decisions on this matter). Often, these factors can be brought together in terms of quality of life issues. If there is a significant impairment overall in the patient's quality of life, then intervention with psychotropic medication may well be indicated.

As in all forms of treatment, the development of a therapeutic alliance with the patient and/or carers is crucial. Educating the patient (and carers) about the disorder and its treatment, together with possible side effects, may be time consuming and require additional input from nursing colleagues, speech and language therapists, particularly if there are significant impairments in communication and understanding. In addition to discussing the nature of the disorder, treatment options, course and prognosis, it is important to explain why psychotropic medication is now indicated, what benefits can be reasonably expected, possible side effects and the likely outcomes if medication is not prescribed.

Some patients and carers need to be reassured that in addition to psychotropic medication, psychosocial factors will continue to be reviewed and any problems in those areas addressed. In other situations, patients and carers have no interest in addressing the psychosocial issues – if the response to psychotropic medication is less favourable than expected, the clinician should continue to gently probe at psychological and environmental factors which may be compromising the management of the patient.

Particularly where there are problems engaging and communicating with patients and/or their carers, objective measures of psychopathology can be useful in monitoring response to medication and progress. Objective signs and symptoms such as aggression and insomnia should be measured at baseline and during the period of prescribing. In addition, standardized assessment tools for the assessment of subjective symptoms such as low mood can be considered.

Increasingly, both in the context of multidisciplinary working and formal shared care agreements between primary and secondary care, medication monitoring protocols are being developed and implemented. For instance, in a patient about to commence neuroleptic medication, baseline measurements would include weight, pulse, blood pressure, ECG, prolactin level, fasting blood sugar and lipid profile, standardized assessments of abnormal movements and cognitive functioning. Again, there is a significant role for nursing in the monitoring of any response to the medication, side effects, specific health education and more general health promotion.

SPECIFIC CLASSES OF MEDICATION

NEUROLEPTICS

Neuroleptics have an established place in the treatment of schizophrenia, mania and other psychotic disorders such as delusional disorder. They are also used for the treatment of anxiety, insomnia and extreme over-arousal/agitation. Perhaps more controversially, they are sometimes prescribed in personality disorders such as dissocial personality disorder and for behavioural problems such as aggression and self-injurious behaviour in the absence of any identifiable mental illness.

Atypical neuroleptics tend to be the drugs of first choice, particularly in functional psychoses such as schizophrenia. They are associated with less troublesome parkinsonian side effects and cognitive impairment. The risk of tardive dyskinesia also appears to be reduced with this group, although it is important to recognize that pharmacologically several of these drugs differ significantly from each other.

Cognitive deficits in schizophrenia can include impaired attention, information processing, serial learning, executive functioning, etc. The atypical neuroleptics olanzapine, risperidone and clozaril have been found to improve the cognitive functioning of some patients although, of course, these drugs may have their own cognitive side effects. Olanzapine may be first choice overall in terms of enhancing cognitive functioning in this group.

Olanzapine or quetiapine are reasonable antipsychotics for psychoses associated with traumatic brain injury as they have fewer extrapyramidal side effects. Their use in the management of agitation and/or aggression in acquired brain injury remains equivocal.

People with Lewy body dementia are frequently difficult to manage. The combination of psychotic symptoms, extrapyramidal signs with frequent falls and hypersensitivity to all types of neuroleptics limits therapeutic options. Clozapine is the most effective drug for psychosis in Parkinson's disease, but the practical limitations of regular blood tests have led to other atypical neuroleptics being considered – quetiapine appears to be the most promising. Drugs such as olanzapine, risperidone and aripiprazole appear limited by an unacceptable motor deterioration.

In Huntington's disease atypical antipsychotics are preferable for treatment of psychosis, so as to avoid exacerbations of motor problems.

In people with dementia, caution has been urged because of the risk of cerebral vascular accidents (CVAs) associated with olanzapine and risperidone. The elderly, those with a personal family history of heart disease or any cardiac abnormalities on examination require ECG monitoring. Olanzapine and risperidone are effective in the management of behavioural problems in this patient group, but because of the above concerns, quetiapine and amisulpiride are being increasingly used. Inappropriate sexual behaviours in patients with dementia are often treated with neuroleptics such as chlorpromazine, risperidone or olanzapine, although there is no good evidence of efficacy for their use in this type of problem behaviour.

Haloperidol and sulpiride are less epileptogenic than other antipsychotics and are therefore the treatment of choice for epilepsy-related psychotic disorders.

In patients with learning disabilities, neuroleptics may be particularly effective in the treatment of severe stereotypies, aggression and self-injurious behaviour. In people with pervasive developmental disorders (with or without learning disabilities) atypical neuroleptics such as sulpiride, risperidone and olanzapine may reduce aggression, self-injurious behaviour and over-activity particularly if associated with over-arousal. In attention deficit hyperkinetic disorder, atypical neuroleptics such as risperidone may improve disruptive behaviours, although it is currently unclear which of the core symptoms (inattention, hyperactivity and impulsivity) are targeted most. Patients with Tourette's syndrome may benefit from traditional neuroleptics, such as haloperidol, or relatively new neuroleptics, such as sulpiride and risperidone.

Recently there has been a growing awareness of certain side effects associated with atypical neuroleptic drugs, including cardiac arrhythmias and dysmetabolic profiles involving abnormalities of glucose and lipid metabolism with associated weight gain. Concerns have also grown regarding the prolactin-elevating properties of some atypicals – quetiapine and aripiprazole appear to be safest in this respect.

ANTIDEPRESSANTS

Antidepressants are indicated for the treatment of depression in addition to some types of anxiety disorders and obsessive compulsive disorder.

Selective serotonin reuptake inhibitors (SSRIs) such as sertraline and escitalopram or serotonin and noradrenaline reuptake inhibitors (SNRIs) such as venlafaxine are recommended as first line treatments for moderate to severe depression because they are relatively low in toxicity in overdose and are better tolerated than tricyclic antidepressants. Higher doses of SSRIs are used for treating obsessive compulsive disorder which can be a comorbid condition in disorders such as Tourette's syndrome or pervasive developmental disorders.

Older adults are generally more susceptible to the anticholinergic effects of antidepressant treatment with tricyclic antidepressants which can precipitate acute confusion. Venlafaxine is contraindicated in people with severe heart disease, and regular monitoring of blood pressure is indicated. Mirtazepine, a noradrenergic and specific serotonergic reuptake antidepressant (NaSSA), may bring about symptom relief in depression faster than other groups of antidepressants not only in older adults but in other patient groups too. In patients with Parkinson's disease who develop comorbid depression, SSRIs are indicated, even if the disease has progressed to include dementia.

Although there is a suggestion that tricyclic antidepressants (and particularly nortriptyline) are more effective in treating post-stroke depression, SSRIs having fewer side effects remain the drugs of first choice. It is important to remember that if all else fails, electroconvulsive therapy has been shown to be safe in the treatment of depression after both a stroke and a traumatic brain injury.

Moclobemide – a reversible monoamine oxidase inhibitor (MAOI) – is recommended in major depression complicating dementia. SSRIs can also be considered for behaviour disorders in people with dementia, for example inappropriate sexual behaviours. SSRIs are less likely to reduce seizure threshold than tricyclic antidepressants which are therefore first choice in patients with epilepsy and suffering from significant depression.

In patients with learning disability, SSRIs should be considered if they present with significant impulse control problems or self-injurious behaviour. In patients with pervasive developmental disorders presenting with significant rituals, regardless of whether the criteria for obsessive compulsive disorder are met, SSRIs can lead to reductions or remission of the ritualistic behaviours. Of course, the core autistic symptoms will remain, but overall the patient's quality of life and general levels of functioning may improve.

MOOD STABILIZERS

Mood stabilizers are used in the prophylaxis of recurrent major depressive disorders and bipolar affective disorder. They are also indicated for the treatment of hypomanic or manic episodes. Finally, lithium sometimes is used as adjunctive treatment in refractory depression.

As carbamazepine and sodium valproate are also anticonvulsants, they have useful mood stabilizing properties in people who may have epilepsy and affective symptomatology. They can also help in the management of people with epilepsy who have behavioural disorders, particularly if the behaviours are linked to seizures (including seizure frequency). Lamotrigine has been shown to have an effect on mood and it is likely that some of the newer generation anticonvulsants also have mood stabilizing actions.

In people with learning disabilities and behavioural problems, mood stabilizers should be considered if the patient has a past history of an affective disorder or the disturbance is cyclical. Carbamazepine is also indicated in the management of aggression. Even in the absence of epilepsy or mental illness, anticonvulsant mood stabilizers may be beneficial in the treatment of aggression, lability of affect and impulsivity in patients with acquired brain damage due to anoxia, trauma, etc.

BENZODIAZEPINES

As in the general population, the role of regular, long-term benzodiazepine medication is limited. Benzodiazepines do have a role to play in the management of over-arousal and agitation leading to aggression, self-injurious behaviour, exhaustion, etc. Lorazepam is often the drug of choice because of its relatively quicker onset of action whilst diazepam can be used if a more prolonged effect is required. In people with intellectual impairment it may be difficult to predict any paradoxical excitatory or disinhibitory reaction and so careful supervision is required when therapy is initiated.

NON-BENZODIAZEPINE ANXIOLYTICS

There is little research evidence regarding the use of buspirone in people with intellectual impairment, but anecdotally it can have a useful role in the management of anxiety and associated problem behaviours. It does not lead to tolerance and dependency and has a more favourable side effect profile in terms of cognitive impairment and hypotonia compared with benzodiazepines.

Beta-blockers appear to have the best evidence supporting their efficacy in treating agitation or aggression associated with acquired brain injury. Usually, however, large doses are required which can lead to significant side effects. Beta-blockers such as propranolol may be considered in people with learning disabilities who are particularly aggressive or when there are significant signs of adrenergic overdrive such as tremor or tachycardia.

HYPNOTICS

As in the general population, benzodiazepines such as temazepam and non-benzodiazepines such as zopiclone can be very effective. With particular reference to melatonin, which is commonly used in paediatrics, there is sufficient evidence for it to be considered in people with intellectual impairment. Seizure control may improve and behavioural problems may diminish in people with severe and profound learning disability who have epilepsy and/or behavioural problems as their sleep pattern improves. It remains unclear at present whether this is due to a direct effect on seizures and problem behaviours, or secondary to the improvement in sleep patterns.

OTHER PSYCHOTROPIC MEDICATION

Anti-androgens and oestrogen are sometimes used for inappropriate sexual behaviours in people with dementia but this remains controversial and should not be considered a first line choice. In people with learning disabilities and similar behaviours anti-androgens, such as cyproterone acetate, and oestrogens are also controversial for similar ethical and moral reasons, but may occasionally have a role to play in their management.

Cholinesterase inhibitors are sometimes used by specialists in the treatment of behavioural disorders associated with dementia. In Alzheimer's disease not only do they lead to an improvement in cognitive function but they also increase adaptive functioning and reduce behavioural problems and caregiver burden. Cholinesterase inhibitors may have a beneficial effect not only on cognitive function in patients with Lewy body dementia, but also on the psychotic and behavioural symptoms. Finally, they also appear to be equally effective in vascular dementia.

Currently there are three main types of cholinesterase inhibitors: rivastigmine, donepezil and galantamine. (Memantine is an NMDA receptor antagonist.) Donepezil can be taken once daily whereas rivastigmine and galantamine need to be taken twice daily. However, rivastigmine is the least likely to cause drug interactions as it does not affect hepatic cytochromes.

Naltrexone is an oral opioid antagonist which may decrease self-injurious behaviour (SIB), acutely – SIB releases endorphins which may lead to positive reinforcement. However, its use in learning disabilities has shown that it is less effective in the long term as SIB is later perpetuated via the dopamine reward system.

Two drugs are licensed in the UK for treatment of ADHD (although initially under specialist supervision). Methylphenidate is a central nervous system stimulant whilst atomoxetine is a noradrenalin reuptake inhibitor. Atomoxetine may have significant advantages over methylphenidate in that it does not lead to weight loss and is also a non-stimulant. It is not yet licensed for use in adults but early signs are promising. Prescribers should be aware of the recent concerns regarding a possible link between atomoxetine and suicidal ideation/behaviour in adolescents. These drugs are effective in reducing the core symptoms of attention deficit hyperkinetic disorder.

OTHER ASPECTS OF PRESCRIBING

COMPLIANCE

Compliance may be improved by simplifying drug dosing schedules and ensuring that patients and carers understand their medication regimes. Most psychotropic drugs only need to be prescribed once or twice daily. The mood stabilizers sodium valproate and carbamazepine also come in modified release preparations – Epilim Chrono and Tegretol Retard respectively. Providing information leaflets, using blister packs or providing, where appropriate, braille labels, are other options. Dossett boxes should also be considered. Liaison and good communication between the patient (or their carer), the prescriber and the pharmacist can often be improved by input from a community nurse.

When compliance is compromised by either cognitive deficits such as poor concentration or memory, or impaired insight and refusal to accept oral medication, depot medication should be considered. Currently only neuroleptic drugs are available in a depot format, and of the six available neuroleptics, only one is an atypical – Risperdal Consta. Disadvantages with Risperdal Consta include the rigid and inflexible dosing regime and difficulties in its administration. The uses of depots are limited to psychotic and behavioural disorders. Advantages include guaranteeing compliance, possibly developing a therapeutic alliance with the nurse who administers the depot, regular follow-ups via the depot clinic (if appropriate), not having to worry about taking oral neuroleptic medication, etc. Disadvantages can include stigma, the inability to 'recall' the drug once administered should side effects develop, occasional discomfort, etc.

TREATMENT RESISTANCE

When faced with treatment resistance in common with all areas of medicine, the clinician should first of all check for compliance. The patient's history, examination and investigation results then need to be reviewed in order to confirm that the diagnosis and treatment are correct. The clinician needs to ensure that a therapeutic dose has been achieved – understandably sub-therapeutic doses are more likely to be used in primary care settings. The wider formulation should be reviewed, for instance, are there ongoing medical problems such as thyroid dysfunction, pain, etc.? Or are adverse psychosocial factors present such as under- or over-stimulation, dysfunctional personal dynamics, etc.? The clinician then needs to consider trying alternative groups of psychotropic medication, for example if an SSRI has been unsuccessful, consider a trial of a RIMA (reversible inhibitor of monoamine oxidase) or tricyclic antidepressant. Finally, augmentation techniques may be necessary, such as adding a mood stabilizer to an antidepressant in treatment-resistant depression.

EMERGENCY TRANQUILLIZATION

When emergency tranquillization is required, essentially there are two groups of psychotropic medications which are considered – neuroleptics and benzodiazepines. The main oral neuroleptics used are haloperidol, olanzapine and risperidone. If intramuscular administration is indicated the neuroleptics of choice are haloperidol and olanzapine. Serious side effects that can be encountered in an acute setting, particularly in neuroleptic-naïve patients, can include significant hypotension, acute dystonias, anticholinergic side effects, cardiac arrhythmias and occasionally neuroleptic malignant syndrome. Organic brain syndromes (which fall within the 'spectrum' of intellectual impairment) have been considered potential risk factors for neuroleptic malignant syndrome. Regardless, it is advisable to have parenteral anticholinergics such as a procyclidine or benzatropine available for parkinsonian side effects.

A benzodiazepine such as lorazepam may be given orally. For intramuscular use, lorazepam or midazolam may be administered. Benzodiazepines may lead to confusion, disinhibition and paradoxical excitatory effects as well as muscle hypotonia. Often the best response to intramuscular medication is obtained by combining a neuroleptic with lorazepam (although there are concerns about using olanzapine and benzodiazepines together). Usually, emergency tranquillization takes place within an accident and emergency department or hospital ward setting. Regardless of whether the patient is in the community or in hospital, risk factors need to be taken into consideration, including staffing levels, appropriate training and a safe and secure environment.

USE OF PRESCRIPTION REQUIRED AS NEEDED MEDICATION (PRN)

Anxiolytic (mainly benzodiazepine) and neuroleptic medication are most frequently used as 'as required' medications. In individuals who are psychotic and over-aroused, consideration needs to be given to administering either extra neuroleptic medication or adding in benzodiazepine medication such as lorazepam or diazepam. It is not good practice usually to treat an individual with two different neuroleptics. Occasionally, however, there may be scope for using a sedative neuroleptic such as clopixol even if the individual is on a different neuroleptic, particularly if alternative sedative drugs such as antihistamines or benzodiazepines cannot be administered. In patients with autism, organic behaviour disorders and other forms of intellectual impairment, PRN medication may be indicated during acute episodes of disturbed behaviour.

Nurses often have a significant role in developing guidelines for the administration of 'as required' medication and monitoring forms for carers to use once the drug has been given. Side effects and any beneficial response, including duration, should be recorded. In this way the prescriber can judge the effectiveness of a current drug at a particular dose. Essentially there are two scenarios in which PRN medication can be considered:

- when there is a sufficiently long escalation which allows for PRN medication to be administered with the aim of preventing a further deterioration, and

- when once an episode of severe disturbed behaviour has commenced, the behaviour usually lasts longer than 30 minutes – in this situation the administration of PRN medication may help bring the episode to an end sooner.

There is usually little role for 'as required' medication when episodes of disturbed behaviour occur suddenly without any warning, last only a few minutes and are not driven by an increase in 'background' anxiety levels. Caution needs to be taken where 'as required' medication is used frequently and regularly as this may indicate an underlying change that needs proper assessment (see Chapter 10 which discusses challenging behaviour).

PSYCHOTROPIC MEDICATION AND BEHAVIOURAL DISORDERS

Intellectual impairment patients may present with significant behavioural disorders which are not obviously underpinned by a functional mental illness. Particularly in the field of learning disabilities and pervasive developmental disorders, various terms have been used to identify these disorders such as challenging behaviour and organic behaviour disorder. The role of psychotropic medication, especially if monitored, is reasonably well established. Concerns have been expressed, however, regarding possible over-prescribing in areas such as learning disability and dementia, mainly because the evidence base for their use in 'pure' behavioural disorders is less robust and side effects may be more common.

Successful reduction or elimination of a particular behaviour is often due to non-specific sedative action which can be associated with additional side effects on cognitive functioning, affect, etc. However, the actions of some psychotropics are more selective and target specific behaviours, for example SSRIs in ritualistic behaviours, and neuroleptics (particularly those which are relatively dopamine 1 receptor selective) in stereotypies. Finally, psychotropic medication and especially neuroleptics are sometimes prescribed when other psychosocial interventions are unavailable because of a lack of resources in these groups.

It is sometimes difficult to differentiate these behavioural disorders from abnormalities of personality, and in particular the Cluster B group of personality disorders (DSM 1V – American Psychiatric Association, 1994). In addition, intellectual impairment can be associated with organic personality disorders such as the frontal lobe syndrome, and enduring personality changes after psychiatric illness, for example schizophrenia, and after catastrophic experiences. All psychotropic drugs are currently licensed for a specific psychiatric disorder, or a small range of such disorders. However, it is common practice for clinicians to use psychotropic drugs off licence in patients with intellectual impairment presenting with behavioural or personality disorders – this is acceptable practice if it can be supported by published research, mainstream professional opinion, patients' best interests, etc. Low dose atypical neuroleptics, SSRIs and mood stabilizers are most often used – the drug of choice may depend on factors such as the presence of comorbid affective symptoms, impulsivity, abnormal EEG or a history of epilepsy.

For some day-to-day clinical decision making the *British National Formulary (BNF)*, produced by the Royal Pharmaceutical Society of Great Britain (in association with the British Medical Association), or local formularies are sufficient. However, the author would recommend, in addition, reference sources such as the electronic Medicines Compendium site on the Internet or authoritative texts such as *The Maudsley Prescribing Guidelines* and Bazire's *Psychotropic Drug Directory* which address more complex clinical issues.

REFERENCES AND RECOMMENDED READING

American Psychiatric Association (1994). *Diagnostic and Statistical Manual of Mental Disorders*, 4th edn. Washington DC: American Psychiatric Association.

Arnold LE. (1993) Clinical pharmacological issues in treating psychiatric disorders of patients with mental retardation. *Annals of Clinical Psychiatry* 5(3):189–97.

Bazire S. (2005) *Psychotropic Drug Directory 2005. The Professional's Pocket Handbook and Aide Memoire*. Fivepin Publishing.

Deb S, Clarke D, Unwin G. (2006) *Using Medication to Manage Behaviour Problems Among Adults with a Learning Disability*. Quick Reference Guide. University of Birmingham.

Dilley M, Fleminger S. (2006) Advances in neuropsychiatry. Clinical implications. *Advances in Psychiatric Treatment* 12(1):23–34. http://emc.medicines.org.uk

Stahl SM. (2000). *Essential Psychopharmacology. Neuroscientific Basis and Practical Applications*, 2nd edn. Cambridge University Press.

Taylor D, Patton C, Kerwin R. (2005) *The Maudsley 2005–2006 Prescribing Guidelines*, 8th edn. Taylor and Francis.

CHAPTER 10
CHALLENGING BEHAVIOUR
Michael Kelly

STUDY AIMS:

1. To understand the concept of the term 'challenging behaviour'.

2. To understand the causes of challenging behaviour.

3. To identify strategies to reduce the problem.

4. To understand the suitability of particular therapeutic interventions used to manage challenging behaviour.

For those unused to dealing with people who have intellectual impairment a major preoccupation is the concern over behaviours that may prove disruptive and difficult to manage. In this chapter we consider such behaviours. Given the numerous impediments already outlined in this book, behaviours exhibited by clients can seriously challenge the ability of services to provide fair and equitable access. The term 'challenging behaviour' has been chosen because that is precisely what such behaviours are − a challenge for those delivering care. Behaviours, which are regarded as challenging, are often those that do not conform to the social norms expected of the people in a given context. The term covers a complex web of interactive processes which in most basic terms involves what the person does, where they do it and how often it is done, as well as how those around that person view the behaviour. As with so many challenges, the appropriate response for caring services is to learn more in order to identify problem solving responses. This chapter thus aims to equip practitioners with knowledge of the tools that can be used to meet the challenge.

Learning Disability and other Intellectual Impairments, Edited by L.L. Clark and P. Griffiths
© 2008 John Wiley & Sons, Ltd

WHAT IS CHALLENGING BEHAVIOUR?

The term 'challenging behaviour' was first used by the Association for Persons with Severe Handicap (TASH) and came into widespread use following the publication of the King's Fund report 'Facing the Challenge' (Blunden and Allen, 1987). The term was adopted in an attempt to remove the stigma from those people within intellectual impairment services who presented with behaviours, which previously would have been described as 'dysfunctional' or 'disordered'. The word 'challenge' was used to illustrate the changes that services would need to make at the point of delivery to meet the needs of these people. The challenge is therefore for the system as opposed to it being a description of the behaviours.

It is difficult to draw up an exact list of behaviours that could be classed as challenging. Judgements vary, not only culturally, but also from service to service. There is a need to prevent misuse of the term by labelling all clients who have behavioural difficulties (Gates, 1996). The shift in emphasis from the individual's behaviour to the service provider encourages a more objective analysis of how services are to meet individual needs within the system. The change allowed for a different understanding of what challenging behaviour was with definitions of the term shifting from operational and 'rule of thumb' (Fleming and Stenfert Kroese, 1993) to a more conceptual and socially inclusive understanding. Emerson's (1995) widely accepted social definition of the term saw challenging behaviour as:

Culturally abnormal behaviour(s) of such an intensity, frequency or duration that the physical safety of the person or others is likely to be placed in serious jeopardy, or behaviour which is likely to seriously limit use of, or result in the person being denied access to, ordinary community facilities.

There are three important components to the Emerson definition. Firstly the challenging behaviour is contextualized within the culture in which it is observed. This allows for current behaviours and our understanding of them to change over time and across the environments in which they are seen. A current example of shifting social evaluations is that of self-harm. This was previously stigmatized and regarded as socially unacceptable, requiring that it be hidden. This makes overt displays of self-harm particularly challenging. There is now a strong health service led initiative in the UK, embodied in National Institute for Clinical Excellence guidelines, to reduce stigma and provide better care for those people who self-harm (NICE, 2004). If successful the extent to which people who self-harm are excluded may be reduced and so may the extent to which the behaviour may be regarded as 'challenging'.

The second aspect of the definition allows for local services to decide how severe the behaviour displayed is by quantifying its intensity, frequency or duration. Although there is some argument that this is too vague it does allow local services to decide on whether they feel they are able to manage the behaviours or not. It also highlights that some behaviours that might be innocuous in isolation become challenging by virtue of their repetition and extent. Thirdly, the definition then focuses on the consequence of such behaviours, by illustrating that many services would not be equipped to deal with these behaviours on a day-to-day basis. What is challenging for some services may not be for others and consequently it is, in part, the services that exclude the person and not their behaviours per se.

Some services, which are unable to meet the needs of patients who display difficult or unusual behaviour, may inappropriately label the patient as being difficult to manage, using the label to excuse poor services and thus avoid the requirement to find a solution. The definition challenging behaviour makes it clear that what makes challenging behaviour challenging is not just the behaviour but the ability of a service to respond and cope.

WHAT CAUSES CHALLENGING BEHAVIOUR?

Focus for the management and treatment of challenging behaviour needs to be centred on the cause of the behaviour rather than the behaviours themselves, i.e. the symptoms of the underlying issue. This can be done by two means. Firstly, knowing the client well and, secondly, having a basic understanding of some of the issues that may cause challenging behaviours.

The underlying causes may be psychological, environmental or they may lie within wider social circumstances or family dynamics. Often the underlying cause is a complex interaction of these factors. Of course 'challenging behaviour' may also have a biological component associated either with behavioural phenotypes resulting from underlying causes of impairment or with the behavioural expression of a symptom of treatable physical or mental illness (see Chapter 2).

PSYCHOLOGICAL

Understanding why a client presents with a challenging behaviour is one of the most widely misunderstood challenges in intellectual impairment services. Simplistic 'diagnoses' such as 'attention seeking' often impede a full understanding. There has been little consideration of 'challenging' behaviour from a psychodynamic point of view. However, one psychological approach does give a framework for interpretation and problem solving which is tangible and potentially beneficial in terms of identifying strategies for positive engagement. Behavioural theories, with their emphasis on reward, may seem to confirm the 'attention seeking' diagnosis on one level and are widely misunderstood. A fuller understanding of this approach removes much of the negativity often associated with challenging behaviours.

There is a general belief that people with intellectual impairment have full conscious control over how they behave. Therefore both the behaviour and an implied intent are judged negatively. However, for all people much behaviour is impulsive and outside direct conscious control. Behavioural theory goes beyond seeking motivations, which will often remain elusive. It sees the behaviour as a learned process that has arisen as a result of an unmet need. The client, unable to express their need, behaves in a way which provokes a response that meets the need (even if this is only partial). Thus a person who 'needs' stimulation and interaction but lacks the skills to initiate constructive interactions may find the attention that ensues from aggressive behaviour (for example) 'rewarding'. Thus what may be a spontaneous outburst of frustration is rewarded which encourages further repetition without a conscious 'plan' ever being formulated.

The A-B-C (Antecedent conditions, Behaviour, Consequence) behavioural model of Operant Conditioning (Skinner, 1953) is used as a framework for understanding the client. Box 10.1 gives a scenario to consider. What are the antecedents which may trigger the behaviours and how might the consequences of it act as reinforcers to encourage the behaviour to worsen in both intensity and frequency?

There are two types of reinforcement: positive and negative. Positive reinforcement occurs when the client experiences a positive experience following their behaviour and tends to increase the frequency of behaviour. In this case John has his lights turned on and receives attention which reduces his fear. Since the behaviour has positive consequences this is rewarding (a positive reinforcement) which tends to encourage it. If response is swifter when behaviour is more extreme the behaviour may be shaped to become more challenging. Negative reinforcement, sometimes referred to as 'punishment', reduces a particular behaviour, as the client avoids something they do not like. However, one of the basic tenets of behaviourism is that reward is a far

BOX 10.1   **JOHN**

John is a client who has intellectual impairment as the result of an acquired brain injury. He has severe communication difficulties. He is afraid of the dark. He has just moved from home to a new community residential unit. John is normally very quiet. However, since moving into his new home he has begun to scream and bang his head on the wall at night time on a regular basis. His family say that this behaviour was previously rare and never so extreme. He usually wakes the other residents and causes bruising to his head. The staff come to his aid and after a considerable period of time John stops screaming and seems to calm down. However, he often repeats the behaviour soon after he is left alone again. ■

more powerful force than punishment. Negative reinforcements (telling the client off for shouting for example) will have little effect compared with the positive effect of attention.

As the unwanted behaviour is something which has been learned then it is something which can be 'unlearned' by the use of positive reinforcement of more acceptable behaviours and lack of reward for the negative ones. So in John's case providing him with a night-light may ultimately stop his behaviours by reducing the need. Such simple solutions may not always suggest themselves and a gradual approach to the desired behaviours must be taken with rewards provided for behaviours that approximate to the desired end state. However, analysis of the situation from a behavioural perspective often suggests potential causes of 'challenging' behaviours because the client finds them rewarding in some way. It also helps to identify aspects of the response of carers that can be modified in order to encourage more positive client behaviours.

ENVIRONMENTAL

Most people have some control over their environment, including the ability to choose where they wish to live, how their home is decorated and when they feel ready to move onwards. People with intellectual impairment generally have less control and are often residing at home with relatives, in community care homes or in other institutional settings. The term 'environment' in a psychological context refers to all those stimuli which are external to the individual and which subsequently influence and shape that individual. This may be the actual physical environment as well as those the person comes into contact with (Gross, 2005).

Challenging behaviour may also be the result of inadequate stimulation in the environment. The behaviour occurs so that the client has an activity in order to stimulate them in a way in which the environment does not – masturbation or self-injurious behaviours may come under this category. The behavioural perspectives above may also be informative in understanding the interaction between the individual and lack of stimulation in the environment. It certainly illustrates why adverse reactions from those around (assumed to be negative stimuli) are often in-effective in modifying behaviour because the reinforcement is less powerful than positive stimuli. Indeed reaction from others may in itself act as a positive reinforcement.

For clients living in care homes the environment can often be sterile and despite efforts otherwise it may not truly simulate a home setting. Often clients move into an already furnished house or room and there is little or no space for personal preferences to be catered for. Usually staff are available to assist with the basic activities of daily living, however, services are often short staffed and meeting even those most fundamental of client needs can be time consuming and demanding. Consequently there may be little or no time to meet non-immediate requirements. If a client is in an environment where others take up staff time they can often feel neglected and uncared for and this may result in behaviours which are either self-stimulating or seen as attention seeking by staff.

The impact of the beliefs that are held by staff on the clients' themselves cannot be underestimated. Low expectations about the potential of an individual mean that adverse behaviours may simply be accepted as inevitable as opposed to challenges to be met. Failure to recognize the 'person' can mean that the need for stimulation is not fully recognized and the power of it as a driver of behaviour may be underestimated. Where possible, it is important to work with the client to determine what kind of positive stimulation can be offered in order to minimize challenging self-stimulating behaviours. Where it is not possible an act of creative understanding of the client's perspective is required in order to generate possible solutions. Labelling behaviours as 'attention seeking' is unhelpful and loses sight of the fact that although the client may want attention it is for a legitimate reason. Staff must work with the individual client in order to determine methods in which their needs can be met in ways that do not require resort to challenging behaviour.

Recall John (Box 10.1) who screamed at night. In John's case staff may perceive his screaming as attention seeking when he knows that staff are busy assisting other clients to bed. This is to some extent true since attention remedies his immediate problem although John is not necessarily aware of the link nor sensitive to the alternative calls on staff time. Having initially responded to the shouts, staff begin to ignore them. Now when John needs attention staff do not respond unless he becomes really upset and bangs his head on the wall as well. He is now having an even more difficult behaviour reinforced. A problem-solving approach might lead them to identify how he could get some stimulation and sense of security during these times when they are busy elsewhere. One potential solution might be giving some sense of human presence through (for example) use of a radio or recorded voice as an 'environmental' intervention. However, because of low expectations they fail to look for either causes or solutions to the challenging behaviour.

SOCIAL FACTORS AND FAMILY LIFE

Negative expectations and beliefs can operate within family environments just as they do in care settings. For many families having a child born with intellectual impairment can have a devastating effect on the family and their understanding of the condition can ultimately have an impact on how they behave around and towards that child. Pagliano et al (1988) reported that many parents felt that their lives were negatively affected by having an intellectually impaired offspring; emotions, time and finances are often stretched and many find the stress of coping too much. In addition to practical frustrations parents must also negotiate a complex social world in which their child is stigmatized and their family not fully accepted as 'normal'. Although the development of the dynamic is different, an intimate carer of a person who becomes intellectually impaired later in life faces similar challenges and indeed may find themselves excluded from areas of life in which they were previously accepted.

Parents, and caregivers alike, may feel frustrated and show anger towards the client. In extreme circumstances this can lead to abuse through physical, verbal or emotional means or through neglect. Clients with intellectual impairment are at greater risk of sexual abuse and exploitation by others (Turk and Brown, 1993; Brown et al, 1994). Although very few people set out to actively abuse someone else the frustration experienced when working with someone with an intellectual impairment may mean that caregivers may fall into the trap of committing abusive acts. Professional carers are also vulnerable in this regard. The impact on the client cannot be underestimated and a client who may have problems with understanding everyday life may find it even harder to comprehend why someone who is caring for them is also abusing them.

Vulnerability in this case covers many areas including the client being a victim of crime, sexual abuse or something less obvious like neglect or financial gain. A better understanding of client vulnerability may be gained by looking at Sobsey's (1994) Ecological Model of Vulnerability. The model suggests a three layer perspective which includes:

1. a microsystem, i.e. the relationship between the abuser and the abused;

2. a macrosystem covering the cultural factors of the situation; and

3. the exosystem where the client resides in an institution or in the community.

The inter-relationship between all three areas is key to understanding why the client is vulnerable and what measures need to be taken to educate or protect them. If a client lives in an environment where their carers regularly abuse them it is then probable that when they enter the wider community they see that behaviour as being an intrinsic part of life. Difficulties with communication may exacerbate the issue, especially when clients are afraid or unable to verbalize what is happening to them. This works at a macrosystems level and impacts on the client's perception of others and indeed on the behaviours they may display.

In order to protect the client from abuse care staff may be tempted to isolate the client from the abusive situation rather than working with the client at addressing the issue, for example if a client has his money taken from him by another client it would be more helpful to enable the client to say 'no', rather than the management of the client's finances being taken over by staff. Although the latter option resolves the issue on one level it disempowers the client from developing the necessary coping skills whilst sending out a signal that staff will manage all aspects of the client's life.

The issue of vulnerability stretches far beyond the environment where the client lives. Brown *et al* (1994) state that only 6% of alleged sex abuse cases against clients with intellectual impairment were prosecuted, indicating the deficiencies in the criminal justice system and local service providers. Reasons for the lack of prosecutions included a low incidence of reporting, social isolation and fear of repercussions.

Consider the case of Mohammed (Box 10.2). Mohammed's case displays many of the issues that challenge not only services but also the family, who are trying their best to lead a normal

BOX 10.2   **MOHAMMED**

Let us meet Mohammed who is of Middle Eastern origin. He lives with his mother, two sisters and wife of five years. He spent most of his life with his family living in an inner city attending a special school. His father died six years ago and shortly after the event changes were noted in his behaviour. He became more withdrawn, began talking to himself, was unable to control his anger and began to hit out at the female members of his family. He was seen by his general practitioner (GP) who prescribed Risperidone to control his behaviour. This was gradually increased to 8 mg daily. ➤

It was felt by the family that he should be married and it was arranged for him to marry his first cousin. She was flown over from the Middle East and moved into his room with him. Two years ago, his brother moved from the family home to live with his new wife and shortly after Mohammed's behaviours intensified beyond the family's control. He began to shout at people in the street, often finding himself in altercations with strangers whilst using public transport. Following one such occasion on a bus he was subsequently placed on Section 136 and was transferred to the local mental health unit where he had his first inpatient contact with mental health services under Section 2 of the Mental Health Act (1983). Whilst on the ward he was observed to have periods of time where he appeared to be talking to someone else and responding actively to voices. He expressed concern that his new wife was trying to poison his food and he knew this as the electrical products in the house were telling him so. He was diagnosed as having schizophrenia and was discharged back into the community on oral Risperidone 6 mg and Risperidone depot 25 mg.

After discharge he was referred to the local Community Mental Health Team and was allocated a community nurse. He discontinued his depot but continued on his oral medication. Since then he has had a further admission under Section 3 of the Mental Health Act (1983) and has had a number of respite admissions to a local mental health unit, which specializes in people with intellectual impairment. The Community Mental Health Team and a psychiatrist from the local Learning Disabilities Team now jointly manage him. He continues on the Risperidone and at times complains of his wife's attempts to poison him. He remains physically abusive to the female members of the household and has threatened to stab his wife on a number of occasions. He regularly hits her.

Having worked closely with the family and using the power of the Care Programme Approach to purchase needed services, the time of a male Middle Eastern speaking support worker was purchased to spend time with Mohammed. It was felt by the team that many of Mohammed's issues centred on the loss of his father and in essence the loss of his brother and own personal space (his room) in such a short space of time. This meant that he was, as the only male left, the head of the household, a responsibility he could not handle, nor were his female family members willing to ascribe to him. His father's death triggered the onset of schizophrenia and his intellectually impaired condition meant that he found it difficult to express himself or cope with the tragic loss of someone he held in such high regard.

The family and the team are currently trying to create better support networks around Mohammed to allow expression of feelings and ventilation of emotions in more constructive and supported ways. ■

life themselves. Joint working between the mental health and learning disabilities team has added differing perspectives to the case and a wider view of the social situation has suggested alternative solutions that encompass the specific social structures and norms within which the client exists.

Mental health problems

Although there is no overwhelming evidence to suggest that there is a strong relationship between mental illness and challenging behaviour (Emerson *et al*, 1999) challenging behaviour itself appears to be the most common reason for people with intellectual impairment to be referred to a psychiatrist (Day, 1985). Emerson *et al* (1999) offer suggestions as possible ways in which challenging behaviours may be associated with mental illness:

1. Challenging behaviours may be an atypical presentation of an underlying mental illness.

2. Challenging behaviours may be a secondary feature of a mental illness or underlying psychiatric symptoms may establish and maintain challenging behaviours.

The difficulty for the family and clinician is to determine which scenario is relevant to their client or family member, whilst noting that behavioural disturbances alone should not be sufficient grounds for a psychiatric diagnosis. The problems surrounding diagnostic overshadowing in people with intellectual impairment remain potentially overwhelming for practitioners.

An example of this difficulty is the identification of mood disorders in this population which is not only hampered by a frequent inability of clients to express themselves but also by the fact that mood disorders may present atypically. Referrals for mood disorders are often instigated after an observed change in behaviour in the client such as an increase in self-injury or aggression. Those with mild or moderate intellectual impairment have a fairly typical presentation of depression and initial assessment can be aided by one of the several well validated screening tools (Hurley, 2006). For the more severely disabled assessment relies more on informants who know the client well and must be based more on behavioural changes in the client's presentation. Many assessment tools for depression rely on self-reporting and many of the diagnostic criteria rely on self-report. Thus a basic level of comprehension and verbal ability is required by the client.

Behavioural changes, often seen as challenging, may be the result of the inability of services and those around the client to identify changes in mood until problems are severe. However, it is all too easy to attribute behaviours to a mood disturbance where another cause is underlying. The case study (Box 10.3) introduces us to Louise and we discover the pertinent reasons for her behaviour.

ASSESSMENT OF CHALLENGING BEHAVIOUR

Assessing clients with an intellectual impairment poses many challenges to the professional, least of all because many people with intellectual impairment may be unable to directly express feelings or articulate the cause of distress. In such instances the observational and deductive abilities of the professional are tested and put to best use. The assessment process is functional and takes a two-pronged approach at comprehension of the underlying causes of the behaviour displayed. Functional assessment is therefore the quest for reasons behind behaviour. It sets out to determine the exact antecedents to the behaviour and the ensuing consequences. The pattern of antecedents and consequences can reveal the functions. (McBrien and Felce, 1992).

Here the purpose of the assessment is to identify the underlying processes that sustain the identified behaviours. Then a constructive approach to intervention focuses on what the individual can do, so that the challenging behaviours may be replaced with more positive and constructive processes. This model is a progression from the historical behavioural approach and

BOX 10.3   LOUISE

Louise is a 22-year-old female living in a group residential home. She has spent much of her life in residential care after she was diagnosed with a severe intellectual impairment when she was younger. She has no family and relies on the staff and other residents for her social network.

In her home there are two support workers on shift during the day and one 'sleeping staff' at night. The home currently has two permanent staff members and many of the workers are employed through temporary agencies. It is usual practice to have a daily handover after every shift, however, in recent months this practice has fallen by the wayside, as the agency staff are not aware of the routines of the previous permanent staff. Usually her learning disability team key worker would visit every three weeks but she was on sick leave for two months. As a result her care was managed by the learning disability 'duty' team, which had different workers regularly.

A month ago it was noticed that Louise was beginning to get restless and found little enjoyment in activities which she would normally have been excited to take part in. Louise began to put her fingers in her anus and smear faeces on surrounding surfaces. Staff considered this to be 'challenging behaviour' or perhaps a 'mood disorder' and began to offer her 'as required' medication on a daily basis, but did not contact any health services. The medication made her drowsy, her appetite decreased and she began to spend more time alone in her room lying on her bed in a foetal position where she continued to 'root and smear'.

After two weeks the staff became very concerned for her after she began screaming in her room and appeared to be in a lot of pain. They took her to the local accident and emergency department where after a simple examination Louise was found to be badly constipated. She was prescribed a course of laxatives. After a few days it was noted by staff that Louise's behaviour was settling and that she was generally less agitated. After a week and a half there were no challenging behaviours noted. ■

consequently develops it by understanding why the person is behaving in a certain way rather than focusing on what it is that they are actually doing.

The behavioural and functional assessment process does not solely focus on the behaviour but takes account of the person, their environment, family and staff. It relies on collaborative working on behalf of all to ensure that a consistent intervention programme is effective. A complete functional assessment should have three phases: **descriptive**, **interpretation** and **verification** (Carr and Wilder, 1998).

The descriptive phase is the most comprehensive part of the assessment process and will give an operational understanding to the behaviour. It should include a thorough description of the behaviour including when it starts, what sets it off, what occurs and what is noted by those working with the client (including observations on the client themselves and the environment). Antecedents and consequences of the behaviour should also be noted.

One of the difficulties in the successful management of challenging behaviours has been the exclusion of direct care staff in the assessment and planning of treatment programmes. Whitworth *et al* (1999) highlight the need for the direct care staff to be actively involved throughout the assessment and treatment process so that all staff have a better and more thorough understanding, not only of the client's issues, but also the reasons why certain treatments are chosen above others and why the client may exhibit behaviours which challenge in the first place. However, staff may have developed a tolerance of challenging behaviour and do not address the issue directly with the client. Proactively encouraging direct care staff or family members to participate in the assessment and planning process empowers them to not only understand the client better, but also take more responsibility for ensuring that care plans are followed through.

The interpretation phase is an attempt by the family and professionals at suggesting hypotheses for the continuation of the identified behaviour whilst the verification phase will test these hypotheses by altering variables and monitoring any changes in the client's behaviour and responses. It is important that the family and all carers are closely involved in this process, as they should be seen as key informants who quite often are able to assist with identifying triggers for behaviours.

Assessment of challenging behaviour must be holistic. Staff conducting the assessment must be mindful that underlying mental or physical health problems may be the focal cause (see Box 10.3 for a cautionary tale). These potential causes must be considered and properly assessed in the search for 'functional' explanations of the behaviour. Evidence of general altered mood or bodily discomfort should always be actively sought from the client and/or carers. More problematic is the potential that abuse is an underlying cause although this is likely to be associated with alteration in mood. Indications of physical or sexual abuse should be noted and if seriously suspected specialist advice sought. A hypothesis as to the cause of the challenging behaviour should be re-examined if behaviour modification is not successful.

In carrying out the assessment staff must judge whether their interventions for the behaviour will have a negative impact on the client. For example, some clients on the autistic spectrum may have repetitive or ritualistic behaviours which, although they may cause some discomfort or be socially unacceptable, may create such anxiety within the client if removed or impeded that they may engage in new and more challenging behaviours. Determining whether to intervene requires a balancing of the risk of the behaviour continuing versus it being stopped.

SEXUALITY

Conservative views about client sexuality are likely to be prevalent amongst clients' parents and care staff (Cuskelly and Bryde, 2004). Personal views can often be expressed to the client who may internalize often conflicting viewpoints, adding further confusion whilst they may also be grappling with trying to understand what is or isn't socially acceptable. Variables affecting staff viewpoints on clients' sexuality varies from the staff age, religious beliefs and even their professional qualifications (Murray and Minnes, 1994) whilst attitudes to sexual behaviour may also be influenced by the actual place of work (McConkey and Ryan, 2001) and the culture within it (Whitworth *et al*, 1999).

For services this presents a dilemma. On one hand there are clients who have sexual needs and on the other there are staff who may feel ill-equipped to cope with or manage meeting that need in a way which is both sensitive and non-judgemental to the client. There is a gap between the perceptions of care managers and direct care staff in relation to inappropriate sexual behaviours (Smith and Willner, 2004). For many care managers there appears to be a better understanding for services to make arrangements to meet client need whilst direct care staff often find managing sexual behaviour on the frontline more challenging. It is perhaps easier to ignore or be more punitive to a client than it is to sit with them and work out what the issues are and identify strategies to help them behave in an appropriate manner.

Clients who publicly masturbate are probably the most frequently encountered forms of challenging sexual behaviour. The dilemma for staff is in trying to meet the needs of the client whilst also ensuring that the behaviour does not have a negative impact on other vulnerable people. At the same time staff must reserve their own judgement of the behaviour. Essentially the goal is to make the person feel that what they are doing is acceptable, but where they are doing it is not. Sensitivity in handling this issue is paramount in preventing unnecessary feelings of guilt and shame in the client which results in the client's sexual health needs not being met. Clients should be encouraged to continue their behaviour in the privacy of their own bedroom, or in the bathroom, and supported in gaining an understanding about the importance of discretion and the needs of other clients. If it is felt that the client is masturbating to relieve boredom staff should work with the client at developing alternative strategies to occupy their time. The education of this client group in areas of sexuality should form part of the client's individual care plan.

RISK MANAGEMENT

The management of clients with challenging behaviour brings with it many associated responsibilities and challenges. Their health, safety and well-being are of utmost importance at all times and sometimes this can be difficult to achieve when the clients' challenging behaviour places themselves or others at risk. Although it is generally accepted that it is impossible to eliminate risk entirely, it is the role of the care professionals to thoroughly assess risk potential and minimize the chances of any potentially dangerous occurrences.

Risk assessment and its management should be performed in *all* health and social care environments that are accessed by the patient, including mainstream acute care (for example general hospital wards). There are five key principles:

1. Risk assessment should be performed on a per client, per member of staff, per activity basis.

2. Risk assessment and management should adopt a person-centred and bio-psychosocial approach.

3. Communication between staff, clients and carers is essential to both good risk assessment and its management.

4. Care planning should be based on the management of risk, and the process should be ongoing.

5. Risk assessment and its management are the responsibility of all who are involved in the care of each client.

These principles centre on the need of services to provide individualized programmes of care and treatment. The ability of services to manage the risk will centre on the quality of their initial and ongoing assessments of both the individual and the environment. Viewing the client in this perspective gives a better picture of the likelihood of unexpected events occurring. It also makes predicting variables more transparent for staff who may intervene to reduce the element of risk at an earlier opportunity.

Although clients who present with challenging behaviours can place others at risk, it is often they themselves who experience negative consequences as a result of their behaviour. The issues of challenging behaviour and vulnerability are linked, as clients who are seen as difficult to manage are more likely to experience abuse from care workers and fellow residents, but also less likely to have their needs met. This is as a result of the staff finding it difficult to work with the client in a productive way leading to unmet health and social needs, for example clients not being allowed on an outing for fear that their behaviour may ruin the event for others. The management process of risk assessment enables staff to identify how the client, as a result of their behaviour, may place themselves at risk of not having their needs met and sets a plan in place to ensure that the likelihood of this occurring is reduced.

The minimization of harm to clients involves a multimodal approach from direct caregivers by ensuring that the clients are aware that they can approach staff for help or for staff to be alert to the high category, taking appropriate steps to minimize the risk. Risk assessment is not only about major incidents but should also focus on less obvious areas of the client's well-being. Many clients in services have problems with communication, and their ability to express needs is often impaired. Nutrition, exercise, mental and physical health should also be addressed alongside risk of self-injurious behaviours, sexually inappropriate behaviours and harm to self or others, either intentionally or accidentally. This is not an exhaustive list and many of the things people do in their daily lives have an element of risk, which is taken for granted as a result of their ability to manage their lives independently. However, when someone has an intellectual impairment, their judgement and ability to assess risk effectively may also be hindered in some way and it is the role of the care professionals to identify the gap between what the client may do and the risk that that activity may place the client or others in.

Completing risk assessments may identify a number of areas where the client or others are at greater risk because of challenging behaviour. Having identified these risks care staff should seek interventions to reduce the risk that avoid restricting the client in their activities of daily living. A positive approach to risk taking should be taken as part of a team approach to manage the risk in a way which reduces the likelihood of harm but at the same time does not allow interventions which may reduce the client's quality of life. This approach is a difficult one which demands much consideration. It requires the staff to take risks themselves in balancing the risk posed by the behaviour versus the risk of intervening. This form of risk management should form part of the longer term care plan where each intervention is considered with an outcome in mind and with back-up plans in place should the interventions fail to help the client. Two of the potential adverse consequences of attempts to avoid risk are longer periods spent in hospital as a result of the lack of specialist placements suited to meet client needs (Watts *et al*, 2000) and the exclusion they face from facilities accessed by the general population.

SEXUAL ABUSE

Although more likely to be victims of abuse, an often neglected area of risk is the management of clients who are perpetrators of sexual abuse. While risk management should consider vulnerability to abuse we do not elaborate on this aspect here since this is not in itself a challenging behaviour exhibited by a client (although abuse can lead to challenging behaviour). Many services simply do not recognize that their clients may be sexually abusing others in their care (Blanchard *et al*, 1999). The home environment and day centres are the most frequent places of abuse (Turk and Brown, 1993). The number of sexual offenders with a diagnosed intellectual impairment varies across studies with several agreeing that there is an over-representation of intellectually impaired people within the sexual offender population (Hayes, 1991; Day, 1993). Although the results vary Lindsay *at al* (2004) indicate that:

It is pointless trying to determine the percentage of sex offenders with intellectual disability. We know the number is significant and we should focus on the most effective way to provide assessment, treatment and management services.

The identification of those clients who are most likely to offend is central to providing help for them whilst protecting others. The identification of likely offenders comes from a thorough initial assessment where a full past history needs to be obtained. Large families (often with absent father), poor impulse control, a history of abuse, behavioural disturbance, relationship issues, sexual naivety and neglect are just some of the factors which contribute to sexual offending with women also being identified as potential offenders (Lindsay *et al*, 2004; Day, 1993). These same authors also identify the presence of a mental illness where there are reduced inhibitions (e.g. bipolar disorder) as a potential contributory factor.

Offenders also present an increased risk to themselves. Reed *et al* (2004) found that clients who have an offending history of any sort are often less likely to be aggressive to others but were significantly more likely to harm themselves. This perhaps reflects some of the inner difficulties faced by clients who may be transferred to more secure settings as a result of their offences. For many clients who have not had the ability to explore their sexuality in a constructive manner their inner confusion and guilt is further compounded by them acting on what they may see as a natural impulse.

The culture within teams can also hinder managing offending behaviour with many workers finding that their confidence and ability to manage risk behaviour is undermined by the attitude of colleagues (Robertson and Clegg, 2002). For many care managers there appears to be a recent shift towards a better understanding of services (Smith and Willner, 2004).The challenge to manage these behaviours does not lie solely with direct care staff but also with the managers who develop policies and are responsible for staff education and training. Enabling staff to raise sensitive issues with their supervisors can lead to a more open environment, where addressing the client's needs holistically is encouraged. This should consequently help staff make better judgements about the management of risk behaviours. Developing their confidence to tackle such issues head on should help staff to work closer with clients in order to discuss and develop care plans which meet all their needs, as far as possible, whilst reducing the potential risk to others.

OTHER INTERVENTIONS

MEDICATION

Much discussion centres on the inability of professionals to distinguish challenging behaviours from symptoms of mental illness while the actual efficacy of drugs to treat challenging behaviours is also called into question. While many neuroleptics are prescribed in an attempt to manage challenging behaviours (Wressell *et al*, 1990) there is little or no evidence to substantiate the effectiveness of neuroleptics for people who have intellectual impairment and no confirmed diagnosis (Brylewski and Duggan, 1999).

Difficulties with using psychotropic medications stem from the numerous and potentially severe extrapyramidal side effects particularly in the face of uncertain diagnosis and benefit. Extrapyramidal side effects are common and include sedation, dystonia (abnormal face and body movements), restlessness, agitation, hyper-salivation, insomnia, constipation and tremors amongst others (*BNF*, 2006). NICE (2002) recommends the use of newer, atypical antipsychotics for the first line treatment of newly diagnosed schizophrenia but many people are still prescribed the older typical medications.

These side effects can impact on the quality of life of an individual and often clients with mental health problems are unable to communicate these issues to staff. The side effects may add to the distress clients may already experience as a result of mental illness or other underlying problems and some side effects such as agitation, restlessness and insomnia may worsen 'challenging' behaviour. Some patients may be further prescribed medication (e.g. sleeping tablets) for what are in fact the neuroleptic side effects.

Some medication is prescribed 'as required' with the choice to medicate the client at a particular time often left to the staff on shift at the time. This decision can be as a result of an observed change in behaviour without an identified cause. There is a general concern that this is an inappropriate method of treatment as often the client may be behaving in a challenging manner for a specific reason. The availability of medication means that no further assessment is undertaken. Interestingly, greater staff–client ratios appear to make no difference to the administration of 'as required' medications (Suresh, 1998).

More recently there has been a decline in the use of neuroleptics but an increase in the use of antidepressants and polypharmacy, where a number of drugs from the same family are prescribed to treat the same condition (McGillivray and McCabe, 2004). These changes in prescribing practices may be as a result of more accurate diagnoses of underlying mental health problems or a general shift from the use of neuroleptics towards antidepressants in the management of behavioural issues. Research in this area is sparse and most studies recommend further investigation to get a better understanding of the increase in polypharmacy prescribing.

The reduction in the use of neuroleptics in clients who have no clear diagnosis of mental illness has shown some positive results, including better engagement with staff and activities, with a general increase in coordination abilities (Ahmed *et al*, 2000). The implication is that better controls should be in place to ensure that the prescription of medication should be monitored and based only on an accurate diagnosis. Effectiveness should be monitored and reviewed by the full team. Medication, although still the centre of much debate and research, has a clear role in the treatment of underlying mental illness in those with intellectual impairment. However, medication alone is not an answer to the management of challenging behaviour and a collaborative team approach, involving other therapeutic interventions, needs to be employed to ensure that medication is not misused or used as a frontline treatment in all cases.

For further information on medication see Chapter 9.

PHYSICAL RESTRAINT/PHYSICAL INTERVENTIONS/HOLDING

In many settings where there are clients who present with challenging behaviours there are times when the risk posed by the client to themselves or others is substantial. At such times care staff are faced with very difficult decisions on how best to manage the behaviour in the safest and most efficient manner. Effective communication with clients and the correct use of medication can make such situations easier to manage and create an open atmosphere where the client can feel comfortable working with care staff. However, sometimes the use of 'talking treatments', behavioural approaches or even medication is insufficient to prevent a risky situation from developing. At these times physical restraint of a patient may have to be considered.

Restraint itself covers a large variety of potential ways of restricting a person's movement and may involve the actual physical use of force, the use of specially designed isolation rooms or the 'over-medication' of a client. Alternatively restraint may be through omission, for example by not allowing a client who is unable to walk access to their wheelchair. Recent press articles (e.g. O'Hara, 2005) have also hinted at the use of mechanical restraints making a comeback in the United Kingdom. A quick search on the Internet shows numerous illegal cases of care homes being investigated for acts such as tying patients to chairs or beds. There is a fine line between restraint and abuse which is easily and often crossed.

Legally, physical restraint may be used in this country but only 'as a last resort and never as a matter of course' (DH, 1999). It should be used in an emergency when there seems to be a real possibility that significant harm would occur if intervention was withheld. Any restraint must be reasonable in the circumstances. It must be the minimum necessary to deal with harm that needs to be prevented (DH, 1999). Physical restraint should never be carried out by people who are not specifically trained to perform it and interventions should be individualized for each client where possible. The risks associated with restraint are great. Serious injury and even death may occur to a client, or staff, when the process of managing an aggressive client goes awry. Many workplaces offer training under headings such as PMVA or the Prevention and Management of Violence and Aggression.

This title illustrates that restraint is part of an overall process which not only looks at the immediate need for physical restraint but the longer term care plan of how particular clients should be managed by the team to reduce the likelihood of incidents occurring. It also places an onus on care teams to look at their policies and procedures in order to evaluate how they can best work as a team so that when incidents do occur there is a process of working with the client that is instigated rather than restraining the client as soon as a difficult situation arises. Initial attempts should be made at talking with the client in an attempt to 'talk them down' from the situation, known as de-escalation. Many clients might react well to being talked gently to by staff and may accept 'time out' or medication to help with how they are feeling at that time.

Outside of specialist settings staff are unlikely to meet such extreme behaviours with any degree of frequency. It is perhaps best to reiterate here that physical restraint is a specialized intervention that must only be performed by those specially trained. However, some of the principles of management can and should be deployed to avoid more extreme behaviours.

DE-ESCALATION TECHNIQUES

De-escalation is a term for any interventions which result in the prevention of an incident. The prevention of a restraint incident begins before the need for restraint is even identified. All clients should have trigger factors identified as part of their care plan. These triggers are situations that may exacerbate their anxieties or behaviour in a way which is likely to need proactive interventions like restraint. Avoidance of triggers may then enable care providers to minimize the risk of an incident occurring.

The success of de-escalation relies on a number of factors including the care providers' ability to remain calm themselves whilst offering reassurance to the client in a way which is not threatening or demeaning to them. Threats of restraint or isolation must be avoided. The aim is to reassure the client that the caregiver is in a position to listen and understand the difficulty that they are in, in a way which will help the client to manage their anxiety and distress in a safe and constructive way. Putting aside the ethical aspects of threatening clients with adverse consequences, the simple fact is that this strategy is unlikely to succeed and indeed is likely to exacerbate the situation.

Some de-escalation attempts to divert a situation from occurring may be:

- communicating with the client to identify what is upsetting them;

- attempting to distract the client or removal of unwanted stimulus;

- making appropriate eye contact with the client and standing in an open posture (without placing yourself at risk);

- speaking softly and clearly without being patronizing or expressing annoyance or anger at the client;

- removal of any 'audience' from the scene;

- offering support and understanding, or 'time out', to allow the client to ventilate their feelings in a productive way;

- maintaining a supportive presence while the crisis persists;

- offering a de-briefing session to the client when they calm down;

- developing a longer term plan, or reviewing current care plans, to minimize the risk of a similar incident occurring again.

CONCLUSION

People with intellectual impairment and challenging behaviours should never be labelled as being 'problematic' or 'difficult'. Although the individual may display challenging behaviours, it is the service which is challenged in meeting that client's needs as opposed to the client being challenging. The behaviour has developed as a result of an unmet need and it is likely that meeting that need will result in a reduction of the behaviour. Stigmatizing someone because of challenging behaviour can lead to marginalization and neglect, the client's needs going unmet and thus reinforcing the reason for negative behaviours. It is always important to praise and highlight the positive aspects and actions of a person and not focus on the negative behaviours.

The concept of challenging behaviours is difficult and care providers need to take time to understand their client group better, as well as gaining a better understanding of the theoretical views around challenging behaviour. Such an understanding should enable workers to value a person even though the person displays challenging behaviour.

REFERENCES AND RECOMMENDED READING

Ahmed Z, Fraser W, Kerr M, Kiernan C, Emerson E, Robertson J, Felce D, Allen D, Baxter H, Thomas J. (2000) Reducing antipsychotic medication in people with a learning disability. *British Journal of Psychiatry* 176:42–6.

Blanchard R, Watson M, Choy A, Dickey R, Klassen P, Kuban N, Feren DJ. (1999) Paedophiles: mental retardation, maternal age and sexual orientation. *Archives of Sexual Behaviour* 28:111–27.

Blunden R, Allen D. (1987) *Facing the Challenge: An Ordinary Life for People with Learning Difficulties and Challenging Behaviour.* King's Fund.

British National Formulary (BNF) (2006) London: RPS Publishing.

Brown H, Turk V, Stein J. (1994) Findings: sexual abuse of adults with learning disabilities. *Social Care Research Findings* 46:46–9.

Brylewski J, Duggan L. (1999) Antipsychotic medication for challenging behaviour in people with intellectual disability: a systematic review of randomized controlled trials. *Journal of Intellectual Disability Research* 43(5):360–71.

Carr J, Wilder D. (1998) *Functional Assessment and Intervention. A Guide to Understanding Problem Behaviour.* Homewood, IL: High Tide.

Cuskelly M, Bryde R. (2004) Attitudes towards the sexuality of adults with an intellectual disability: parents, support staff, and a community sample. *Journal of Intellectual and Developmental Disability* 29(3): 255–64.

Day K. (1985) Psychiatric disorder in the middle aged and the elderly mentally handicapped. *British Journal of Psychiatry.* 147:660–7.

Day K. (1993) Crime and mental retardation: a review. In: Howell K, Hollin CR (eds), *Clinical Approaches to the Mentally Disordered Offender* John Wiley & Sons, Ltd: Chichester, 111–44.

Department of Health and Welsh Office (1999) *Code of Practice: Mental Health Act 1983*, 3rd edn. London: The Stationery Office.

Emerson E. (1995) *Challenging Behaviour: Analysis and Intervention in People with Learning Disabilities.* Cambridge: Cambridge University Press.

Emerson E, Moss S, Kiernan C. (1999) The relationship between challenging behaviour and psychiatric disorders in people with severe developmental disabilities. In: Bouras N (ed.), *Psychiatric and Behavioural Disorders in Developmental Disabilities and Mental Retardation.* Cambridge: Cambridge University Press, 38–48.

Fleming I, Stenfert Kroese B. (eds) (1993) *People with Learning Disability and Severe Challenging Behaviour – New Developments in Services and Therapy.* Manchester: Manchester University Press.

Gates B. (1996) Issues of reliability and validity in measurement of challenging behaviour (behavioural difficulties) in learning disability: a discussion of implications for nursing research and practice. *Journal of Clinical Nursing* 5:7–12.

Gross R. (2005) *Psychology. The Science of Mind and Behaviour*, 5th edn. London: Hodder Arnold, 907pp.

Harris J, Allen D, Cornick M, Jefferson A, Mills R. (1996) *Physical Interventions: A Policy Framework.* Plymouth: BILD Publications.

Hayes S. (1991) Sex offenders. *Australia and New Zealand Journal of Developmental Disabilities (Journal of Intellectual and Developmental Disabilities)* 17:220–7.

Hurley AD. (2006) Mood disorders in intellectual disability. *Current Opinion in Psychiatry* 19:465–9.

Lindsay WR, Smith AH, Quinn K, Anderson A, Smith A, Allan R, Law J. (2004) Women with intellectual disability who have offended: characteristics and outcome. *Journal of Intellectual Disability Research* 48(6):580–90.

McBrien K, Felce D. (1992) *Working with People who have a Severe Learning Disability and Challenging Behaviour: A Practical Handbook on the Behavioural Approach.* Avon: BILD Publications.

McConkey R, Ryan D. (2001) Experiences of staff in dealing with client sexuality in services for teenagers and adults with intellectual disability. *Journal of Intellectual Disability Research* 45(1):83–7.

McGillivray JA, McCabe MP. (2004) Pharmacological management of challenging behaviour of individuals with intellectual disability. *Research in Developmental Disabilities* 25:523–37.

Murray JL, Minnes PM. (1994) Staff attitudes toward the sexuality of persons with intellectual disability. *Australian and New Zealand Journal of Developmental Disabilities* 19:45–52.

National Institute for Clinical Excellence (2002) *Guidance on the Use of Newer (Atypical) Antipsychotic Drugs for the Treatment of Schizophrenia.* London: NICE. Also available at: http://www.nice.org.uk/page. aspx?o=TA043guidance

National Institute for Clinical Excellence (2004). *Self Harm. The Short-term Physical and Psychological Management and Secondary Prevention of Self-harm in Primary and Secondary Care.* London: NICE. Also available at: http://www.nice.org.uk/page.aspx?o=cg016niceguideline

O'Hara M. (2005) Straitjacket may be brought back into NHS. *Guardian Newspapers* February 2. Retrieved September 22, 2006, from: http://www.guardian.co.uk/uk_news/story/0,,1403666,00.html

Pagliano P, Gannon P, Patching W, Parker J, Ainge D, Berry P. (1988) Living with disabled intellectually handicapped persons. In: Fraser WI, Hussell CGI. (eds), *Key Issues in Mental Retardation Research.* London: Routledge, 171–80.

Reed S, Russell A, Xenitidis K, Murphy D. (2004) People with learning disabilities in a low secure in-patient unit: comparison of offenders and non-offenders. *British Journal of Psychiatry* 185:499–504.

Robertson J, Clegg J. (2002) Dilemmas in the community risk management of sexually offensive behaviour. *British Journal of Learning Disabilities* 30:171–5.

Skinner BF. (1953) *Science and Human Behaviour.* New York: Macmillan.

Smith M, Willner P. (2004) Psychological factors in risk assessment and management of inappropriate sexual behaviour by men with intellectual disabilities. *Journal of Applied Research in Intellectual Disabilities* 17:285–97.

Sobsey D. (1994) *Violence and Abuse in the Lives of People with Disabilities – The End of Silent Acceptance?* Baltimore, MD: Paul H Brookes.

Suresh T. (1998) 'As required' neuroleptics: Have these drugs a place in the management of challenging behaviour in intellectual disability? *Journal of Intellectual Disability Research* 42(6):500–4.

Turk V, Brown H. (1993) The sexual abuse of adults with learning disabilities: Results of a 2-year incidence survey. *Mental Handicap Research* 6:193–216.

Watts RV, Richold P, Berney TP. (2000) Delay in the discharge of psychiatric in-patients with learning disabilities. *Psychiatric Bulletin* 24:179–81.

Whitworth D, Harris P, Jones R. (1999) Staff culture and the management of challenging behaviours in people with learning disabilities. *Mental Health Care* 2(11):376–8.

Wressell SE, Tyrer SP, Berney TP. (1990) Reduction in antipsychotic drug dosage in mentally handicapped patients. A hospital study. *British Journal of Psychiatry* 157:101–6.

CHAPTER 11
CONSENT AND CAPACITY

Alison Hobden and Simon Mills

STUDY AIMS:

1. To explore the principles of consent.

2. To understand the legal framework for consent in the UK.

3. To consider issues raised in managing care with and for people with intellectual impairment.

In this chapter we consider the legal framework and issues that arise in relation to consent for people with intellectual impairment. Consent, as defined by the *Oxford English Dictionary* is the voluntary agreement to or acquiescence by one person in what another proposes or desires – compliance. In essence, consent is permission by a client for professionals to touch, question, examine or deliver care to a client. Many things happen in health care that, without consent, would be unlawful. For example, patients are cut with scalpels, injected with needles and subjected to potentially harmful X-ray. Without consent, any of these things would be a crime.

Any competent adult has the right to govern who touches their person, and therefore consent is required to any such action (Dimond, 2005). Philosophically, consent has its roots in the idea that everyone has the right of autonomy, which should be respected. In more legal terms, consent is often viewed as a defence against litigation that might otherwise ensue. When a patient consents to an intervention, they cannot subsequently assert that they were assaulted. For the purposes of the law, consent is valid when three criteria are met:

- The consent is based on sufficient relevant information.

- The consent is voluntary.

- The consent is given by someone with the capacity to give consent.

Learning Disability and other Intellectual Impairments, Edited by L.L. Clark and P. Griffiths
© 2008 John Wiley & Sons, Ltd

THE HEALTHCARE PROFESSIONAL AND CONSENT

According to the law, a healthcare professional is bound by the giving (or withholding) of consent by a patient. Respecting a patient's decision may be easy when a patient is seen to make a rational decision about health care. At the other end of the spectrum there are certain times when it is impossible to ask the patient their view (such as if the patient is unconscious) and a decision must then be based on what is perceived to be a patient's 'best interests'. The most problematic area is patients that lie between these two states, where they may be able to communicate a decision regarding their health care but there is uncertainty as to what extent they understand the implications of the decision they are making. This often arises when caring for people with intellectual impairments because the health professional is unsure of the rationale for treatment.

Anyone who is in a position to lawfully give consent may also withhold it. The law recognizes that a fundamental corollary of the right to give consent is the right to say 'no', and to be left alone. The law furthermore recognizes that once a refusal meets the criteria for giving consent (that is to say, the refusal is voluntary, informed and comes from someone with the capacity to refuse), then it is binding on healthcare practitioners.

Refusal to consent to treatment need not be for reasons that the treating healthcare professionals regard as rational or sensible. None the less, the refusal is binding. Judges in the United Kingdom have concluded that the right to refuse treatment 'is not limited to decisions which others might regard as sensible. It exists notwithstanding that the reasons for making the choice are rational, irrational, unknown or even non-existent.' 'Competent adults . . . are generally at liberty to refuse medical treatment even at the risk of death.'

In general, the law requires that consent be given in a particular form. However, there are some specific exceptions, for instance consent to clinical research must be given in writing. In the normal everyday clinical setting, consent may be given in any one of two recognized ways. Consent may be:

- implied or

- expressed either orally or in writing.

All forms of consent are equally valid but written consent is often seen as providing the best evidence that consent has in fact been obtained should any dispute subsequently arise. In general, the greater the risk associated with a procedure, the more likely we are to want to have written consent.

IMPLIED CONSENT

Implied consent is best described as 'actions speaking louder than (or instead) of words'. Therefore, implied consent is where patients present themselves in such a manner as to suggest that they are consenting to a particular healthcare intervention. For example, the patient who presents at a clinic to have a blood sample taken and who, without being asked, rolls up their sleeve, is giving an implied consent to the blood sample being taken. Indeed, either or both of the patient's actions (turning up to the clinic and baring their arm) suggest the patient's consent to the procedure.

One danger with implied consent is that healthcare professionals may make an assumption based on the patient's actions and this assumption may well be wrong. It is therefore advisable to verbally verify the patient's understanding before proceeding: in this way, the consent is taken into the realms of 'express consent'.

EXPRESS CONSENT

Express consent is more formal than implied consent because the patient articulates, through the spoken or written word, the fact that he or she is consenting to a proposed course of action. For example, a general practitioner might ask a patient's permission to carry out an intimate examination where consent might be given (or withheld) orally. In a more structured setting, such as a preoperative protocol, the patient's consent to the operation will most commonly be recorded in writing, using a preprinted form into which relevant information, such as the patient's name is inserted.

In pure legal terms, there is no significant difference between express consent obtained orally and that obtained in writing: written consent is not 'more valid' than oral consent or implied consent. Many simple interventions are carried out after obtaining verbal consent. A problem may arise, however, where there is a dispute about the terms of any consent. Where consent was given orally then what was said may come down to the 'patient's word' against that of the healthcare professional. In general, for low risk interventions, such disputes are rare.

However, as the associated risks of an intervention increase, so the responsible healthcare professional will want to satisfy themselves that the patient understands the risks and benefits of the proposed treatment. For example, merely because the patient has turned up at the hospital with an overnight bag it cannot be assumed that they are giving consent to complex heart surgery. Similarly with the increasing complexity of a procedure so the complexity of the consent process also grows. With this the desirability of recording consent in writing (including the precise terms of that consent) becomes apparent. Obtaining and recording written consent is also more likely to ensure that mutual understanding regarding treatment is secured.

It is important to note that the validity of consent is not based on the form of consent obtained, but on the process by which it is obtained and whether all of the components of valid consent are present. The UK Department of Health produces specimen forms of consent, all of which require a health professional to discuss with the patient in mainstream hospital or clinic environment (excluding mental health settings), the benefits of the proposed treatments, and the likely associated risks involved. There are four consent forms available (available for internet download – see Internet Resources below):

- Form 1 – Patient agreement to investigation or treatment

- Form 2 – Parental agreement to investigation or treatment for a child or young person

- Form 3 – Patient/parental agreement to investigation or treatment (procedures where consciousness is not impaired)

- Form 4 – Form for adults who are unable to consent to investigation or treatment.

When using Form 4 the health professional who will be carrying out the procedure will sign the form themselves stating that in their opinion the procedure is in the patient's 'best interests'. Under no circumstances can a parent, spouse or paid carer of an unconscious or intellectually impaired adult sign this under current law. Thus while the law provides that parents can consent for children it does not provide for *anyone* to consent on behalf of another adult. Rather it allows for circumstances where care may be given to someone who is *unable* to give consent because it is deemed to be in their best interests.

CONSEQUENCES OF ACTING WITHOUT CONSENT

Acting without consent is a breach of duty of care towards our patients, and there are two categories of legal consequence:

• An action in assault or trespass on the person

• An action in negligence.

Historically, the more common action for acting without consent was 'trespass to the person' (sometimes referred to as assault or battery), but with the passage of time the more common legal action is negligence. In recent years the approach of the law has been to regard a failure to obtain proper consent as negligence, save for the most exceptional of circumstances. In modern times, this is only likely to arise where a patient has been fundamentally misled by the clinician, for example about what is to be done or who is to do it (e.g., where a doctor lies about his qualifications) or where there was a total absence of consent (e.g., where a non-consenting Jehovah's Witness is subjected to a forced blood transfusion).

In order to win a negligence action, a person has to prove each and every one of three things:

• A duty of care

• Breach of the duty of care

• That the patient was harmed by the breach of the duty of care.

In general, there is no problem in proving the duty of care. When a patient is cared for by a healthcare professional, there is a duty of care. The standard of care (or in other words, the expected level of disclosure of information when obtaining consent) is discussed below. Finally, in order to prove harm, the patient must show that the failure to obtain proper consent caused the patient to suffer harm, for instance by consenting to undergo an operation that the patient would not have undergone had they been adequately informed about the risks or side effects from which they are now suffering as a result of the procedure.

Where consent is fully voluntary and informed and the patient has the capacity to consent, no legal action can arise. Where the patient says that a proper explanation of treatment was not given or that the information that was given was not understood by them then, assuming that the negligence tests are satisfied or that the facts are serious enough to ground a trespass action, the patient can lay a claim against the clinician that they have not fulfilled their duty of care towards the patient (Dimond, 2005).

Alongside legal consequences, there is also the issue of trust within the professional clinician–patient relationship. If a patient has expressed a wish to undergo certain treatment they then have the right to expect the clinician to carry out that treatment and not, for example, to change the patient's therapy without discussion. Failure to have a proper basis for consent could lead to a permanent breakdown in the working relationship. It is therefore sufficient to say that consent is important from both a legal and ethical viewpoint.

In order to ensure that valid consent has been obtained from patients there are a number of models available to guide the health professional through the process and they include both 'legal' and the other 'ethical' components of what constitutes proper and valid consent to medical treatment.

THE LEGAL MODEL OF CONSENT

Healthcare professionals are required to ensure that three legal criteria have been met in order to satisfy a claim that consent was obtained. The standard legal model for consent breaks the process down into three components, namely:

- Voluntariness – the patient should give or withhold consent voluntarily
- Information – the patient should have the necessary information with which to take the decision
- Capacity – the patient should have sufficient capacity to take the decision.

VOLUNTARINESS

Consent is a voluntary process. A person must be acting free of pressure, coercion and inducements. Some scenarios may suggest the absence of free will. Some writers have argued that the nature of medical treatment is such that, once on the 'treadmill of treatment', particularly in the hospital setting, patients are never truly free to choose (McLean, 1999). All patients will be under the influence of certain external factors that may serve to limit choice. So a patient can only choose from the options put in front of them by the medical team caring for them, this may be limited by the severity of their disease in terms of travelling to receive a treatment elsewhere. The clinician's role is, in part, to help maximize the patient's freedom of choice.

The fact that consent, in order to be valid, must be voluntary means in turn that it should be given (or withheld) free from undue pressure or coercion. A patient should be free to make his own treatment decision and should not be placed under pressure from a healthcare practitioner. However, the question arises as to the concept that a patient should not be placed under 'undue pressure', which means that there is a certain degree of pressure that could be deemed permissible. For example, does the emphasis of the benefits of the best available treatment, while stressing the negative aspects of a less successful treatment, constitute the application of undue pressure? Beauchamp and Childress (2001) suggest three influencing forces to which people are susceptible: coercion, manipulation and persuasion. People with intellectual impairments may be particularly vulnerable to any or all of these.

In coercion, the 'coercer' uses some threat of a negative outcome if a proposed choice is not taken, for example 'if you do not give up smoking, you will not be placed on the waiting list for a heart transplant' or 'this treatment is your only real hope'. In coercing a patient the health professional negates their autonomy and consequently places them in a position whereby they feel that they can only choose one option. Persuasion has similar features, but its defining characteristic is that reasons rather than threats are deployed to lead a patient to a desired outcome. For example, 'most people choose procedure A', which carries the underlying subtext that therefore no reasonable person would choose procedure B or any other option. In manipulation, a person is led to the desired choice, not through reasoning or threats, but through misinformation, incomplete information or by withholding the truth.

There may be circumstances in which practitioners use elements of these approaches in clinical practice. There may be times when a professional might be judged not to have fulfilled their duty to their patient unless they successfully advocate and bring about a particular course of action, such as agreeing to a lifesaving blood transfusion. At this point it is useful to consider a patient whom we know is choosing a course of action that is going to cause them harm (smoking for example), it is easy to see that there is a professional obligation to promote outcomes for the patient that would benefit them and so smoking cessation is suggested to them. It may therefore be argued that it is not unreasonable to try and persuade that person to stop smoking, even if in doing so, we 'chip away' at the patient's freedom to make an untrammelled choice.

All these factors apply to people with intellectual impairment as much as anyone else although it may be that the range of options offered to them may differ. Professionals should also be mindful that they may be more susceptible to forms of pressures such as coercion as they invest undue authority in others. However, the most significant issues arise when considering an individual's ability to make *informed* choices based on information given.

INFORMED CONSENT

In order to make a decision, a certain amount of information needs to be given in a manner that is relevant and comprehensible to the individual and on the basis of which the patient can reach a decision: so called 'informed consent'. People are entitled to receive information that is appropriate, relevant and through such channels that enable them to make a decision about their health care. The term 'appropriate' means that the information should be presented in a way that the patient can understand. It would not, by way of example, be appropriate for a doctor to use the English language to inform an elderly woman from the Indian sub-continent whose only language was Urdu about a proposed surgical procedure, the information might be both relevant and exhaustive, but it would not be appropriate. Similarly it would not be appropriate to rely on written information to give detailed information to a person with intellectual impairment who cannot read. To say that the information must be relevant is simply to say that it should relate to the decision that must be made by the patient.

Where problems arise in the area of delivering information to patients it is problematic to establish a standard form, according to which a patient is sufficiently informed. In other words it is difficult to establish when informed consent actually informed. Looking at the legal answers to this issue, two strands of thought have emerged:

- The 'professional' standard – a patient is informed once they have been given such information as the reasonable doctor would provide.

- The 'reasonable patient' standard – a patient is informed once they have been given such information as the reasonable patient would wish to know.

BOX 11.1   THE SIDAWAY CASE (UK)

Mrs Sidaway suffered from recurrent neck and shoulder pain, and her surgeon recommended that she had a spinal operation to relieve the pain. She was advised that there was a risk of nerve root damage to the nerve root but not of the small risk (1–2%) of spinal cord damage. The operation was competently performed but her spinal cord was damaged leaving Mrs Sidaway severely disabled. She sued her surgeon on the grounds that he had breached his duty of care by not informing her of this risk.

Mrs Sidaway lost the case and the House of Lords ultimately upheld that decision. They applied the 'professional' standard test: the non-disclosure of the risk was not negligent because a responsible body of neurosurgeons had confirmed in evidence that they would not have disclosed this risk to their patient. ■

BOX 11.2   THE PEARCE CASE (UK)

Mrs Pearce was expecting her sixth child and was two weeks past her expected date of delivery. She requested that her obstetrician induce her or carry out a caesarean section. Her doctor advised against this for a number of reasons but did not mention the small increased risk (0.1–0.2%) which was associated with going past her expected date of her baby dying 'in utero'. The baby did die 'in utero' approximately one week later. Mrs Pearce sued on the basis that she had not been fully informed of the risks associated with leaving the pregnancy to continue.

Mrs Pearce lost her case, the court once more applied the professional standard. The risk of death was a small one and one that doctors did not regard as significant, so the failure to disclose was reasonable. Non-disclosure was in this case considered a reasonable and logical course of action. Doctors were only required to explain significant risks that would affect the judgement of a reasonable patient, and to take into account relevant considerations (such as the patient's emotional and physical state) when deciding how much to tell a patient of the risks involved. ■

BOX 11.3   THE ROGERS CASE (AUSTRALIA)

This case is an example of the reasonable patient standard. A patient, who was blind in one eye, was considering an operation to restore the sight in the affected eye. The patient was not told that there was a 1 in 10000 risk that the sight in the good eye could be affected and he could be left totally blind. This is exactly what happened.

The doctor attempted to defend the case by reference to the 'professional' standard: the risk, although a serious one, was extremely rare and most doctors did not warn about it. However, the court preferred to take a 'reasonable patient' approach and to say that no matter what the professional standard was, the risk of blindness was a material risk to which the 'reasonable patient' would attach importance, and so the patient should have been warned. The patient won the case. ■

In the United Kingdom and in Ireland, the 'professional' (or 'reasonable doctor') standard is the norm, while the 'reasonable patient' approach has become the norm in many Commonwealth countries (such as Australia and Canada) and in the United States of America. In order to further explore the idea of informed consent and these differing standards, some key legal cases will be explored.

A third approach, aside from the 'professional' and 'reasonable patient' approaches, that could be brought to bear on informed consent is that of the 'subjective standard'. Beauchamp and Childress (2001) suggest that when giving information clinicians should by all means provide information in a quantity deemed appropriate by the relevant professional and/or in a quantity sufficient for the reasonable person to comprehend, but the clinician is also under an obligation to make that information applicable to the particular patient to whom the information is being given. This element of information giving has been highlighted in a number of legal cases, including the case of *Chester* v. *Afshar*. In that case, the information that was given met the 'professional' standard, and the 'reasonable patient' standard, but what was different here, and which resulted in the patient winning the case, was that the information did not take into account the patient as an individual and the information was not tailored to her needs. This has significant implications when considering consent from people with intellectual impairments.

Ethical models of consent have also been suggested. Beauchamp and Childress (2001) propose that informed consent can be broken down into two different definitions. The first centres on the process of respecting autonomous choices (as discussed), but also they say that a second definition of informed consent can be used that considers consent in terms of the principle of informed consent as a social standard or institutional rule. In this case, informed consent is determined by a legal authorization to consent. That is so that a child, for example, might authorize a certain procedure but under the legal definitions of consent, they are not able to consent to the treatment, but they are autonomously authorizing the procedure. Some might say that this is giving informed consent but, in general, institutional or legal authorizations are not held in the same regard as going through the more rigorous process of informed consent that concentrates on this principle of autonomy.

CAPACITY TO CONSENT

In order for consent to be valid, it must be voluntary and based on sufficient relevant information. The final component of valid consent is capacity (or competency). Consent can only be gained from someone who is capable, in a legal context, of making a decision. Capacity refers to distinct qualities: the first is age (adults are free to give and withhold consent; the rights of under-18s and more particularly under-16s are more limited), while the second is that of 'mental capacity'.

Put at its most basic, mental capacity is concerned with an individual's ability to comprehend information and to make a decision as a consequence of that information. A person who lacks mental capacity may not be able to understand any information or have only a limited capacity to do so, or may only be able to comprehend information if presented in a certain way. Clinicians must be able to assess mental capacity as part of the consent process, subsequently a number of different bodies have attempted to define when a person possesses mental capacity. Clearly this issue is of great concern in relation to people with intellectual impairment.

DEFINITIONS AND APPROACHES TO MENTAL CAPACITY

The Mental Capacity Act 2005 (UK) states (Section 2(1)) that a person lacks mental capacity if at the material time he or she is unable to make a decision for him or herself in relation to the matter because of an impairment of, or a disturbance in the functioning of, the mind or brain. The act goes on to state (Section 2(2)) that it does not matter if the impairment or disturbance is of a permanent or temporary nature. The act further states (Section 3) that a person is unable to make a decision due to lack of mental capacity, when he is unable to:

- *understand* the information relevant to the decision;
- *retain* that information;
- *use or weigh* that information as part of the process of making the decision;
- *communicate* his decision (whether by talking, using sign language or any other means).

A person is not to be regarded as unable to understand the information relevant to a decision if they are able to understand an explanation of it given to them in a way that is appropriate to their individual circumstances, for example by utilizing simple language, visual aids or any other appropriate means. The fact that a person is able to retain the information relevant to a decision for only a short period of time does not prevent them from being able to make the decision. The information relevant to a decision includes information about the reasonably foreseeable consequences of either giving or withholding consent, or in failing to reach a decision at all.

The US President's Commission on Bioethics (1983) took a different approach in stating that any determination of the capacity must relate to the individual abilities of a patient, the requirements of the task at hand, and the consequences which are likely to be the result of such decision. According to the President's Commission (1995) decision-making capacity requires, to greater or lesser degree, that the person has possession of a set of values and goals, the ability to communicate and to understand information as well as the ability to reason and to deliberate about one's choices.

Beauchamp and Childress (2001) suggest some other standards that might be used to determine a lack of competence or capacity. These include situations whereby the person has an inability to express or communicate a preference or choice, to comprehend their situation and its consequences or relevant information supplied. In addition, they may have an inability to give a rational reason (although some supporting reasons may be given) coupled with an inability to give risk/benefit-related reasons (although some rational supporting reasons may be supplied), consequently this will render them unable to reach a reasonable decision (as judged, for example, by a reasonable person standard).

What is clear from all of these definitions is the idea that capacity is function specific. It relates to the capacity of a particular person to make a particular decision. Thus, a person may be competent to make certain decisions but not others. For example, we might feel satisfied that a person with severe learning disabilities is able to make a decision regarding what clothes to wear, but not about whether or not to undergo a heart transplant.

Mental capacity is a vital part of informed consent and the decision-making capacity of an individual might fluctuate in certain circumstances, with a disease process such as early stage dementia. In other circumstances the mental capacity of a patient will be comparatively static (for example, in moderate intellectual impairment due to a genetically acquired learning disability), but the patient may none the less be able to take certain decisions. The very nature of the cognitive state of a patient with intellectual impairment renders it likely that there will be some impairment in mental capacity. It is important, then, that healthcare professionals have a subtle understanding of the principles of capacity and its role in maximizing the autonomy of the intellectually impaired patient.

Beauchamp and Childress (2001) point out that it is rarely possible to have fully informed consent. That is to say that the process is rarely fully voluntary, fully informed nor does the patient often have full capacity to understand the process. However, in spite of this, we do not simply throw out this notion of informed consent, but instead the way in which we obtain consent should allow the person to maximize voluntariness, information and capacity in all the circumstances of the particular patient's case. Within this, we can take into account temporary factors that might alter a patient's capacity at a given moment in time, but would still facilitate the process of consent at a given point in time.

THE LEGAL TEST

Many of the most problematic cases in consent generally, and in the area of capacity specifically, arise in circumstances where a patient wishes to refuse a treatment. Clinicians often believe that the refusal of an intervention is for reasons that appear to be less than wholly rational. Competent adults have the same right to refuse treatment as they do to consent to it, including the right to take their own discharge from hospital, for example. As we have observed, competent adults have the right to refuse treatment or to demand that treatment already in being be withdrawn. This right cannot be over-ruled even if the choice will result in serious harm or even death for the patient. It is important to note that the law always presumes that a person possesses capacity and it is always for the person that asserts a lack of capacity to prove the fact.

Broadly speaking, the starting approach of the courts is that the test for competency requires two questions be asked of the patient: can (or could) the patient comprehend and retain the information and can (or could) they weigh up the information to make a decision? This test has been refined in two legal cases: *Re C (Adult: refusal of medical treatment)* and *Re MB (An adult: medical treatment)*.

The question in *Re C* was whether C had the mental capacity to refuse treatment (which the doctors did not believe to be the case). After considering the evidence, the court ruled that he was competent to make this decision because he was able to comprehend and retain the information given to him, able to believe that information and also to weigh it up in order to make a choice even though it was acknowledged that his general capacity was impaired by the presence of schizophrenia. From this, we can see that the presence of a mental disorder does not inherently render someone incompetent to make a decision (see the discussion of 'functional capacity' below).

The courts reached a different decision in the case of MB but reaffirmed the same basic principles.

Refusal of treatment can be distressing for the healthcare practitioner, especially given that most practitioners will advocate treatment that is intended to be beneficial to the patient.

BOX 11.4   C

C was a patient with a diagnosis of paranoid schizophrenia and detained in hospital following the stabbing of his girlfriend. He was diagnosed, subsequent to his admission, as having gangrene in his right foot and was moved to an NHS hospital for treatment. There the surgeons considered that C's life was in immediate danger unless he underwent a below knee amputation. C consented to more conservative treatment but refused to consent to the amputation and sought an injunction to prevent the doctors from carrying out the procedure in the future. The courts supported C's refusal of treatment, notwithstanding his psychiatric diagnosis. ■

BOX 11.5	MB

MB was 40 weeks pregnant and required a caesarean section in order to safely deliver her baby, which was in the breech position. She suffered from a needle phobia and because of this had previously refused to have blood tests during the pregnancy. She initially consented to the operation, but panicked when they tried to start the operation, and subsequently withdrew her consent. She eventually went into labour naturally but still required the caesarean section and the hospital applied to the court to be allowed to operate. The doctors' request to the court was upheld and the operation was carried out.

The court reaffirmed that a doctor could only intervene if it was shown that the patient lacked capacity to make that decision. For MB, her fear of needles occupied her thinking at the critical point and rendered her incapable of making any decision. On the basis of this, the doctors were granted permission to carry out the operation, using reasonable force if necessary. The courts, however, emphasized that they would only intervene in such cases where a clear case regarding the capacity of the patient could be shown. ■

However, taking into account these two cases, we can see that patients, even where they were not (in the classical sense) of fully sound mind, have the right to refuse treatment, and that right cannot be over-ruled solely on the basis that healthcare professionals disagree with either the decision or the apparent basis on which that decision has been reached. These decisions add greater weight to the need to properly assess the capacity of the patient to take any decision facing the patient and to recognize that patients with intellectual impairment may well have the capacity to both give and withhold consent to medical or surgical treatment.

Following on from the decisions in *Re C and Re MB*, the courts have laid down the broad legal principles regarding the criteria to determine capacity:

1. The person is unable to understand and retain the information pertinent to the proposed treatment. This has special relevance if the information pertains to the likely outcomes regarding refusal of treatment.

2. The person is unable to use the information to inform their decision making process.

FLUCTUATIONS IN COMPETENCE

The competent patient has a right to make the wrong decision, even for reasons that may be irrational or non-existent to health professionals. This 'right to be wrong' was highlighted perfectly in the case of *Re C* (discussed in greater detail below) where a patient's decision to refuse treatment was initially deemed irrational and therefore a symptom of his incompetence, only for further investigation to demonstrate that notwithstanding the unorthodox nature of the patient's reasoning, he was in fact competent. The mere presence of emotional responses such as that of panic or irrationality does not in itself indicate incompetence, although it may be a symptom of it. A patient who requires an emergency appendectomy but who is refusing to consent to it might be assumed to be panicking and therefore to be incompetent to make the decision. It is easy to assume that such a decision must be the result of incompetence, but is important that it is recognized that such an outlook may also reflect prejudice or unconsciously (but firmly) held beliefs about what is the right course of action.

Equally, fear can hinder a person's ability to make a decision, but once more, it is important to look behind the response and to assess the patient. A patient may decline a procedure, as they believe it will be very painful and they do not want to experience pain, this fear might be groundless and arise because the patient has not been properly informed. Through careful explanations of the procedure and the options for pain relief, the patient's fear may be allayed and they consent to the treatment. Other temporary factors such as shock, drugs and confusion may erode someone's competence. As Hendrick (2000) points out, as caregivers we must satisfy ourselves that this is truly the case.

There are times when a person's capacity to consent to or refuse treatment may fluctuate within an episode of care for clinical reasons. In some psychiatric conditions or for people with dementia capacity may vary in accordance with period of relapse and remission. There are some steps that can be taken to maximize decision-making capacity where that capacity is hampered, but not obliterated, by illness:

- Treat underlying conditions that may be impairing soundness of mind or decision-making capacity, such as infections or the presence of depression.

- Recognize that a patient's mental powers may fluctuate and that any impairment may be temporary. Delaying or repeating an assessment may be appropriate.

- Consider that apparent deficiencies in mental functioning may in fact be deficiencies in the power of communication, such as dysphasia after a stroke, and attempt to overcome those hurdles.

- Conduct the assessment, where possible in circumstances and surroundings where the patient feels most comfortable. Consider whether the presence of a third party might help or hinder matters (British Medical Association, 2004).

FUNCTIONAL CAPACITY

Mental capacity may be 'function specific'. Clinicians should be wary of labelling patients as 'lacking capacity' or 'incompetent' for the purposes of all treatment decisions. This approach is sometimes known as a 'status' approach to competence. Using this view (now largely displaced by the functional view of consent) a patient is held to be incompetent by reason of their status, that is, they have dementia so they are considered to have no capacity to give consent; however, in reality their capacity may fluctuate. Status notwithstanding, there may be some decisions that the patient can take. Let us consider the case of Emma (Box 11.6) to demonstrate this.

Before her discharge, there is a case conference whereby a key worker questions if Emma is still going to be able to prepare her own meals, now that she was deemed incompetent to consent to this surgery. It should be easy to see that the answer to the key worker's question should be 'yes'. If Emma was making rational decisions about her choice of food prior to her surgery, there is nothing about the surgery that would cause her capacity in that respect to be diminished. Emma should therefore be allowed to prepare meals with the same level of assistance as that prior to her operation.

BOX 11.6   EMMA

Emma is a 34-year-old woman with Down syndrome; she is able to wash and dress independently and to prepare simple meals for herself. She lives in assisted housing where carers help her with her shopping and assist in preparing more complex meals. Recently Emma underwent an emergency appendectomy without her express consent, having been deemed to lack capacity, as she did not appear to comprehend the likely outcome should she continue to decline treatment. The appendectomy was performed on the basis of necessity and acting in Emma's best interests. Emma has now recovered from the surgery and is returning back to her assisted housing. ■

CONSENT TO SEXUAL RELATIONS AND CONTRACEPTION

The Home Office in their report *Setting the Boundaries: Reforming the Law on Sex Offences* (2000) states that it is an offence to engage in sexual activity with someone who lacks capacity to consent to sex and when determining capacity to consent, whilst all the usual requirements for consent need to be met, specifically, when consenting to sex, someone should understand:

• that sex is not part of personal care;

• the relationship between vaginal sex and pregnancy;

• the risk of transmission of HIV/AIDS with anal sex.

The Law Commission (2000) report, *Mental Capacity*, has also proposed that in terms of sexual activity for any non-consensual sexual offence, a person should be regarded as lacking capacity to consent to an act if at the material time they are unable by reason of mental disability to make a decision themselves on whether to consent to the act; or if they are unable to communicate their decision on that matter. 'Valuing People' (DH, 2001) identifies that people with learning disabilities have the same opportunities as the general population, including the right to have meaningful relationships, and should be supported in so doing. However, staff need to be mindful of their duty of care and the individual's capacity to consent.

Some people with an intellectual impairment may be able to take quite complicated anti-conception precautions, whilst others may not. The issue of preventing pregnancy raises particular challenges in someone who is unable to take responsibility for her (and in this discussion, it will almost always be a female patient) contraception and who would be unable to care for an infant. In these circumstances it is not unusual to encounter the request that someone who has an intellectual impairment is sterilized in order to prevent a pregnancy from taking place.

The preference for contraception in the sexually active patient would always be to use the least invasive, yet still effective, method of contraception (in preference the use of condoms whereby pregnancy is prevented and sexually shared diseases kept to a minimum). However, there may be scenarios where a patient cannot manage a simple contraceptive regime, where three-monthly depot contraceptive regimes are burdensome and upsetting for the patient and

---

BOX 11.7   **RE B (A MINOR) (WARDSHIP: STERILIZATION)**

B was a 17-year-old girl who had a mental age of five or six. She had no understanding of the causative relation between sexual intercourse and pregnancy. It was felt that she would not be able to cope with pregnancy or childbirth, and that any child born to her would have to be taken into care. Other forms of contraception were unsuitable owing to other medication that she was taking. The Local Authority requested that she was made a ward of court and that the court would grant leave in order for her to undergo the operation.

B was a minor (under 18), however the court believed that waiting until she was 18 would not alter her capacity to consent to this operation. On the basis of this and of the reality that she would not be able to cope with the repercussions of a pregnancy, the right to carry out the sterilization in B's best interests was granted. ■

BOX 11.8   **RE F (MENTAL PATIENT: STERILIZATION)**

F was a 35-year-old woman in an institution who had an intellectual impairment and who had formed a sexual relationship with a male patient. F had the mental age of a small child and the hospital staff believed that she would not be able to cope with a pregnancy. The doctors were granted the right to undertake sterilization. ■

---

where implant methods are not indicated or suitable. In such situations, sterilization may be considered but can only be approved by the law courts. Three decisions of the courts are examined in order to highlight the considerations that are applied before the compulsory sterilization of an intellectually impaired patient will be considered.

However, it is not automatically the case that a court will direct the sterilization of an intellectually impaired person in circumstances where it is argued that the patient's 'best interests' would be served by sterilization. In the cases of *Re S (Adult patient: sterilisation)* – where sterilization was sought to help a patient with distressingly painful periods – and *Re A (Medical treatment: male sterilisation)* – where the mother of a man with Down syndrome applied for him to undergo a vasectomy – the courts refused permission for the operations to be carried out on the basis that they were not in the patient's best interests. Another element that sometimes comes into play with court decisions on compulsory sterilization is whether the sterilization proposed would also be consistent with good medical practice, if it would not, then it is less likely to be approved by the courts.

There are those who are critical of compulsory sterilization. McClean (1999) argues that compulsory sterilization does nothing to protect patients from sexual exploitation and indeed may even, by removing the possibility of pregnancy, make the patient more susceptible to exploitation.

Sterilization does not mean that they will not be vulnerable to sexual assault, unsuitable liaisons or sexually transmitted diseases. All it does is ensure that no conception takes place, reinforcing the . . . suggestion that the actual reasons for the non-consensual sterilisations are not the same as those that are overtly given . . . It is clear that the 'best interests' test will be met where there is a congruence of clinical recommendation, parental support and judicial inclination.

It is clear that courts will not lightly contemplate sterilization and it is obvious too that the decision to sterilize the patient who lacks mental capacity raises issues of 'best interests'.

ACTING IN THE ABSENCE OF CONSENT

Broadly speaking, where an adult cannot consent to treatment, there is no one who can consent in his or her stead. With children, parents will be surrogate decision makers, but for adults there is no such convenient repository of authority where the adult has lost the power to consent. A patient may not be able to consent for a variety of reasons, for instance the patient who cannot consent because they lack any capacity, for example, due to infancy or coma, or the patient who may be competent to consent to some things, but not to others (patients such as Emma in the example in Box 11.6). In such cases, two principles are generally relied upon, although they are often described separately, the twin principles of 'necessity' and 'best interests' can often overlap. A patient may require treatment as a matter of necessity, but whatever treatment is provided should be provided in the patient's best interests. Two cases are described (Box 11.9 and Box 11.10) in order to demonstrate the concepts of necessity and best principles.

In this case, the key factor to be considered is time. If John is not treated with haste, he is likely to die as a result of the blood loss from his injury. There is no time to formally assess John's mental capacity and to establish if he would or would not want surgery to be undertaken so the decision is made to take John to theatre. The operation to repair John's femur is being performed because John 'needs it' and so this is known as the 'principle of necessity'. The treatment provided is also within John's 'best interests'.

BOX 11.9

John is a 35-year-old man who has been knocked off his motorcycle. He is brought into the accident and emergency department of the hospital in a semi-conscious state. He has a fractured femur and appears to have lost a significant amount of blood through his injuries. His conscious state is deteriorating and it is vital that the surgery is carried out as soon as possible. The staff are unable to obtain any coherent response from John regarding his treatment and the decision is made to operate on John before it is too late to save his life. ■

BOX 11.10   KHALDA

Khalda is a 35-year-old woman with Down syndrome, who also suffers from clinical depression. Due to her genetic condition, she has had swallowing difficulties since birth. Khalda should have a puréed diet but she enjoys, and is often found eating, 'normal food'. As a result, she suffers recurrent chest infections due to aspiration of food and she has also been found choking on solid food. The frequency of her chest infections is increasing, the consultant learning disability psychiatrist (who also looks after her general health care) proposes a referral for the insertion of a gastrostomy tube (enabling feeding directly into her stomach) which would be 'inserted for her own safety'. Other carers, including her Community Psychiatric Nurse (CPN), social worker and parents who have all known Khalda for a number of years, disagree with this decision, reasoning that eating is one of Khalda's few pleasurable activities and that she should be allowed to continue with this, even if she is putting herself at an increased risk of ill health, or even death. ■

This is a conflict of two types of 'best interests': best medical interests and the best 'personal interests' of a patient. The psychiatrist who has taken advice from the gastroenterologist has a sound clinical rationale for advising that a gastrostomy tube is inserted. This is deemed to be acting in her best 'medical interests'; however, her carers are aware of how much Khalda enjoys eating and feel that she should be allowed to continue to do this and so are advocating what they believe is in her 'best interests'. In this case, both the psychiatrist's and the gastroenterologist's decisions were over-ruled, Khalda did not have a gastrostomy tube inserted. In this case it should be noted that 'best interests' exist in isolation from necessity. The distinction between 'best medical interests' and 'best personal interests' is an important one.

There are formal legal structures that allow decision-making authority to be vested somewhere other than with the incompetent patient. A patient may be made a ward of court, in which scenario the courts have ultimate decision-making authority. However, the most recent addition to the armoury is the Mental Capacity Act 2005 (discussed above), which although passed by Parliament is only expected to come into force some time in 2007. The act allows for the creation of Lasting Powers of Attorney (LPA), by which a patient can transfer decision-making authority (including authority over healthcare decisions) to another person, which power will be activated when the patient loses mental capacity. The act also allows (Sections 25 and 25) for the creation of Advance Directives, which allow a person to make plans for future care and treatment decisions. Of further relevance is the creation (Section 45) of a new Court of Protection which will determine legal issues relating to mentally incompetent persons but the question still remains – on what basis will (or should) decisions be taken concerning the treatment of mentally incapacitated patients who cannot consent to treatment? There are two tests generally proposed:

• Best interests

• Substituted judgement.

BEST INTERESTS

As we have already noted, the best interests test is that preferred in the United Kingdom and Ireland. In the application of this test, a third party (such as the court or clinicians acting in concert with a patient's family) will make a decision concerning the patient through a process of weighing up different options and deciding which one will produce the greatest net gain for the patient. So, a court might take a decision that sterilization is in a patient's best interests or that, as in the *Anthony Bland* case, which concerned a survivor of the Hillsborough disaster who lived but in a persistent vegetative state, life-sustaining treatment can be withdrawn.

Best interests are related to the doctrine of necessity, but they have wider implications: it seems to be the case that best interests treatment can include non-necessary treatment (for example, in the *Bland* case, it was not 'necessary' that the man be allowed to die, but was none the less found to be in his 'best interests').

Properly applied the best interests test has a number of elements which include consultation with family members (which may give insight into the values and wishes of the patient), an assessment of medical best interests (the risks and benefits of available medical treatment), a wider assessment of holistic best interests, including social and spiritual considerations and the acceptability from a medical point of view, of any proposed treatment. Where a proposed course of treatment for an incapacitated patient is consistent with the test of best interests then even though there has been no consent that treatment will be lawful.

SUBSTITUTED JUDGEMENT

'Substituted judgement' involves attempting to make a decision that *the patient* would choose if he were competent. This is an effort to acknowledge that the person has a right to make an autonomous decision, notwithstanding that he is incapable of doing so, and to give expression to the patient's own autonomy. The problem here is that because the person cannot exercise that right to make a decision, another competent individual is – in effect – making the decision, albeit that the claim is made that the decision represents a 'best guess' at the patient's wishes.

Advance directives – or 'living wills' – are an example of how substituted judgement could work (although strictly speaking, they are not substituted judgement). Where a patient cannot give a contemporaneous treatment decision, then regard may be had to the patient's prior expression of wishes and that past expression may – if it envisaged the present circumstances – be applied to the present treatment decision. However, it is not clear either that advance directives work as they are intended (Fagerlin and Schneider, 2004) or that that substituted judgement really comes close to establishing a patient's autonomous wishes (Elliott, 1998). Chief among the criticisms is that it is impossible for me to really know what it is like to be you and to know what you would want, now that you are lacking mental capacity, perhaps even in a coma. The proxy decision maker is dealing with a patient who at some point had capacity, and at that time made (or may only have hinted at) an autonomous decision about how they wanted to be treated. Achieving clarity in the decision, while remembering that the sick do not reason in the same way as the well, may not be possible.

CONCLUSION

There are few easy answers in relation to consent. A key lesson from this chapter is that for many individuals with intellectual impairment there is no single answer. The ability for an individual to give consent depends upon the information that is given to them and how it is conveyed. It depends upon their understanding and the competence to make the decision. An individual may be competent to make decisions about some things but not others – either due to the complexity of the decision or their understanding of the consequences. Perhaps one of the most crucial messages to practitioners, especially those in fields other than mental health where many of the same arguments are rehearsed, is that consent cannot be given for another adult. Reliance on the agreement or indeed acquiescing to the urgings of carers does not protect practitioners from consideration of the *client's* ability to consent or the appropriateness of acting with it.

REFERENCES, RESOURCES AND RECOMMENDED READING

Beauchamp T, Childress J. (2001) *Principles of Biomedical Ethics*, 5th edn. Oxford.

British Medical Association and The Law Society (2004) *Assessment of Mental Capacity*, 2nd edn. BMJ Books.

Chester *v*. Afshar, House of Lords (2004) UKHL 41, (2005) 1 AC 134 (2004) 4 A11 ER 587, (2004) 3 WLR 927, (2005) PIQR 173, (2005) PIQR P12,81 BMLR 1,14 October 2004.

Department of Health (2001) *Valuing People: A New Strategy for Learning Disability for the 21st Century*. London: DH.

Dimond B (2005) *Legal Aspects of Nursing*, 4th edn. Glasgow: Pearson Education.

Elliott C. (1998) Patients doubtfully capable or incapable of consent. In: Kuhse H, Singer P. (eds), *A Companion to Bioethics*. Blackwell.

Evans D, Fitzgerald M. (2002) Reasons for physically restraining patients and residents: a systematic review and content analysis. *International Journal of Nursing Studies* 39:735–43.

Fagerlin A, Schneider CE. (2004) Enough: The failure of the living will. *Hastings Center Report* 34(2): 30–42. Available online: www.thehastingscenter.org/pdf/publications/hcr_mar_apr_2004_enough.pdf (Last accessed December 2006).

Hendrick J. (2000) *Law and Ethics in Nursing and Health Care*. Cheltenham: Stanley Thornes.

Home Office (2000) *Setting the Boundaries. Volume I Reforming the Law on Sex Offences*. London: The Stationery Office.

McLean S. (1999) *Old Law, New Medicine*. Pandora.

Mental Capacity Act 2005. www.opsi.gov.uk/acts2005/20050009.htm

National Patient Safety Agency (2004) Understanding the patient safety issues for people with learning disabilities.

Pearce and another *v*. United Bristol Healthcare NHS Trust, Court of Appeal, Civil Division, 48 BMLR 118, 20 May 1998.

The Law Commission Report (1995) *Mental Capacity*. Report No 231.

United States President's Commission for the Study of Ethical Problems in Medicine and Biomedical and Behavioural Research (1983). *Making Health Care Decisions*. Washington.

Internet Resources

NHS Consent forms

http://www.dh.gov.uk/PolicyAndGuidance/HealthAndSocialCareTopics/Consent/ConsentGeneral Information/fs/en (Last accessed December 18, 2006)

Legal Cases

Airedale N.H.S. Trust v. Bland [1993] AC 789

Chester v. Afshar [2004] 3 WLR 927

Pearce and another v. United Bristol Healthcare NHS Trust [1998] AC 48 BMLR 118

Re B (A minor)(Wardship: sterilisation) [1988] AC 199

Re C (Adult: refusal of medical treatment) [1994] 1 WLR 290

Re F (Mental patient: sterilisation) [1990] 2 AC 1

Re MB (An adult: medical treatment) [1997] 2 FLR 426

Rogers v. *Whitaker* (1992) 175 CLR 479

Sidaway v. *Board of Governors of the Bethlem Hospital and the Maudsley Hospital* [1985] 1 AC871

CHAPTER 12
THE FUTURE OF SERVICES FOR INTELLECTUAL IMPAIRMENT

Peter Griffiths, Rob Winterhalder, Louise L. Clark and Allan Hicks

STUDY AIMS:

1. To develop a brief overview of the policy context and guidelines including legislation and National Service Frameworks (NSF).

2. To identify the necessity for cross agency working for people with intellectual impairment and some of the problems associated with such an approach.

3. To look at the advantages of a Care Programme Approach (CPA) in relation to adults who have intellectual impairment and complex issues.

4. To identify the challenges of implementing CPA.

5. To present contrasting views on the future of services for people with intellectual impairment and explore the implications.

All systems, as they become outmoded and outdated, stagnate and cease to provide the type of treatment and care that is required in contemporary society. The particular forms of treatment and training that we provide at this point in time may very quickly be seen as inappropriate to future needs. It is crucial, however, not to confuse change with progress – to demonstrate that the development of intellectual impairment services is indeed progress, ideological and philosophical arguments will be insufficient.

Learning Disability and other Intellectual Impairments, Edited by L.L. Clark and P. Griffiths
© 2008 John Wiley & Sons, Ltd

Historically, major changes in service provision have been driven by financial pressures and idealistic philosophies of care, as seen with the process of deinstitutionalization and community care in the fields of learning disabilities and mental health. These two processes can be interlinked and sometimes explain why insufficient resources have been allocated to meet the health needs of groups whose morbidity has been grossly underestimated. Any move towards the development of intellectual impairment services may run similar risks, which must be avoided if service gaps are to be closed and service delivery enhanced.

The history of learning disability service developments during the last 30 years may provide an insight into the challenges ahead for the concept of intellectual impairment services. Even now, there has been little or no evaluation of the effectiveness and costs of the multitude of service delivery models in learning disability. The different clinical groups which come together under the term intellectual impairment do, however, seem to have several factors in common in addition to the common needs outlined in Chapter 1 of this book, namely fragmented services, lack of cohesive public policy planning, and blurred interfaces with other health and social care services.

This can be illustrated by the lack of a joined up approach in most localities between Old Age Mental Health and learning disability services. The assessment and management of dementia in people with learning disabilities is met by specialist memory clinics, which are run by Old Age Mental Health services whilst the mental health needs of this patient group are met by specialist learning disability services, but rarely do the two services work together. The gaps in commissioning and service delivery are further compounded by significant cultural differences in service provision between LD and elderly services. People with learning disabilities often experience significant problems adapting with a move from an LD to an elderly service, which in turn can lead to loss of skills and development of mental health problems such as depression or anxiety. The development of intellectual impairment services may help remove some of these barriers and facilitate the exchange of good models of working practice.

A robust analysis of both current need and shortfalls in service delivery is central to any progress in the development of intellectual impairment services. It will also require an understanding of competing policy developments and allocation of resources. If the concept of intellectual impairment is to be translated into a reality in terms of service delivery, existing services will need to be dismantled and reassembled to form a novel service to meet the complex health and social care needs of this group. An understanding of the current strategic directions in commissioning will help inform how intellectual impairment services could be developed and aligned within the broader healthcare service.

NATIONAL SERVICE FRAMEWORKS

The National Service Frameworks (NSF) are long-term strategies for improving specific areas of care. In the context of intellectual impairment the three most relevant are those for older people, mental health and long-term conditions. There is no NSF for learning disabilities. Instead, a White Paper, commonly referred to as *Valuing People* (DH, 2001b) has provided guidance. However, it focuses primarily on health promotion and accessing mainstream services. It fails to address meaningfully how to meet the mental health and challenging behaviour needs of people with learning disability.

The NSF for Older People (DH, 2001a) addresses the treatment of dementia. It emphasizes the importance of a shared single assessment process, the development of locally agreed shared care protocols and also the development of intermediate care to prevent and reduce prolonged hospital admissions. It acknowledges the need for NHS continuing care beds as well as forging greater links with primary care. Whilst intellectual impairment services may embrace some of these strategic concepts, there is little else within this NSF which lends itself to care organized according to the concept of intellectual impairment.

The NSF for Mental Health (DH,1999) sets out seven standards of which standards 4 and 5 address services for people with severe mental illness. Schizophrenia is considered in terms of disability, but there is no focus on learning disability, developmental disorder, acquired brain injury services or other related services. It does emphasize the need to commission local specialist mental health services through a unified local commissioning process. Health authorities, under the aegis of regional specialized services commissioning groups, retain a responsibility for commissioning specialist mental health services.

The NSF which most closely reflects the strategic directions implicit in the concept of an intellectual impairment service (and also its operation) is the *NSF for Long-term Conditions* (DH, 2005), which focuses mainly on neurological disorders but which can be applied to all long-term conditions. Conditions present at birth, for example cerebral palsy, and others associated with various degrees of learning disability are specifically mentioned within the NSF. It acknowledges that people with long-term neurological conditions can be affected by a range of different problems in the areas of motor function, sphincter control, sensory impairments, cognitive behavioural difficulties, communication problems and psychosocial and emotional functioning.

It actively encourages commissioners to use this NSF in planning service developments for people with other long-term conditions, which could include those with intellectual impairment. Targets specified within the NSF include improving health outcomes for conditions by offering a personalized care plan for vulnerable people most at risk, reducing emergency bed admissions by 5% by 2008 through improved care in primary care and community settings, and improving access to services following GP referrals to hospital treatment including all diagnostic procedures and tests. Therefore one aim overall is to reduce the number of hospital admissions.

Eleven quality requirements are set. These include a person-centred service, early recognition, prompt diagnosis and treatment, acute management, rehabilitation, provision of appropriate equipment and accommodation, personal care and support, supporting family and carers, and providing services in hospital or other health and social care settings. Again, many of these quality requirements could be, and should be, encompassed within an intellectual impairment service. Integrated assessment and care planning in the context of interdisciplinary working seems to be favoured over multidisciplinary working, although it acknowledges that different modes may be appropriate depending on the setting and the patient's needs.

Implementing the NSF for long-term conditions requires coordinating service commissioning and delivery, taking into account that some services are commissioned locally, whereas others are through specialized commissioning arrangements. It proposes the establishment of *neuroscience networks* to coordinate the planning, commissioning and provision of services. These networks will need to engage all stakeholders including clinical and other staff, commissioners, managers, voluntary organizations, service users and their carers. They will also need to work across traditional service boundaries in models of care whilst having clear leadership, management and accountability arrangements.

The aims of such networks are to integrate care, improve clinical outcomes and experiences for people using health and social care services, and be cost effective whilst ensuring equity of service provision. It suggests a model in which a *network board* would have representation from all key stakeholders. In addition, *managed network clinical groups* would be able to advise the network board. These groups could enable clinicians to work collaboratively to provide access to a wide range of services, support each other through training in the development of clinical skills and improve quality of care through systematic audit and evaluation of clinical practice.

STRATEGIC AND COMMISSIONING MODELS

In the UK all services are now working in a mixed care economy with multiple providers from public and private or voluntary sectors. Stakeholders include service users, the private and voluntary sectors, local authorities, health organizations – primary care trusts and hospital trusts. Service delivery takes place within multidisciplinary and multi-agency frameworks, and there is an increasing move towards integration particularly of health and social care services. Integration is not solely confined to service provision but can include commissioning. There are many questions that need to be addressed such as whether intellectual impairment services are commissioned at a secondary or tertiary care level and whether they should be jointly commissioned, in which case the lead agency would need to be identified. Regardless of this, intellectual impairment services will need to be underpinned by both clinical service delivery and academic services for ongoing research.

One of the challenges with the concept of intellectual impairment is the diverse needs of the people that the term encompasses, ranging from the developmental disorders group to the acquired brain injury/dementia group. Whilst a life span approach might fit comfortably with the developmental disorders group, it might not resonate so well with the dementia group. It is also unclear, particularly if such a service were developed on a locality basis, whether it would sit alone or within an existing service such as a mental health service.

Advantages to this approach could include having access to local community and hospital-based facilities, being able to advise and support other mental health teams, and avoidance of disputes such as whether the patient's primary problem was due to cognitive impairment or mental illness. However, for patients with severe mental illness and challenging behaviour, local inpatient services would be unlikely to manage this patient group, necessitating transfer to costly out of borough units often in the private sector. Further, by locating a service within the mental health specialty, there is a risk that concomitant physical health needs remain relatively neglected.

A competing model akin to a tertiary care service will be that of a sub-regional service – this would provide a full range of services in a range of settings to meet the health and social care needs of the various clinical groups within the intellectual impairment spectrum. It should theoretically lead to lower management costs, and higher levels of expertise, within a coherent framework of policy and organization. However, this model does not guarantee access to services in the local community, and runs the risk of being perceived as elitist and potentially difficult to access by primary and secondary care services.

Although the Department of Health guidance has designated the rehabilitation for adults with acquired brain injury and complex disorder services as specialized, there appears to be little coherence nationally on how to provide these services (in keeping with LD and elderly care services). In some areas this has led to the development of specialist centres with outreach-type rehabilitation services. In other areas 'virtual' teams are being considered. Tensions often exist between primary care trusts and local authorities around the funding and service provisions for people with acquired brain injury. Patients with acquired brain injury may find themselves within physical disability services where staff do not have the prerequisite skills and experience for 'cognitive' rehabilitation. The Department of Health has also identified early dementia services as 'more specialized' but clearly states that they should continue within specialist mental health NHS trusts.

Intellectual impairment could be considered in the future as a 'specialized' service in commissioning terms. The Department of Health defines specialist services as those with low patient numbers but which need a critical mass of patients to make treatment centres cost effective. It acknowledges the challenges for these services including training specialist staff, supporting high quality research, making the best use of scarce resources like expertise or high tech equipment. A large number of services are already commissioned as specialist services and have their own definition set. These sets include descriptions of the model of service provided, lists of relevant national guidelines, any national databases containing health outcomes information, details regarding finance and identifying activity levels and service gaps. Specific issues which are considered to be important for that particular service are also highlighted.

The following case introduces Doris (see Box 12.1). The study highlights some of the multiple and complex issues which may present in patients who have intellectual impairment. The problems associated with a multi-agency, multidisciplinary but mainstream approach to the management of care of people like Doris are explored.

BOX 12.1 DORIS

Doris is a 46-year-old woman who lives in a staffed group home with five other residents in a London borough which is run by a private social care company. She has Down syndrome, a moderate level of intellectual impairment and spent her early years in an institution for the 'mentally handicapped' until it was closed down in 1995. Doris then moved into her present home with other individuals who all have differing levels of intellectual impairment and dissimilar needs. Doris was diagnosed as having schizophrenia in her twenties and has been admitted to acute psychiatric services on a few occasions since leaving her long-stay hospital despite taking regular medication. Doris has hypothyroidism for which she takes thyroxin; she also suffers regularly from constipation and is clinically obese. In addition to this she is hypertensive although is not taking medication for this currently.

Until recently she was seen by the local Community Learning Disability team who administered her depot injections. Six months ago she was referred to the Community Mental Health team as the role of what remained of the local learning disability nursing team had changed in accordance with government policy to become more involved with health promotion and facilitation. Mental health issues in this geographic area for people with known learning disabilities are now all dealt with in mainstream psychiatry.

Staff in the group home have noticed that Doris has become very forgetful and confused lately but much of this was originally ascribed to the fact that Doris's day centre had closed and she was now at home all day long with little to interest her and the absence of many of her friends. The next time that the CPN visits, the staff mention their concerns over Doris's declining mental health status. ■

ASSESSMENT

Prior to the changed role of the learning disability community team Doris would have been assessed and managed by them with referrals made to outside agencies if necessary. The question of who should now assess Doris does not have a straightforward answer because of the complexity of both her physical and mental health problems and the interplay that these conditions will have upon one another.

Throughout this book the complexity of assessment has been raised. Assessment may be problematic owing to diagnostic overshadowing between intellectual impairment, schizophrenia and the possible presence of dementia or depression. The presence of a thyroid condition and hypertension may further complicate the diagnostic process. A comprehensive bio-psychosocial approach is needed in both the assessment and care planning process. However, the suitability of generic services, whether it be in generic older adult mental health care or the acute adult environment, must be questioned for individuals like Doris. It is known that mental health problems in adults with intellectual impairment often go undetected. With the demise of many specialist mental health services for people with intellectual impairment the assessment process may be extremely problematic for the professional who is either inexperienced or untrained in working with adults who have intellectual impairments.

The psychiatric formulation process is further complicated in patients with intellectual impairment because of reliance on care staff for information and patient history as well as in the Mental State Examination (MSE) process. In the case of patients with intellectual impairment the clinician must substantially alter the MSE (Andrew *et al*, 2001a). The MSE acts as a monitoring tool and can give confirmation of the carers' observations and reports but 'abnormal' behaviour in a person with an intellectual impairment may be normal within the context of the impairment and thus of little additional significance.

Clinical assessment of mental health status in some patients with intellectual impairment may be compared with that of child psychiatry whereby the patient is seldom able to furnish the clinician with the necessary details and therefore carers are important in the process (Andrew *et al*, 2001b). Comparisons are also made with the psychiatry of the generic older adult in that there may be multiple medical conditions present in addition to polypharmacy, which may alter the patient's presentation. Doris presents a complex picture, in terms of her physical and mental health and her developmental level.

High rates of acquiescence in certain interview situations may be problematic in the interview process, including a tendency to agree with the viewpoints of others and an increased incidence of recalling the words most recently spoken (Sigelman *et al*, 1982). Difficulties with comprehension, attention and the capacity to formulate and express responses may all affect the diagnostic interview (Krose *et al*, 2000).

Distinguishing between behavioural disturbance and psychiatric disorders in people with intellectual impairment is problematic, and empirical as well as conceptual factors relating to the nature of these disorders undermines both the reliability and validity of the standard diagnostic process in a person with intellectual impairment (Krose *et al*, 2000).The problems cited in relation to MSE could consequently have a bearing on the formulation process and skew Doris's diagnosis (for further discussion see Chapter 8). Several mental health screening tools for this population are now available including The Psychopathology Instrument for Mentally Retarded Adults (PIMRA, Matson *et al*, 1984), The Diagnostic Assessment for the Severely Handicapped (DASH, Matson *et al*, 1991) and the Reiss Screen (Reiss, 1988). Psychiatric Assessment Schedule for Adults with Development Disabilities (PAS-ADD, Moss 2002) is popular within the United

Kingdom but does require specially trained nurses to carry this out in conjunction with the patient's carer.

Cases such as that of Doris (Box 12.1) also emphasize that often the picture and assessment process is further clouded by physical health problems. Such assessments are often not performed when care is managed by mental health services. Physical health assessment should be particularly stringent in patients with intellectual impairment. Many physical symptoms may be masked for a myriad of reasons including communication problems, challenging behaviour, lack of carer expertise and knowledge in the detection of physical decline. Such symptoms and the disorders that they represent may have gone unnoticed for long periods of time and coping behaviours in the patient can sometimes be the result of chronic physical pain or discomfort. Common examples of this include 'head banging' for the communication and relief of tooth, ear and headaches, 'rooting and smearing' of faeces to relieve the symptoms of constipation or faecal impaction, and urinary incontinence when the patient has a long-term undiagnosed urinary tract infection.

CARE PROGRAMME APPROACH (CPA)

The complexity of Doris's situation means that there is a very real danger that her needs may be overlooked or her problems not properly managed. The Care Programme Approach (CPA) is a person-centred approach to care management which may solve many of the potential problems. Not only is a mental and physical Health Action Plan (HAP) developed but other issues such as housing, finances, employment and daily living skills are also addressed. Risk assessment and the management of challenging behaviour are also integral to the CPA process. One of the concerns of using CPA is the focus that it has on the individual's mental health, however, this may also be viewed as an advantage. It does provide single, accountable care with cross agency communication and has good access to mainstream NHS care. There are two levels of CPA, the one most commonly used in patients with intellectual impairment is the standard level. The enhanced level of CPA involves intensive case management.

There is certainly a case for the use of the CPA in the overall management of Doris's case. The use of CPA is now becoming more widespread where clients have intellectual impairment and additional mental health problems (even in instances where the client is not subject to section 117 aftercare under the 1983 Mental Health Act). This particular approach ensures that any plan is based on a specialist psychiatric assessment, the outcome of such being then linked to the appropriate level of CPA.

Valuing People (DH, 2001b) promotes the use of CPA in circumstances where the client with a known learning disability has additional and complex mental health problems. Doris has reached a point whereby a crisis situation is a possibility and a full assessment and care strategy is essential. By utilizing this approach it would be possible to include members of specialist mental health/ learning disability teams (if they were available in any given geographic area) as part of the multi-agency/multidisciplinary group who would plan and oversee Doris's care. The National Service Framework (NSF) for Mental Health (DH, 1999) states that patients should be offered referral to specialist services for assessment and treatment if necessary and specialist psychiatry is certainly indicated in this complex case. The core CPA team members might include the following:

- Specialist psychiatrist; learning disabilities

- Learning disability community nurse (health facilitation role, if available)

- Community psychiatric nurse
- Medical specialist (thyroid)
- Dementia nurse specialist
- Speech & language therapist
- Social worker
- Key worker (from group home)
- General practitioner
- District nurse
- Occupational therapist.

One individual from the group must be allocated as its coordinator. Their role is to act as a link between the client and the services and agencies involved. They must monitor the care plan and arrange regular reviews in addition to emergency meetings where necessary. Issues raised by the team would revolve around a bio-psychosocial approach to Doris's life. This should be person centred and involve forward planning as well as assessment of the immediate issues. Doris should be involved as fully as possible in the development of the care plan.

However, the success of the CPA approach depends upon the existence of some degree of specialist input which is currently being threatened. CPA, far from providing a rationale for the dismantling of specialist services, provides a rationale for their continued existence as they provide a key tool to ensure the effectiveness of mainstream services for the physical and mental health care of people with intellectual impairments.

SOCIAL CARE

Doris's social care will be overseen and purchased by the local social services department under the direction of a social worker. In many cases people like Doris may not have an identified individual and will fall under the umbrella of the 'duty' social worker. This situation is often far from ideal as the client and professional do not know each other and it is often only a crisis situation that will bring them into contact. Care for older adults with intellectual impairment is not defined as a specialist subject either within or outside the mainstream health or social services arenas. Therefore there is no obvious fit between Doris's needs and available specialist facilities. Due to the nature of Doris's current placement (i.e. a social care home with no qualified staff) a move to a more specialized environment with the presence of qualified nursing care would certainly be indicated if the decline continues. But the procurement of such placements is problematic with many nursing homes being wary of taking patients with complex health issues and intellectual impairment.

Doris's day care provision has been withdrawn. This is not an uncommon scenario with the switch from traditional day care services towards a more community-based model of service. Anecdotal evidence would suggest that the young and more able people with intellectual impairment will be considered for employment opportunities whereas older adults will be 'retired' from day services, thus removing them from long-term friendships and a routine and purpose in their lives. This may exacerbate feelings of loneliness and isolation and lead to mental health problems in these older individuals. Social services need to work closely with the rest of the multi-agency team in order to achieve the most suitable placement for both day and residential services.

Social care priorities include:

1. Suitable residential accommodation with similar house-mates (i.e. similar levels of impairment, adaptive functioning, ages and shared experiences).

2. Meaningful day service provision that caters for the older adult with additional mental and physical health problems.

3. Early interventions by both health and social care professionals when decline is noticed in older patients.

4. Adequate education and training of social care staff (both statutory and private sectors) in the specific care of older adults with intellectual impairment.

5. Maintenance of long-term relationships with family and friends.

6. Regular daily routines (often based around reminiscence and reality orientation) and involvement with the larger community.

7. Multidisciplinary and multi-agency working and a person-centred approach to assessment, care management and ongoing evaluation using CPA if necessary.

The points made regarding the care needs of Doris also raise questions about the needs of a significant group of people with an intellectual impairment, those with a dementia not linked to another intellectual impairment such as Down syndrome. Working with Doris illustrates the difficulty in providing an integrated approach which addresses her needs, particularly when financial or organization imperatives mean that services are withdrawn or changed in scope. Doris is suffering from a number of challenges to her health both physical and mental. Multiple pathology and complex patterns of behaviour arising from different stimuli are a hallmark of older people suffering from different forms of dementia. To meet their needs services must firstly accept that one person or service is unlikely to have the knowledge and skills to meet all of a person's needs. That said there are challenges to working jointly across organizational and service barriers.

THE PROBLEMS OF JOINT WORKING

In many areas of the UK social services departments have taken the lead for learning disability services. However, this seemingly enlightened step towards providing holistic care has not been without its problems. Medical, nursing and allied health professionals have expressed difficulties in being managed by social services staff and the philosophies of the two statutory services do vary. The different professional philosophies of the groups involved can generate tensions. A major argument surrounds the debate about whether 'intellectual impairments' in themselves are wholly a social care issue and should therefore have social care as their lead agency.

A social care lead is in line with policy (*Valuing People*, DH, 2001b) but is often criticized by health professionals because of the complexity of both physical and mental health issues that are prevalent in people who have learning disabilities. Their critique has a number of premises, which have become recurring themes in this book. A totally social model of care will do little to ensure that a bio-psychosocial approach to care planning is followed. Many health professionals object to the social care community's push away from a medical model of care that is now prevalent. They have struggled to move along with government plans whereby learning disability community teams should be mainly concerned with health facilitation towards mainstream NHS services and health promotion of their client group.

Mainstream NHS services are ill-prepared or ill-equipped to care for people with intellectual impairment especially if there are additional problems such as mental health issues or behavioural problems. Specialist expertise is needed but is not available routinely. Learning disability specialist support is rare while for other intellectual impairments it may be non-existent. Much of the caseload of a learning disability community nurse will consist of patients who have additional mental health problems. Some in mainstream community mental health services may feel that it is not within their remit to take on people with learning disabilities. This may be for a variety of reasons which include already overstretched caseloads and an appreciation that such patients may be extremely complex to manage. This may mask a negative view on the worth of providing care to such clients or a perception that they lack expertise and experience in this area.

Existing health professional expertise has been questioned by the government in its attempt to move towards the social model of care and mainstream NHS service provision. Doctors, nurses and allied health professions working in learning disability services have reported feeling undervalued and surplus to requirements in the government's future plans. They, like many generic health practitioners, recognize that with the demise of specialist health services much expertise may be lost and added pressure will be placed on already overstretched mainstream services. This has resulted in 'delaying tactics' in the shift towards the vision outlined in *Valuing People* (DH, 2001b).

A SINGLE OVERARCHING SPECIALITY: A DEBATE

The following dialogue is between two of the authors of this chapter. Rob Winterhalder (R) is a consultant psychiatrist specializing in people with learning disabilities who have concurrent mental health problems. Louise Clark (L) has a nursing background and is a lecturer in intellectual impairment. Their conversation represents some of the varying opinions that health professionals have as to where the future of services for people with intellectual impairment should go and what particular service models would be beneficial. Interestingly, although having made the assumption that they had very different views on service provision, they do find many areas of common ground. The conversation also touches on the educational needs of professionals working in the area.

L: Rob, I know that you have concerns surrounding the broader terminology of intellectual impairment'?

R: *Yes, essentially this relates to my belief that the commonalities of the various groups in terms of all sharing some level of cognitive impairment is outweighed by their differences. I do believe that it is necessary to share skills and knowledge across the umbrella of intellectual impairment, this could be achieved through joint clinics, shared care protocols and the development of appropriate courses and training. This would still need to be supported by a comprehensive commissioning strategy but would avoid all the pitfalls involved in radically restructuring services in health, social services, and the private and voluntary sectors. Any changes in pre- and post-registration training in the various disciplines would also be more manageable.*

L: True, but within each group there are multiple differences – we know this within learning disability services alone.

R: *That's my point! Learning disabilities (together with other developmental disorders) have the philosophy of enabling habilitation as opposed to dependence, which is prevalent in some of the other services.*

L: I disagree! Mental health doesn't look towards a model of dependency, for example, in terms of 'risk taking' there is usually a positive approach adopted. You have just endorsed my point; if the various sectors involved in the management and care of people with intellectual impairment stand alone in terms of both expertise and funding then they will be unable to share skills and knowledge and will also be merely a series of small minority groups of services which will attract neither government attention nor funding.

R: *The clinical needs in terms of screening, investigations, management, etc., are very different in the neurodevelopmental disorders groups compared with the acquired brain injury/dementia group. The underlying aetiologies are obviously very different as are associated psychiatric comorbidities and emotional/psychological needs in these two groups. Even when there is an overlap in aetiology, e.g. brain trauma which could lead to learning disability, acquired brain injury or dementia, any associated behavioural or psychiatric problems tend to present differently in these three clinical settings, and require different therapeutic approaches and contrasting courses and prognoses.*

L: Can you elaborate on that one because as I see it they all share the commonality of having cognitive deficit and services which predominately have unqualified or minimally trained staff and inadequate government funding?

R: *I think everyone would agree that virtually all the patient groups encompassed within the term intellectual impairment are supported by staff who have the least training, and yet they have the highest health morbidity. In the field of learning disabilities, at least, the government is making a commitment to people with learning disabilities through the creation of the learning disability awards framework (LDAF) which ultimately aims to ensure that all carers working within learning disability services undergo training and reach a certain set of standards in order to help them meet the social and healthcare needs of their patients/clients.*

L: Rob, you're quoting a basic qualification for social care staff in only one area of intellectual impairment which is only relevant in the social care sector. What about the fact that we are training fewer learning disability nurses than ever before and those health professionals working in mainstream services (who are supposed to be the primary contact for care for people with intellectual impairment) are only minimally acquainted with the speciality? Furthermore, is it right that intellectual impairment services should lie predominantly within social care with local authorities taking the lead in the area and in many cases actually managing the clinicians and staff who work in health care for these patients and clients?

R: *I totally agree that it seems ludicrous that the local authority should take the lead in commissioning for health services and even directly manage clinicians and other healthcare staff. To compound the matter further there are often significant gaps between commissioning, management and clinical practice which results in ill-informed commissioning at a strategic level. Without a clinical background it becomes difficult for commissioners and managers to even begin to understand the complexities of a patient group's healthcare needs and how best to meet them.*

L: I think that this issue represents an opinion that I have long held in that we should be investing in health professionals from all disciplines and considering them for management routes if they show such flair in that direction. I don't just mean 'make them a manager' I refer to sponsoring them through MBAs (Master of Business Administration), or similar qualifications.

R: *Getting into issues at the coal-face is extremely problematic, in addition to being subject to market forces (especially in relation to employment) and I do think that the manager or commissioner who has a clinical background is much more suited to coping with such issues, as well as often more able to generate respect and the concurrence of staff teams.*

L: Very true! Not to mention the small matter of economics. Given the government's supposition that people with intellectual impairment are simply a variant of the 'human condition' it reduces the necessity for them to provide specialist services and thereby saves a massive amount of money in the process. However, I do strongly believe that the wider umbrella of 'intellectual impairment' is important, not least in relation to cross–intelligence of services and a bigger and louder voice to fight for funding!

R: *That's all very well and I am not opposed to the concept of 'cross-intelligence' of services, but I would worry about the dilution of all specialties within a much larger intellectual impairment service. For instance, I run a learning disability epilepsy service with my nursing colleagues and I firmly believe that my patients receive a high calibre service which I would not want to see disappear. I am confident that this type of service is sustainable within either a learning disability service or a larger neurodevelopmental disorder service, as long as it is clearly linked in at both a service and commissioning level with mainstream adult neurology and paediatric services.*

L: Don't get me wrong. I'm not promoting total services, simply a broader umbrella, which has smaller specialties within it, really no different from the mental health model which incorporates separate services such as eating disorders, EMI, acute, substance abuse, etc.

R: *But Louise, training is different.*

L: Yes, but currently nurses, in particular, come into all areas across the spectrum of intellectual impairment from all branches of the nursing register and I do feel that this is by far the most ideal model as a huge myriad of specialties are essential in the care of patients from all branches of intellectual impairment. I certainly have advocated the development of a post-registration qualification in the broader subject of 'intellectual impairment' as well as in individual specialties within the group.

R: *I would certainly be in agreement regarding deficiencies in nurse training – particularly in relation to learning disabilities and mental health. The reasons for this are multifactorial: first of all I believe that an insufficient number of suitably high calibre students are attracted. Secondly, the curriculum is heavily orientated towards social models of care which results in nurses qualifying without a basic understanding of the scientific basis of disease and its treatment. Thirdly, many nurses become disillusioned and leave the profession because their skills and roles are undervalued or misunderstood particularly by managers and commissioning. Finally, particularly in learning disability services, there is no coherent national framework for nurses which clearly identifies their clinical roles and remits. These issues are interlinked and are compounded further when service managers are from non-health backgrounds or the lead agency (in management or commissioning terms) is, for example, the local authority.*

Ultimately then, these contrasting views on the need for a specialism lead to closely aligned positions, where we agree on the priorities. Services across intellectual impairment have much to learn from each other and the broad 'umbrella' of the specialty may be a useful one, however, the individual specialities need to be retained within the broader framework. In terms of specific services there is an argument in favour of services for 'Developmental disorders', which includes autism and related conditions, the hyperkinetic disorders and other genetic conditions which result in cognitive impairment.

The commissioning of services must be addressed by closing the gap between commissioners, managers and clinicians. Clinicians should be involved in the commissioning process. The education and training needs of both health and social care staff working in intellectual impairment services must be addressed. There is certainly a case for a post-registration qualification in intellectual impairment for nurses from the Adult and Mental Health branches of nursing as a greater skill base is needed.

The model of an intellectual impairment service might be similar to that of mental health, for example dementia services, developmental disorder services, epilepsy clinics, inpatient and reha-bilitation for acquired brain injury, outreach services for cognitive impairment to include clients with long-term mental health problems whereby cognition is affected. The broader focus of the service might also allow for some degree of specialism to emerge in general practice for primary care of people with impaired communication.

Shaping the Future: A Vision for Learning Disability Nursing (2006) has been recently released by the UK Learning Disability Consultant Nurse Network. It gives a clear direction for the future of this particular part of the nursing register. It recognizes that behavioural overshadowing in these clients may act as a barrier to diagnosis as can the complexities of physical and mental health problems. The document therefore suggests that learning disability nurses should continue to promote and maintain the health status of their clients and be involved in the education of mainstream health professionals.

In many ways the *Vision for Learning Disability Nursing* (2006) builds on *Valuing People* but it also urges nurses working in this area to become more actively involved in research and educa-tion in addition to becoming more politically aware and to look at their own input to the public health arena. This particular message is one that could well be applied across many other special-ties within intellectual impairment; there is certainly less research carried out in these particular fields of nursing, this ultimately leads our more 'hi-tech' colleagues to believe that intellectual impairment nursing is of a lower professional status.

The intrinsic notion of the learning disability healthcare professional being there to enable mainstream health care through facilitation is an admirable one. However, this should not be as a replacement for the community learning disability teams (CLDN). However, there is certainly an argument for a new model of specialist outreach or community team that will have a diverse skill mix in the general area of intellectual impairment and will cater for people with learning disability, acquired brain injury, long-term and severe mental health problems where cognition is affected. Ideally these professionals would act as facilitators to primary care and acute services but would also have links to developmental disorder services, where epilepsy services would sit but which would also be available to any patient with intellectual impairment for whatever reason.

A MANIFESTO FOR THE FUTURE

Current services for people with intellectual impairments, limited as they are to people with learning disabilities, are now aimed towards mainstream health services supported by minimal specialist provision and social care support. A number of issues must be addressed as a matter of urgency. In this section we offer a manifesto for the future, which we believe identifies necessary steps to be taken if the quality of health care for people with intellectual impairment is to be maintained and enhanced in the future.

Primary care services need to address the skill mix within their teams. Employing specialists with knowledge and experience may not always be practical and so greater links need to be formed with both community mental health and what remains of community learning disability teams. The use of CPA is essential in the management of people who have intellectual impairment and complex physical and mental health issues. Generic healthcare professionals need to be both aware and involved in this process. Acute inpatient services for both physical and mental health must have access to specialist advice when caring for clients with intellectual impairment. Ideally, each trust should employ an intellectual impairment nurse adviser who can not only help with practical advice but also liaise with outside agencies which may be able to give support.

As specialist mental health units for intellectual impairment/learning disability are lost it is important to ensure that specialist psychiatry is not also lost. These professionals are highly adept at understanding the relationship between behavioural and mental health issues in their patients as well as in the complex interplay that physical health problems may have on both diagnosis and treatment.

Education and training for doctors, nurses and allied health professionals must incorporate the assessment, care and management of people with intellectual impairment at both pre- and post-registration levels. This must be addressed by the professional bodies so that the universities can include the subject to a greater extent in their undergraduate curricula in addition to planning for postgraduate and post-registration courses.

Just as there is a case for some generic professionals (Adult and Mental Health) to undertake more in-depth post-registration courses in intellectual impairment, many learning disability specialists may lack skills in physical care and could benefit from additional study in generic care.

CLOSING THOUGHTS

The concept of intellectual impairment has yet to be embraced widely by clinicians, managers and commissioners – only time will tell whether it will be translated into a reality in terms of service organization and clinical specialty. However, few would disagree that some of its underlying principles behind the arguments deployed here, such as the sharing of knowledge and expertise, the dismantling of barriers to effective care, and a greater integration of health and local authority services with the private and voluntary sectors for people with intellectual impairment, merit serious discussion. Such consideration needs to be at a national level and involve a strategic commissioning approach in order to bring about any meaningful and lasting change.

Currently patients with intellectual impairment have their health needs met by a variety of health services including paediatrics, learning disabilities, physical disabilities, acute hospitals, child and adolescent mental health services, adult mental health services (generic, neuropsychiatry, rehabilitation), elderly mental health services, neurology and, of course, primary care. Any restructuring towards a full 'intellectual impairment' service will need to divert resources from at least some of these existing services whilst also ensuring that a meaningful interface is retained with mainstream services. As well as community and inpatient services, day hospital and respite care services will need to be reviewed.

In addition to health services, local authorities would have to realign teams, services, boundaries, eligibility criteria. This would apply particularly to their learning disability, physical disabilities, child and families, and elderly teams. The private/voluntary sector equally would have to readjust in terms of any commissioning arrangements, contracts, and service delivery. This would have to include the provision of specialist residential schemes, independent supported living initiatives, day services and other types of specialist community support.

Within health services, health professionals would need to develop an extensive knowledge of developmental, neuropsychiatric and degenerative disorders. This would have major implications for training in psychiatry, nursing, clinical psychology, professions allied to medicine and beyond. Similar issues might apply to social work training. Relevant postgraduate training schemes in the various disciplines would need to change course curricula and training, including student placements. There would also be significant implications for the training needs of staff in the private/voluntary sector.

Can this happen? Should it happen? The enthusiasm of those who contributed to writing this book and that of you, the reader, who has made the effort to read this, suggests that there is hope. We, the authors, disagree with each other as to whether or not an all encompassing specialty of intellectual impairment is a necessary part of the solution. But we agree that a wider knowledge and understanding of the issues, challenges and solutions is vital. If the diverse needs of people who fall under the 'banner' of 'intellectual impairment' are to be met then changes from the current state of affairs are necessary.

If the people that are brought together by this label share one thing in common it is the potential to be marginalized within the healthcare system. If, at times, the tone of some of this discussion has seemed negative it is because we recognize the pitfalls in the way ahead and the danger that isolated pockets of excellence and expertise may be lost in the struggle to integrate care in the mainstream. This book could never hope to fill all the gaps in knowledge or provision but we hope it goes some way towards outlining the necessary expertise and provides a useful framework for identifying the way forward.

REFERENCES AND RECOMMENDED READING

Andrew S, Levitas S, DesNoyers Hurley A, Pary R. (2001a) The Mental Status Examination in patients with mental retardation and developmental disabilities. *Mental Health Aspects of Developmental Disabilities* 4(1).

Andrew S, Levitas S, Silva Van R. (2001b). Mental health clinical assessment of persons with mental retardation and developmental disabilities: History. *Mental Health Aspects of Developmental Disabilities* 4(1).

Brown RI. (1984) The field of developmental handicap – the development of rehabilitation education. In: *Integrated Programmes for Handicapped Adolescents and Adults*. London: Croom Helm, 1–22.

Department of Health (1998) *Commissioning in the New NHS*. London: DH.

Department of Health (1999) *Modern Standards and Service Models. National Service Framework for Mental Health*. London: DH.

Department of Health (2001a) *National Service Framework for Older People*. London: DH.

Department of Health (2001b) *Valuing People: A New Strategy for Learning Disability for the 21ˢᵗ Century*. London: DH.

Department of Health (2005) *National Service Framework for Long-term Conditions*. London: DH.

Krose B, Dewhurst D, Holmes G. (2000) Diagnosis and drugs: help or hindrance when people with learning disabilities have psychological problems? *British Journal of Learning Disabilities* 29(1):26–33.

Matson JL, Kazdin AE, Senatore V. (1984) Psychometric properties of the psychopathology instrument for mentally retarded adults (PIMRA). *American Journal of Mental Retardation* 5:881–9.

Matson JL, Gardner WI, Coe DA, Sovner RR. (1991) A scale for evaluating emotional disorders in severely and profoundly mentally retarded persons: development of the Diagnostic Assessment for the Severely Handicapped (DASH) scale. *British Journal of Psychiatry* 159:404–9.

Moss S. (2002) *PAS-ADD Schedules*. Brighton: Pavilion.

Reiss S. (1988) *Reiss Screen for Maladaptive Behaviours*. Worthington, Ohio: IDS.

Sigelman CK, Budd EC, Winer JL, Scoenrock CJ, Martin PW. (1982) Evaluating alternative techniques of questioning mentally retarded persons. *American Journal of Mental Deficiency* 86:511–8.

UK Learning Disability Consultant Nurse Network (2006) *Shaping the Future: A Vision for Learning Disability Nursing*. UKLDCNN.

Index

Learning Disability and other Intellectual Impairments, Edited by L.L. Clark and P. Griffiths
© 2008 John Wiley & Sons, Ltd